THE BRAIN AND HEARING

Hearing Disturbances Associated with Local Brain Lesions

Neuropsychology
A Series of Special Research Reports
Under the Editorship of A. R. Luria

1972 • THE BRAIN AND HEARING: Hearing Disturbances Associated with Local Brain Lesions
A. V. Baru and T. A. Karaseva

THE BRAIN AND HEARING

Hearing Disturbances Associated with Local Brain Lesions

A. V. Baru
Laboratory of the Physiology of Hearing
Pavlov Institute of Physiology
Academy of Sciences of the USSR
Leningrad, USSR

and

T. A. Karaseva
Department of Nervous Diseases
Sechenov First Moscow Medical Institute
Moscow, USSR

Translated from Russian by Basil Haigh

CONSULTANTS BUREAU • NEW YORK-LONDON • 1972

Anna Vladimirovna Baru was born in 1922 and was graduated in 1947 from the Pavlov First Leningrad Medical Institute with the degree of Candidate of Medical Sciences. She holds the post of Senior Researcher in the Laboratory of the Physiology of Hearing at the Pavlov Institute of Physiology, Academy of Sciences of the USSR. Her field of research is the neurophysiology and physiology of hearing.

Tat'yana Aleksandrovna Karaseva was born in 1936 and was graduated in 1960 from the Sechenov First Moscow Medical Institute with the degree of Candidate of Medical Sciences. She worked for a number of years under Prof. A. R. Luria's direction in the Laboratory of Neuropsychology, Burdenko Institute of Neurosurgery, Academy of Medical Sciences of the USSR. At present she is a member of the Department of Nervous Diseases, Sechenov First Moscow Medical Institute. Her field of research is the pathology of the cerebral cortex and hemispheric dominance.

The original Russian text, published by Moscow University Press in 1971, has been revised and corrected by the authors for the present edition. This translation is published under an agreement with Mezhdunarodnaya Kniga, the Soviet book export agency.

THE BRAIN AND HEARING
MOZG I SLUKH
МОЗГ И СЛУХ
А. В. БАРУ, Т. А. КАРАСЕВА

Library of Congress Catalog Card Number 72-82624
ISBN 0-306-10876-3

A Division of Plenum Publishing Corporation
227 West 17th Street, New York, N.Y. 10011

United Kingdom edition published by Consultants Bureau, London
A Division of Plenum Publishing Company, Ltd.
Davis House (4th Floor), 8 Scrubs Lane, Harlesden, London, NW10 6SE, England

Printed in the United States of America

Introduction

One of the ways in which the cerebral organization of sensory systems in general, and the auditory system in particular, can be investigated is by studying defects of the perception and discrimination of acoustic stimuli resulting from destruction of different parts of the auditory system by a pathological focus in them or by their surgical removal.

The disturbances accompanying lesions of the peripheral part of the auditory system (disturbances of sound conduction, disturbances arising in the hair cells of the cochlea) are well known. It is much more difficult to determine the character of disturbances specific for lesions of the central parts of the auditory system and, in particular, of the auditory cortex.

Types of visual disturbances in man associated with lesions of the visual cortex – homonymous hemianopia with preservation of central vision in unilateral lesions and cortical blindness in bilateral lesions – are described in the neurological literature (Brower, 1936).

The visual agnosias found in lesions of the secondary visual areas and inferior temporal zones of the human and animal cortex are also well known.

Analogous facts showing that destruction of the parietal cortex disturbs complex (epicritic) forms of sensation but leaves more elementary sensation (protopathic) intact are described by Head.

What types of acoustic analysis cannot take place in the absence of the auditory cortex?

Investigations have shown that certain areas of the left temporal cortex in man are connected with phonemic hearing, while areas of the right temporal cortex are associated with musical hearing. However, it is not definitely known what operations in the processing of acoustic information are disturbed by lesions of the auditory cortex, nor is it known whether defects in the detection and diagnosis of the physical properties of elementary acoustic stimuli lie at the basis of disturbances of complex integrative functions such as the discrimination of speech or the appreciation of music.

The monograph now presented to the reader is based on the results of investigations conducted for several years in G. V. Gershuni's laboratory with the aim of establishing the temporal characteristics of activity of the auditory system using psychophysical, electrophysiological, and behavioral techniques.

The study of the detection and discrimination of stimuli as functions of their duration has revealed the special importance of the auditory cortex in the identification of stimuli whose essential characteristics are transitional phenomena: short duration of exposure, measurement of time, and successive replacement of components.

This monograph describes the results of an investigation to study the thresholds of detection of acoustic stimuli of varied duration in patients with pathological foci in the auditory cortex and other parts of the brain, and also the results of observations on patients with lesions of the central parts of the auditory system at different levels. The state of some other types of auditory analysis in these patients is also examined.

Having regard to the main purpose of this book, which is to discover the role of the auditory cortex in the perception of acoustic stimuli of varied duration, and because of the absence of any adequate survey in the Russian literature of the state of auditory function in patients with central lesions of the auditory system, the results of investigations of auditory function in these patients are first described in a survey of the literature. No attempt is made to give a detailed description of the structure of the auditory system, but in order to clarify some problems concerned with those disturbances of function in lesions of the temporal cortex which are discussed in the book a brief schematic account of the structure of the auditory system is essential. The problem of sensory aphasia, its diagnosis and classification, likewise does not receive detailed treatment, and discussion is limited to the relationship between sensory speech defects and disturbances of hearing.

The results described in the book and also the examination and comparisons of the known facts concerning the state of auditory function in patients with central lesions of the auditory system described in the literature shed some light on the mechanisms of auditory perception in man and may be of assistance in the topical diagnosis of local brain lesions.

Contents

CHAPTER 1

Disturbances of Hearing Due to Lesions of the Central Parts of the Auditory System (a Review of the Literature)

STRUCTURE OF THE AUDITORY SYSTEM

The auditory system in man and animals is complex and consists of the following components: a sound-conducting apparatus (the outer and middle ear), the organ of Corti with its hair cells (receptor cells) in the cochlear canal of the inner ear, and a number of interconnected nuclei – the spiral ganglion, the cochlear group of nuclei, the superior olive and the trapezoid body, the inferior colliculi, the medial geniculate body, and the auditory cortex. For a detailed account of the anatomy of the auditory systems, see Ramon y Cajal (1909), Rasmussen (1964), and Crosby, Humphrey, and Lauer (1962).

The first neuron of the auditory system consists of cells of the spiral ganglion of the cochlea (ganglion spiralis, ganglion Cortii). It lies at the base of the pyramidal lamina of the cochlea and in man consists of 29,000–30,000 bipolar cells (Guild, 1932). The peripheral processes of these cells run in radial and spiral bundles to the receptor cells of the organ of Corti. Two types of hair cells are described: inner and outer. It was previously considered (Lorente de Nô, 1933) that one inner hair cell is innervated by one or two radial fibers, and one outer spiral fiber innervates many outer hair cells. However, Spoendlin (1968) found that 80% of nerve fibers are connected with the inner hair cells and, consequently, to each hair cell there must be about 12 nerve fibers.

The central fibers of the bipolar cells of the spiral ganglion form the cochlear branch of the VIII cranial nerve which enters the internal auditory meatus, where it joins the vestibular branch to form the trunk of the VIII nerve. The auditory nerve enters the brain stem at the level of the inferior border of the pons in the region of the cerebellopontine angle laterally to the descending root of the trigeminal nerve and above the retro-olivary fissure. Here the two branches of the VIII nerve separate again.

The lateral or posterior cochlear branch, running laterally from the inferior cerebellar peduncle, terminates in two nuclei of the medulla: the ventral (nucleus cochlearis ventralis), lying between the restiform body and the cerebellum, and the dorsal (nucleus cochlearis dorsalis or tuberculum acusticum), located on the postero-lateral surface of the restiform body. The structure of the cochlear nuclei is described in detail by Ramon y Cajal (1909), Lorente de Nô (1933), Rasmussen (1964), Harrison and Warr (1962), and Harrison and Irving (1965).

The first relay in the auditory pathway takes place in the cochlear nuclei. Cells of the cochlear nuclei are neurons of the second order, the axons of which form the contralateral and ipsilateral ascending tracts. Some fibers leaving the ventral cochlear nucleus terminate in the medial and lateral nuclei of the superior olive of the same side, but most of the fibers forming the system of the trapezoid body cross to the opposite side, run along the border between the tegmentum and the base of the brain, and terminate in the nuclei of the trapezoid body and the nuclei of the superior olivary complex, where the lateral lemniscus arises. Some fibers of the trapezoid body are not interrupted in the superior olivary nuclei but run in the lateral lemniscus and terminate in its nuclei and in the inferior colliculi, while solitary fibers may also terminate in the medial geniculate bodies. Collaterals from the cells of the trapezoid body run to the nuclei of the VI cranial nerve, cells of the reticular formation, and the motor nucleus of the trigeminal nerve.

Some axons of cells of the cochlear nuclei (neurons of the second order) run along the floor of the 4th ventricle as the white striae of Monakow (striae acusticae, striae medullares ventriculi quarti), cross to the opposite side, and join the lateral lemniscus at the level of the superior olive. Other fibers of the crossed auditory pathway also arise from the cochlear nuclei, but the fibers of the second order neurons run deeply on the opposite side to form Held's decussation or the stria intermedia, after which they climb to the level of the superior olive where, without relaying, they enter the lateral lemniscus. Decussation of the auditory pathway at this level in man is incomplete. The nuclei of the superior olive are an important relay station of the ascending auditory tract. Many fibers of the trapezoid body terminate on the nuclei of the superior olivary complex. This complex consists of five nuclei: the medial or accessory olive, the lateral olive, an S-shaped segment, the medial and lateral preolivary nuclei, and the retro-olivary group; the last forms part of the system of the descending auditory pathway.

An additional decussation of the ascending auditory pathway is formed by fibers from the S-shaped complex of the superior olive. The S-shaped complex receives fibers from the ipsilateral cochlear nuclei; axons of the cells of the S-shaped complex of the superior olive run into both lateral leminisci in equal proportions. Both lateral lemnisci also are connected by Probst's commissure.

The lateral lemniscus is thus formed by fibers of the superior olive of the same side, fibers of the dorsal and intermediate striae acusticae, axons of cells of the contralateral olive, and fibers of the trapezoid body. It runs forward and upward from the olive toward the inferior colliculi. Among its fibers there are groups of cells: the ventral, intermediate, and dorsal nuclei of the lateral lemniscus.

Some fibers in the lateral lemniscus terminate on cells of the inferior colliculi, while others do not relay in the inferior colliculi but continue into the medial geniculate body.

The lateral lemniscus is a common path for the axons of second- and third-order neurons; it contains fibers from the ipsilateral cochlea and, to a greater degree, fibers of the contralateral cochlea. Some second order neurons relay on cells of the nuclei of the lateral lemniscus. Most of the axons reach the inferior colliculus as axons of third-order neurons, but a few fibers are formed by processes of second-order neurons. Some fibers of the lateral lemniscus penetrate into the nuclei of the inferior colliculus, while others surround it like a cup to form its capsule. According to Ramon y Cajal many fibers of the lateral lemniscus do not relay in the inferior colliculus but run on to the medial geniculate body. However, later investigations (Wollard and Harpman, 1940) have shown that most fibers of the lateral lemniscus relay in the inferior colliculi.

The inferior colliculi are the most important structures of the auditory system at the subcortical level (the largest in volume and in the number and density of their cells). Cells of the inferior colliculi are mainly concentrations of fourth-order neurons, but neurons of the third and fifth orders are also represented there. The structure of the inferior colliculi has been described by Zvorykin (1963), Ramon y Cajal (1909), Morest (1964), and Levin (1959).

Most fibers of the inferior colliculus form its brachium. The inferior colliculus has both ipsilateral and contralateral connections. The ipsilateral projections are more numerous; they run in the lateral part of the brachium. Most fibers from the inferior colliculus terminate in the medial geniculate body on the same side. A few fibers terminate in the parabrachial region and in the interstitial nucleus (the parabrachial region extends from the rostral pole of the inferior colliculus to the caudal pole of the medial geniculate body medially to the brachia of the inferior colliculi). A few fibers also run into the lateral region of the posterior thalamic group. Some fibers of the inferior colliculi run through the commissure into the contralateral colliculus; many fibers relay there, and the relayed and unbroken fibers run in the brachium of the inferior colliculi and terminate in the medial geniculate body. A small group of fibers reaches the nuclei of the pons and forms the tectopontine tract. Some fibers run toward the superior colliculi. The medial geniculate body is the next relay in the ascending auditory pathway. Its structure has been investigated by Ramon y Cajal (1909), Morest (1964, 1965), Levin (1961), and Sychowa (1962).

Ramon y Cajal (1911) and Sychowa (1962) found that all fibers of the ascending auditory pathway relay in the medial geniculate body. Gudden's commissure connects the two geniculate bodies.

Fibers of the auditory pathway arising from cells of the medial geniculate body initially lie close to the ventral bundles of thalamocortical fibers running from the ventrolateral nucleus

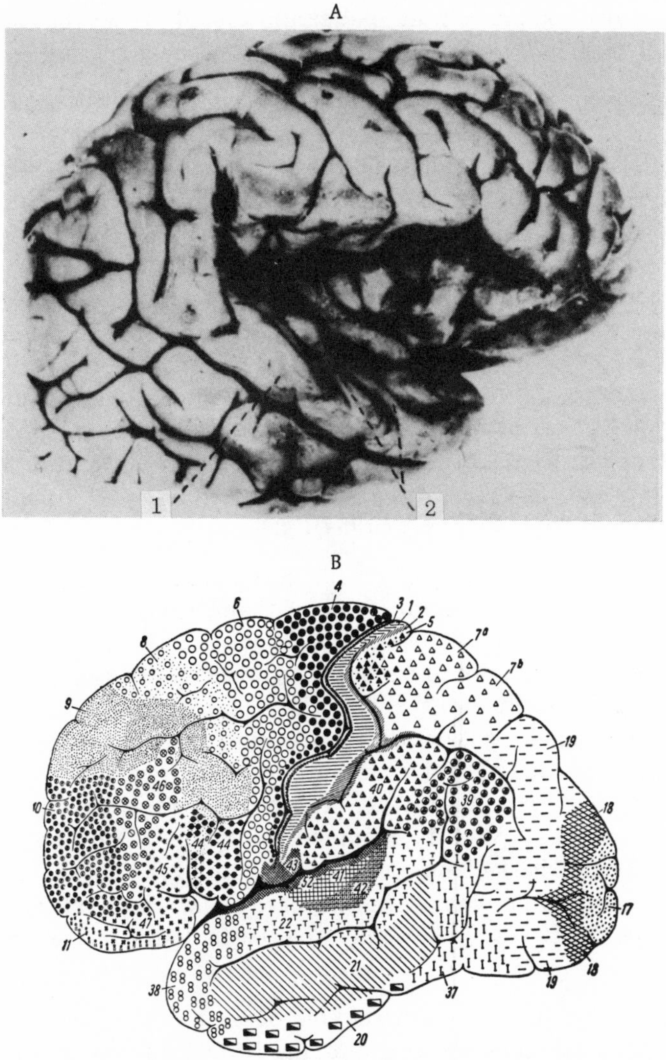

Fig. 1. A) topography of the cortical auditory area in man after separation of the edges of the lateral cerebral fissure (the fissure of Sylvius). Superior temporal gyrus (1) and transverse gyri (2) can be seen in this figure; B) cytoarchitectonic map of the superior temporal subregion (after Brodmann).

of the thalamus, but later they enter the ventral portion of the internal capsule above the lateral geniculate body, follow a sublenticular course, approach the claustrum closely from the lateral side, and then radiate fanwise to form the acoustic radiation.

Anatomical investigations by Flechsig (1920), Venderovich (1916), and Poljak (1932) showed that the central auditory pathway in man terminates in the region of the transverse gyri of the temporal lobe. According to Monakow and Zachler (1914), it terminates in the whole of the superior and even in the middle temporal gyri. Arutyunova (1954) studied secondary degeneration of cells of the medial geniculate body in the presence of pathological foci in various parts of the temporal lobe and found that the central auditory pathway terminates in cortical areas 41, 42, 41/42, and to some extent, 22, on the inferior wall of the sylvian fissure in the region of Heschl's gyrus and the superior temporal gyrus (Fig. 1). Most fibers of the acoustic radiation run to area 41, fewer fibers to area 42, while area 22 receives fibers mainly from areas 41 and 42 (Peele, 1954).

The transverse gyri (2-3) lie in the anterior portion of the superior temporal subregion. One of them, Heschl's gyrus, is the most marked, although it is very variable in size and position. Much of Heschl's gyrus is occupied by area 41. It has the typical coniocortical structure of receptor cortical areas, and consists of 6 layers with most of its cells in afferent layer IV. Area 42 forms a horseshoe around area 41. In this area, the granular layer IV is much narrower than in area 41. The middle two-thirds of the superior temporal gyrus is occupied by area 22. Morphologically and functionally it is closely connected with areas 41 and 42. The granular layer IV is narrow in this area also. Area TD of Economo or area 41/42 of Blinkov may also be included in the auditory system.

Differentiation of the structure of the auditory cortex in man begins at the 4th month of intrauterine life. By 6 months it contains all the layers, and by the age of 2 years all the adult features are present, i.e., the cortical lamina is converted into a six-layered cortex (Arutyunova, 1954). In the process of growth and differentiation area 41 increases in size much more than the medial geniculate body and area 22. This emphasizes the importance of the primary projection area for the higher forms of nervous activity in man (Blinkov, 1955).

The auditory cortex has numerous connections with other regions of the brain. Through the posterior parts of the corpus callosum, one cortical area is connected with the homonymous area of the opposite side. Connections of the auditory cortex with areas 21, 8, 18, 19, 6, 44, 43, and 37 have been demonstrated (Peele, 1954).

Two bundles of fibers (uncinate and arcuate) connect the temporal lobe with the frontal lobe. The uncinate bundle enters the external capsule and the capsula extreme, while the arcuate bundle enters the wall of the hemisphere between the lateral angle of the lateral ventricle and the surface of the frontal and parietal lobes, above the Sylvian fissure (Blinkov and Brazovskaya, 1957). Descending pathways to all lower levels of the auditory system leave the auditory cortex (Rasmussen, 1964).

The auditory cortex increases considerably in size during evolutionary development. According to Blinkov and Zvorykin (1950), for instance, in man the primary auditory area is 53 times larger than in monkeys, whereas the medial geniculate body is only 5.5 times larger. The auditory cortex in man differs considerably in its structure from that of animals. As the work of Blinkov (1955) showed, Heschl's gyrus is absent in lower monkeys, poorly developed in the anthropoid apes, but very large in man. The cytoarchitectonics of the auditory cortex is completely different in type in man. Area 41 is considerably larger. It accounts for 9.9% of the total area of the superior temporal subregion, whereas in monkeys it occupies only between 1 and 5% of this subregion. Area 41 in man is more highly differentiated and is subdivided into subareas which are absent in monkeys.

It is clear from this description that certain structural features distinguishing the auditory system are of great importance to the topical diagnosis of injury to its central portions. Symptoms connected with an accompanying lesion of structures lying next to auditory formations are very important for clinical diagnosis. For example, the combination of auditory and vestibular disturbances in acoustic neurinomas or systemic disturbances with tumors located in the floor of the 4th ventricle have been fully described in textbooks of otoneurology (Blagoveshchenskaya, 1962; Zhukovich, 1966; Tsimmerman, 1967).

So far as the problem of the character of disturbances of auditory function in central lesions is concerned, it is essential to realize that the fibers in the auditory nerve run in a compact bundle; in the medulla and pons the ascending auditory pathway consists of independent bundles side by side. In the lateral lemniscus and in that part of the ascending pathway which lies between the inferior colliculi and the medial geniculate body, and also in the lateral genu of the internal capsule, it runs once again as a single common bundle. It must therefore be expected that a pathological focus of any character (tumor, hemorrhage), if situated in those parts in which the auditory pathway is a compact bundle, must give rise to more severe disturbances of hearing.

The presence of several levels of relays and commissures makes for wide representation in all auditory nuclei above the cochlear inflow from the right and left cochleas. Consequently, whereas the auditory nerve contains fibers from the organ of Corti on one side only, the lateral lemniscus and other parts of the ascending auditory pathway contain both crossed and uncrossed fibers. Complete unilateral deafness is therefore possible only as the result of destruction of the auditory nerve or of the organ of Corti. A unilateral lesion of all structures located higher than the cochlear nuclei can give rise only to partial diminution of hearing. Moreover, it can be expected that a diminution of hearing of varying severity can be found as the result of changes on the side of the lesion and also on the contralateral side.

The comparative importance of the direct and crossed auditory pathways has been assessed in anatomical and physiological investigations.

The work of Flechsig (1920) and Bekhterev (1905, 1907) showed originally that the auditory cortex in man receives many fibers from the opposite ear.

Electrophysiological investigations show that the primary responses recorded from the cortical projection area have higher amplitude and lower threshold intensities if the sound is conducted to the ear contralateral to the investigated hemisphere than to the ipsilateral ear (Gershuni, 1940; Bremer and Dow, 1939; Bremer, 1943; Tunturi, 1946, 1952; Rosenzweig, 1951).

The leading role of the crossed auditory pathways is also clear from the results of an investigation by Penfield and Erickson (1945), who showed that electrical stimulation of the auditory cortex in man gives the sensation of the ringing of a bell, whistling, buzzing, droning, or tapping, and these sounds are projected to the ear contralateral to the stimulated hemisphere.

LESIONS OF THE CENTRAL BRAIN STEM

Most workers who have studied disturbances of hearing in lesions of the central portions of the auditory system state that the methods used nowadays to test hearing in otiatric practice* (determination of discrimination of whispered and conversational speech, tuning-fork tests, threshold tonal audiometry with air and bone conduction, Schwabach's test, tests of equalization or "recruiting" of loudness, investigation of differential thresholds of intensity and the lateralization of sound in Weber's test) provide a sufficiently accurate method of differentiating between a loss of hearing through injury to the sound-conducting apparatus of the ear and a loss of hearing due to disturbance of the sound-receiving apparatus of the cochlea of the inner ear. However, despite all these tests it is impossible to distinguish syndromes of disturbances characteristic of lesions of the central portions of the auditory system.

Disturbances of hearing discovered with the aid of these "classical" methods of investigation are frequently identical regardless of whether the pathological process is in the cochlea, the root of the auditory nerve, or the central nervous system (Gol'din, 1951; Blagoveshchenskaya, 1962; Wildhagen 1954; Bocca and Calearo, 1963; Matzker, 1965; Zhukovich, 1966; Tsimmerman, 1967).

The diagnosis of these lesions is largely based on other accompanying symptoms: vestibular, neurological, ophthalmological.

Blagoveshchenskaya (1962) holds more optimistic views on the possibility of diagnosis of lesions affecting the central portion of the auditory system on the basis of hearing disturbances.

By making use of published data and the results of her own investigations she distinguishes the following levels of lesions of

*For a full account of methods used in clinical practice to investigate hearing, which many authors describe as "classical methods of investigation," see: Gershuni (1959), Blagoveshchenskaya (1962), Zhukovich (1966), and Hirsch (1952).

the auditory system:

1. root lesions;
2. lesions at the level of the nuclei and tracts of the medulla and pons;
3. lesions at the level of the mesencephalon and geniculate bodies;
4. lesions of the internal capsule and temporal lobes.

The character of hearing disturbances in root lesions and in lesions affecting the mesencephalon and diencephalon, and also the results of comparison of hearing disturbances with the character of vestibular disorders and other neurological findings are fully described in textbooks of special otoneurology (Blagoveshchenskaya, 1962; Zhukovich, 1966).

Some general principles governing disturbances of the functions of the central parts of the auditory system depending on the level of the lesion can be distinguished from the published data.

The main symptom of a lesion of the auditory system, namely impairment of hearing at different frequencies, diminishes in importance as the site of the lesion moves closer to the cortical part and away from the peripheral part of the auditory system.

Various degrees of impairment of hearing from complete unilateral deafness (Blagoveshchenskaya, 1962), from an impairment of hearing less marked at low frequencies and increasing toward higher frequencies (Wildhagen, 1954) to a combination of slight impairment of hearing detectable by audiometry with gross disturbances of speech discrimination (Jerger, 1960, 1964; Citron et al., 1963) have been described in lesions of the VIII nerve.

If the pathological process is localized in the brain-stem portions of the auditory system or in the mesencephalon or diencephalon, all degrees of impairment of hearing have been described from the mildest, unilateral, to a very severe, bilateral, increase in the thresholds of audibility, but total unilateral or bilateral deafness has never been observed in this condition (Krassing, 1950; Greiner et al., 1956; Saltzman, 1952; Ladyzhenskaya, 1960; Arnold, 1951; Pötzl, 1946).

The increases in the thresholds discovered in diseases of the brain stem apply mainly to the homolateral ear (Goodman, 1957; Wildhagen, 1954; Bittrich, 1956).

Some workers consider that audiograms of parabolic shape, resulting from impairment of hearing at low and high frequencies, are characteristic of lesions of the brain stem (Appaix et al., 1957; Jatho, 1954; Greiner et al., 1957).

Lesions of all the central parts of the auditory system are characterized by absence of sound lateralization in Weber's test despite asymmetry of the thresholds of audibility, shortening of bone conduction, and absence of the rapid increase in loudness phenomenon. However, Greiner and coworkers (1957) have recently detected positive recruitment in brain-stem lesions, which they associate with disturbances in the cochlea resulting from the involvement of the efferent pathways of the auditory system, through which the system of the inner ear is controlled by the higher centers (Thiebaut et al., 1956; Pfaltz, 1963), in the pathological process.

Besides these general manifestations, lesions of the central portions of the auditory system also exhibit a certain specificity. For example, the most characteristic feature of a lesion of the VIII nerve is rapid adaptation of hearing, so that during 60 sec of continuous action of a sound the auditory threshold may rise by 40-50 dB (Jerger, 1960b).

Dissociation between a gross disturbance of the discrimination of speech and the slight changes discovered by tonal audiometry is regarded as characteristic of lesions of the brain-stem portions (Blagoveshchenskaya, 1965; Jerger, 1960; Tsimmerman, 1967).

The use of additional methods of investigation of hearing, in conjunction with the "classical" methods, led to the distinction of special hearing disorders characteristic of diencephalic lesions (Arnold, 1946, 1951; Stockert and Fresser, 1954; Stockert, 1954; Pötzl, 1946b; Rabending, 1959). In patients with a lesion in the thalamus, these workers observed neglibible impairment of hearing in the ear contralateral to the focus, a disturbance of pitch perception, acoustic allesthesia,* and central diplacusis† a disturbance of the temporal relationship between the perception of stimuli by the left and right ears. The patients likewise could not distinguish between chords and individual sounds, they could not recognize simple melodies which they knew before, and they could not distinguish or reproduce rhythms.

The form of speech disorders in these patients is of special interest. They did not understand speech in noisy rooms or if several people spoke simultaneously, but they understood phrases perfectly well during ordinary conversation.

These authors thus consider that central auditory lesions are characterized by dissociation between the very slight lowering of the auditory threshold and the marked disorders at levels above the threshold.

The results of the investigation of hearing in patients with cortical lesions will be examined in the next section.

LESIONS OF THE TEMPORAL LOBE

The first experimental results showing that the cortical center of hearing is located in the temporal lobe were obtained by Ferrier (1876). He showed that unilateral destruction of the superior part of the temporal lobe in monkeys caused impairment of hearing which was more marked on the opposite side, and that bilateral destruction of this region was accompanied by marked deafness although other forms of sensation (vision, olfaction, taste) remained intact.

Similar results were obtained on other species of animals by Munk (1881) and by Luciani and Sepilli (1866). Despite the fact that some results of these investigations were not subsequently confirmed, they provided an impetus for research into the state of the hearing function in animals after injuries to central portions of the auditory system.

*By central allesthesia is meant a distortion of perception of the acoustic image through 180°.

†Diplacusis means absence of fusion of the acoustic image, in which the patient hears the stimulus separately in time and modified in tone with the left and right ear.

Simultaneously with these investigations, Broca (1861) published his anatomical studies showing that aphemia (now called motor aphasia) is the result of injury to the inferior frontal gyrus of the left hemisphere in man.

Wernicke (1874) showed that a localized lesion of the lateral portion of the superior temporal region in the left hemisphere, which he described as the speech-hearing area, causes a disturbance of the understanding of speech.

When he described the syndrome of sensory aphasia, Wernicke considered that this type of speech disorder, which he observed in lesions of the posterior third of the first temporal gyrus of the left temporal lobe, is due to a disturbance of hearing in the speech region of the tone scale, i.e., that it is a purely auditory disturbance.

As a result of many investigations in recent years the character of the speech disturbance in patients with temporal lesions has been described (Luria, 1947, 1962; Orfinskaya, 1958; Bein, 1948, 1964; Tonkonogii, 1968; Lebedinskii, 1941; Nielsen, 1946; Goldstein, 1948; Penfield and Roberts, 1959; Kleist, 1934; Marie, 1906; Head, 1926). As a result of these investigations, an orderly theory of the aphasias was developed, a classification of the aphasias was drawn up, and their topical-diagnostic significance was examined.

Sensory aphasia was shown to arise when a lesion is present in the left (in right-handed persons) temporal lobe. In sensory aphasia the lesion is found particularly often in the posterior third of the superior temporal gyrus (the posterior zone of area 22). Narrow localization is not found in every case, for the character and intensity of the aphasic manifestations are determined not only by the site of the lesion, but also by its extent and by other factors: the character of the process, the patient's general condition, and, in particular, the state of vascularization of the brain, the patient's age, and so on.

The preservation of speech or the transient nature of the speech disturbances after excision of localized parts of the speech areas of the cortex for temporal epilepsy has been described by Penfield and Roberts (1959).

Consequently, the localization of a pathological focus in certain zones of the left temporal lobe does not necessarily mean that it will give rise to marked disturbances of speech, and a focus in the right temporal lobe will not, in general, be accompanied by a disturbance of the perception of speech. For these reasons the diagnosis of lesions of the temporal lobe can be very difficult (Popov, 1959; Shimanskii, 1959). To determine the localization of a pathological process it is often necessary to resort to electroencephalography, arteriography, and ventriculography. However, besides these techniques, the development of precise otoneurological methods of diagnosis is of great importance.

Investigation of the state of hearing in patients with lesions of the temporal lobe has been conducted in two directions. In the first, the object was to determine whether disturbances of auditory function lie at the basis of the speech disturbance in the aphasias, and in the second, attempts were made to find diagnostic tests capable of revealing the localization of pathological foci in the temporal lobe despite the absence or trivial nature of the aphasic syndrome.

There are so many papers describing results of the investigation of hearing in individual patients or small groups of patients with temporal lobe lesions that it is impossible to enumerate them fully, and for this reason we shall merely describe those results which were obtained by the investigation of comparatively large groups of patients and, in particular, those in which the site of the lesion was verified in sufficient detail, largely by histological methods.

Auditory Thresholds in Patients with Temporal Lobe Lesions

The results of investigation of the acuity of hearing in patients with lesions of the temporal cortex are highly contradictory. The literature contains a few reports of an impairment of hearing in some patients with a unilateral lesion of the temporal cortex.

Cushing (1921) investigated 59 patients with tumors of the temporal lobe and found slight impairment of hearing in only 7 patients.

Grahe (1932) described 21 patients with a unilateral lesion of the temporal cortex, observed by himself and by other writers, and noted a transient disturbance of hearing in nearly all the patients.

Kolodny (1928) noted a slight impairment of hearing in only 3 of 38 patients with temporal lobe tumors.

Bozzi (1929) tested the hearing of 82 patients with temporal lobe tumors and found hypoacusia in only 7 cases: in 5 of these patients the impairment was bilateral, in 1 patient it was observed in the homolateral ear relative to the pathological focus, and in the other patient it was in the contralateral ear.

Dandy (1933) studied 8 patients after unilateral right or left hemispherectomy and observed impairment of hearing on the side opposite to the operation in only 1 patient. This patient's hearing was fully restored after 4 months. In all these patients the investigation was carried out with tuning forks.

Phillippides and Greiner (1950) used pure-tone audiometry and described two patients with unilateral extirpation of the temporal lobe; in both patients they found impairment of hearing in the ear contralateral to the operation. Similar results were obtained by Santos and Correa (1957) in two patients also after hemispherectomy.

The workers cited above give the result of single observations even in cases when the number of patients under observation was large (Cushing, 1921; Kolodny, 1928; Bozzi, 1929), and impairment of hearing is not characteristic of the whole group of patients studied, but merely of individual patients and it evidently cannot be reliably concluded that the observed impairment of hearing was in fact due to a peripheral lesion of the auditory system.

A higher percentage of hearing disturbances in temporal lesions was described by Shileiko (1940), Wildhagen (1954), and Street (1957).

Z. I. Shileiko investigated 47 patients with temporal lobe tumors and observed an impairment of hearing in 49%, bilateral in the majority of cases. In nearly all her patients, regardless of the site of the tumor, the impairment of hearing was more marked at low frequencies.

Wildhagen (1954) investigated 120 patients with tumors variously located in the cerebral hemispheres, including the temporal lobe, the cerebellum, the ventricular system, and the cerebello-pontine angle. In 75% of these patients he observed impairment of hearing, but only in patients with tumors of the cerebello-pontine angle could he demonstrate a regular impairment of hearing, more marked in the direction from low to high frequencies. In all the other cases it was impossible to differentiate the site of the tumor on the basis of the audiograms.

Street (1957) investigated the thresholds of audibility of pure tone in the range from 125 Hz to 12 kHz in 90 patients, aged from 19 to 70 years, with marked aphasia (regardless of its etiology – whether vascular, traumatic, or neoplastic). In 88% of the patients he found a varied degree of impairment of hearing, bilateral in 68% of the group and unilateral in 32%. In some patients the impairment of hearing was observed at low frequencies, and in others at high frequencies. Naturally, Street did not possess audiometric data for these patients before the beginning of the disease, but the subjects themselves had not previously noticed any appreciable impairment of hearing.

The acuity of hearing was investigated in 73 persons in a free acoustic field by Terr, Goetzinger, and Rousey (1958). After correction for loss of hearing due to age, these workers found no significant differences between the thresholds of audibility within the range from 125 to 2000 Hz between patients with temporal aphasia and patients with lesions of the other parts of the cerebral cortex. There was likewise no difference between the results of audiometric testing of the right and left ears in each group of patients, or between the results of measurement in patients with lesions of the dominant and subdominant hemispheres, These workers found some impairment of hearing at low frequencies below 125 Hz and high frequencies of 4–8 kHz.*

*In some investigations a similar impairment of hearing was observed in patients with tumors of the parietal lobe and also with a cystic tumor of the frontal lobe (Matzker, 1965).

Some impairment of hearing at high frequencies in patients with temporal epilepsy as the result of atrophy was also described by Sinha (1959).

Impairment of hearing was thus observed in only a few patients, and as the results of the tests described above show, those workers who consider that removal or destruction of the temporal lobe by a pathological process leads to impairment of hearing have not been able to correlate the character of these disturbances with a particular localization, extent, or etiology of the pathological process.

A correction for the patient's age was not introduced in all investigations carried out to assess the degree of impairment of hearing. It must also be taken into account that, for obvious reasons, no audiograms were obtained from the patients before the disease began, and some degree of impairment of hearing could be attributable to previous illnesses.

The attempt made by Pialoux (1962) to distinguish certain types of audiograms characteristic of lesions of the auditory cortex from those characteristic of lesions of the auditory system at other levels proved unsuccessful.

Most authors, whether describing single changes examined in detail and verified at autopsy or describing extensive series of cases, have been unable to establish a permanent impairment of hearing in patients with unilateral lesions of the temporal lobe or even after its removal.

Morrell (1935) cites a patient described by Bonhoeffer (1915): a 47-year old physician with destruction of the auditory radiation in the left hemisphere, subsequently verified at autopsy, who exhibited verbal deafness, although hearing at all frequencies was completely intact when tested in both the right and left ear.

Henschen (1918) cites the results of observations on the patient Clara Nielsen, (aged 54 years), in whom the right temporal lobe, including the transverse temporal gyri, was completely destroyed, yet no disturbance of hearing could be found. The results of Morrell's own observations also indicate the complete preservation of hearing after destruction of the right or left temporal lobe.

Integrity of hearing at different frequencies after complete removal of one hemisphere was also observed by Greiner, Kantzer, and Rohmer (1951) and by Brunetti (1961).

No decrease in the absolute thresholds likewise was observed during an investigation of 115 patients with traumatic lesions of the temporal lobe by Alekseenko and coworkers (1948). King (1958) found normal thresholds during tonal audiometry in cases of unilateral hemispherectomy (for infantile hemiplegia) both before and after the operation. In these patients King observed a contralateral loss of the hearing of speech after removal of the left hemisphere.

The integrity of tonal hearing in unilateral lesions of the temporal lobe likewise has been reported by many investigators (Shmar'yan, 1937, 1949; Undrits, 1963; Blagoveshchenskaya, 1962; Clark et al., 1938; Greiner et al., 1951; Stockert, 1954; Schubert and Panse, 1953; Bocca et al., 1954; De Sa, 1958; Jerger, 1960b; Alajouanine et al., 1955; Schankweiler, 1966).

It can be concluded from these investigations that unilateral destruction or extirpation of the temporal lobe does not result in any marked decrease in hearing specific for a lesion with a particular localization. However, since each ear is connected with both the left and the right temporal lobes, the role of the auditory cortex in the detection of acoustic stimuli can only be assessed on the basis of tests carried out on patients with total bilateral destruction of the temporal lobes. Very few observations on patients with total bilateral destruction of the auditory cortex, confirmed histologically, have been described. Henschen (1920) publishes the results of 9 clinical–anatomical observations on patients with bilateral destruction of the transverse temporal gyri. All these patients had total deafness. Deafness following bilateral lesions of the auditory cortex has been described by Bekhterev (1905), Bramwell (1927), Misch (1928), Pfeifer (1936), Lhermitte (1936), and Clark and Russell (1938). Bramwell (1927) describes a 62-year-old woman with mitral stenosis who developed a focus of softening in the left temporal region as the result of embolism on the left middle cerebral artery, accompanied by sensory aphasia. Twelve days after the first stroke she had a second in the opposite temporal region, and she became totally deaf. At autopsy an extensive lesion of the left hemisphere was found, involving the greater part of the left temporal lobe, while on the right the lesion was more local and included the supramarginal gyri and the superior and posterior parts of the left superior temporal gyrus.

A similar case was described by Misch (1928). In a patient with septic endocarditis embolism of the vessels of the left temporal region caused sensory aphasia and hemiplegia, but hearing remained completely intact. After the onset of cerebral changes on the right side, leading to destruction of the cortex of the medial part of the anterior transverse gyrus, total deafness ensued. In both cases the patients died a very short time after the second stroke (10–30 days), so that the deafness described by these workers was observed in the acute stage of the stroke.

No new cases of total deafness in bilateral lesions of the auditory cortex have been published. On the other hand, Lemoyne and Mahoudea (1959) made clinical and anatomical observations on a patient with audioverbal agnosia. Tonal audiometry revealed slight bilateral impairment of hearing in this patient. The differential thresholds of intensity, measured by the Lüscher – Zwislocki method, were indistinguishable from the results of measurement of healthy subjects. However this patient could not recognize music and did not understand speech addressed to him. At autopsy almost complete bilateral destruction of the acoustic radiation was found.

Deafness likewise has not been observed in cases of bilateral lesions of the temporal lobe confirmed at autopsy (Heilbronner, 1910; Wohlfart et al., 1952; Hansen and Reske-Nielsen, 1963).

Larsell (1961) and Ranson and Clark (1959), on the basis of their findings, also deny that total deafness develops after bilateral destruction of the transverse temporal gyri and acoustic radiation in man.

This contradiction in the results of investigation into the state of hearing of patients with bilateral lesions of the auditory cortex can be explained by the fact that methods used to investigate hearing at the beginning of this century were very imperfect.

In this connection it cannot fail to be observed that in more recent investigations of hearing by tonal audiometry no new cases of deafness associated with bilateral lesions of the temporal lobe have been described.

In many investigations no detailed microscopic study of the brain at all levels of the auditory system was made. Moreover, in the cases described by the authors cited above the diseases causing destruction of the temporal cortex were different (tumors, vascular diseases, Pick's disease), and this could mean that the subcortical structures were involved to a different degree in the pathological process. For example, Greiner, Kantzer, and Rohmer (1951) noted the absence of disturbances of hearing on tonal audiometry in one patient after total extirpation of the temporal lobe against the background of quietness and of masking noise, and normal differential thresholds of intensity. In another patient in whom deafness was observed, but whose ability to speak spontaneously was unimpaired, a symmetrical vascular lesion was found at autopsy in the external capsule, isolating the insular cortex and the submarginal cortex on the upper surface of the middle part of the superior temporal gyrus on both sides. In addition, a small part of the projection fibers connected with the lower border of the central gyrus was damaged. As a result, total degeneration of the medial geniculate bodies, the medial part of the lentiform nucleus, and the nucleus centralis medialis was observed in the thalamus. Degeneration of the greater part of the nucleus ventralis and base of the pulvinar also was found. Despite the deafness, the patient was still able to speak spontaneously. These workers attribute the deafness observed in this patient to the total degeneration of the medial geniculate bodies.

The state of the acuity of hearing in man after bilateral destruction of the auditory cortex is thus not yet finally settled.

Differential sensation in patients with lesions of the auditory cortex has received much less investigation.

Schubert and Panse (1953) gave a detailed account of the results of an investigation of a patient with a unilateral wound of the left temporal region in whom hearing was unimpaired, and the thresholds of discrimination of sound intensity on days when his general condition was good were indistinguishable from the normal values, and the thresholds of discrimination of sound frequency also were normal. However, this patient exhibited an increased tendency toward auditory fatigue, accompanied by a marked increase in the differential thresholds.

Great fluctuations in auditory thresholds in children with sensory alalia are also mentioned by Traugott (1946). He calls this phenomenon temporal acupathia and explains it by the instability of auditory attention.

Differential thresholds of intensity investigated by Zhukovich and Khortseva (1964) by the Lüscher – Zwislocki method in 4 patients with a pathological focus in the temporal cortex were indistinguishable from those measured in patients with lesions in the frontal or parietal lobes, with tumors of the mesencephalon or diencephalon, or with tumors of the posterior cranial fossa.

Boiko (1966) investigated the differentiation of intensity by the same method in patients with different forms of temporal aphasia and found no consistent changes in differential sensitivity. In some patients she observed much lower values than normally of the minimal distinguishable changes of intensity (just as in diseases of the cochlea), while in other patients with a pathological focus in the same situation the differentiation of intensity was much greater than that characteristically found in subjects with normal hearing.

Swischer (1967) observed a temporary decrease in the differential thresholds of intensity of long acoustic stimuli for up to 3 weeks after removal of a large part of the left temporal cortex including Heschl's gyrus for the operative treatment of temporal epilepsy. The mean level of the differential thresholds of intensity was 0.68 dB, compared with 0.98-1.98 dB before the operation in these patients and in patients undergoing operation but leaving Heschl's gyrus intact, and also in the control group, i.e., it was very little different from the corresponding values in healthy untrained subjects. The absence of changes in differential thresholds of intensity of long acoustic stimuli in patients with sensory acoustic aphasia resulting from vascular diseases has also been described by Baru and Vasserman (1968). The level of the differential thresholds in their patients was 1.6 ±0.2 dB.

Discrimination between two tonal stimuli by frequency in patients with sensory aphasia likewise shows no significant difference from the results of tests on healthy persons or on patients with motor aphasia. Two patients with sensory aphasia, as Traugott, Kaidanova, and Meierson (1967) showed, distinguished a tone of 200 Hz from tones of 205 and 210 Hz. However, these workers state that the differentiation of acoustic stimuli by these patients took longer to develop than differentiation of visual and tactile stimuli. Acoustic differentiation also was formed more slowly in patients with sensory aphasia than in patients with motor aphasia. No disturbances of other subthreshold audiological tests have been described in patients with injury to the auditory cortex.

Jerger (1960) finds that although their thresholds of audibility in the right and left ears are the same, patients with cortical lesions show negative recruitment on the side opposite to the lesion. To balance the loudness of subthreshold tone, a sound of higher intensity had to be applied to the ear opposite to the lesion.

The results obtained by most investigators thus suggest that the absolute and differential thresholds of frequency and intensity are not significantly disturbed by unilateral destruction of the auditory cortex, or even after total removal of one temporal lobe. Convincing data on the state of hearing after bilateral destruction of the auditory cortex are not yet sufficiently available.

Since the extent of the destruction varies considerably in different patients, since subcortical structures may be involved, since secondary changes (hypertensive, for example) cannot be ruled out, and also since the state of hearing before the beginning of the disease is as a rule unknown, the results of animal experiments are of great importance to the determination of the state of auditory function after unilateral and, in particular, after bilateral extirpation of the auditory cortex.

Experiments on animals have shown that after extensive bilateral ablations of the temporal cortex in cats, dogs, and monkeys not only can conditioned reflexes be formed to acoustic stimuli, but these stimuli can also be distinguished in frequency and intensity (Babkin, 1911; Mering, 1952, 1962; Khananashvili, 1965; Belenkov, 1965; Kalinina, 1962; Sosenkov, 1963; Mosidze, 1965; Tunturi, 1955).

Quantitative investigations, with measurements of absolute thresholds and also of differential thresholds of frequency and intensity, likewise revealed no significant increase in the thresholds after extensive bilateral ablation of the temporal cortex* in cats and dogs when stimuli of the usual duration, i.e., of the order of 1 sec or more, were used (Baru, 1964, 1966, 1967b; Kryter and Ades, 1943; Stroughton and Neff, 1950; Raab and Ades, 1946; Rosenzweig, 1946; Butler, Diamond, and Neff, 1957; Goldberg and Neff, 1961; Thompson, 1960).

Slight disturbances of frequency discrimination described during tests on dogs (Allen, 1945) and cats (Meyer and Woolsey, 1952), as Thompson (1960) showed, are due to the nature of the techniques used by these workers and the mode of presentation of the stimuli.

Somewhat different results were obtained by investigation of differential thresholds of frequency in monkeys (Massopust et al., 1967). After bilateral extirpation of the auditory projection cortex, like other investigators they found no increase in the differential thresholds. However, bilateral extirpation of the auditory association area as well as the projection area in the temporal lobe caused an increase in the differential thresholds to a frequency of 100 Hz from 7 to 20 Hz.

The published evidence thus shows that removal of the auditory projection area (and also the adjacent areas of the temporal cortex) in animals or injury to and removal of the temporal cortex in man does not cause any significant disturbance of the detection and the discrimination of the frequency and intensity of single tonal stimuli such as are used in ordinary behavioral and audiometric tests.

Examination of the results of the investigations cited above shows that new methods of testing are required both for the diagnosis of central auditory lesions and for the determination of their nature.

At the present time, besides methods used previously, four independent lines of development can be identified in the study of the functions of the temporal cortex.

*Extensive ablation of the temporal cortex included the whole middle ectosylvian gyrus, the superior part of the anterior and the superior, middle, and inferior parts of the posterior ectosylvian gyri, the superior part of the anterior and posterior sylvian gyri, and also the insulo-temporal cortex.

1. Investigation of the ability to distinguish the meaning of verbal communications when the extent of information contained in them is reduced (Bocca, Calearo, and Cassinari, 1954; Calearo and Antonelli, 1963; Bocca and Calearo, 1963).

2. Investigation of the perception of binaurally presented stimuli. In this case two independent problems can be examined:

a) the lateralization of the sound and localization of the source of sound in space (Matzker, 1957, 1959; Arnold, 1946, 1951; Sanchez-Longo and Forster, 1958);

b) investigation of the possibility of binaural summation or integration.

3. Analysis of the state of musical abilities, perception of complex sounds, rhythm, the time of perception, and the phenomena of auditory fatigue (Luria, 1962; Semernitskaya, 1945; Arnold, 1951; Stockert, 1951, 1954; Rabending, 1959; Kimura, 1964; Schankweiler, 1966; Feuchtwanger, 1930).

4. An independent line of research is the investigation of the neurodynamics in temporal lesions. Workers using the conditioned-reflex method have investigated the interaction between excitation and inhibition, and trace phenomena in the central nervous system (Traugott, 1947; Shmidt and Sukhovskaya, 1954; Kaidanova and Meierson, 1961; Stolyarova-Kabelyanskaya, 1961).

Perception of Speech when the Excess of Information Is Reduced

Although a number of investigators (Undrits, 1963; Blagoveshchenskaya, 1965) have found a definite dissociation between intact hearing of pure tone and a disturbance of the intelligibility of speech in patients with lesions of the central zones of the auditory system, subthreshold verbal audiometry has proved to be insufficiently reliable as a test for the diagnosis of temporal lobe lesions.

Good results were obtained by Bocca and his coworkers by the use of spoken stimuli for the diagnosis of temporal lobe lesions when the excess of information contained in the spoken words was reduced by filtration, by compression in time, by periodic interruption, or by the addition of interference in the shape of a dictated text or a noise background applied to the same ear as that receiving the speech, or to the opposite ear.

The first monaural test suggested by Bocca, Calearo, and Cassinari (1954) consisted of testing the intelligibility of speech when verbal material (disyllabic words, phrases composed of disyllabic words, passed through a low-frequency filter which removed all frequencies above 800 Hz from the spectrum of the phonetic material) was applied separately to the left or right ear by means of a telephone.

While the ability to understand the verbal communication was generally reduced, its intelligibility was significantly worse when it was applied to the ear contralateral to the affected temporal lobe, whether the focus was in the left or the right hemisphere. Bocca's second monaural test (Bocca, 1951; Calearo and Antonelli, 1963) consisted of investigating the intelligibility of interrupted speech in which the frequency of the interruption ranged from 2 to 20/sec. In the third test (Bocca and Calearo, 1963), accelerated speech was used: instead of normal speech (140 words per minute in Italian), mechanically accelerated speech with a speed of 250-340 words per minute was presented monaurally. The fourth monaural test consisted of the identification of normal speech during the simultaneous presentation of interfering speech applied to the same ear (Bocca and Calearo, 1963).

In all these tests a decrease in the intelligibility of speech was clearly observed in the ear contralateral to the affected temporal lobe, regardless of whether the lesion was in the left or right hemisphere. Tests of a similar character with analogous results have also been described by Tato and Quiros (1960), Quist-Hansen and Strömsnes (1960), Harris, Haines and Meyers (1960), and others. A disturbance of the recognition of speech during the masking action of noise has also been demonstrated by Mounier-Kuhn and Lafon (1962).

Binaural Hearing in Temporal Lobe Lesions

A method frequently used to locate lesions of the auditory system at its various levels is to examine the state of the patient's binaural hearing.

The use of binaural tests is based on the fact that, starting from the level of the superior olives, there is interaction between the afferent impulses from the two symmetrical receptor fields of the auditory system when sound is conducted to both ears. If the auditory system is injured at a certain level, the character or the comparison of the excitation patterns arising from symmetrical areas of the auditory system may be disturbed.

The integrity of binaural hearing can be demonstrated by testing:

1. the lateralization of sounds and the localization of the source of sound in space;
2. the possibility of binaural summation or integration;
3. the identification of speech and music under conditions when the useful signal is applied to one ear and noise to the other.

One feature of the integrity of binaural hearing in patients is their ability to localize a sound in space. This phenomenon has been investigated in healthy subjects and in patients both in the form of lateralization, i.e., identifying the movement of the acoustic image in response to a change in the intensity of one of the binaurally presented stimuli, a change in the time interval between them, or from the phase difference between the sound waves reaching both ears, and also in the form of determining the localization of a sound in a free acoustic field.

The quantitative characteristics of the ability of the healthy human subject to localize a source of sound have been described by Rozenzweig (1951). By the use of Vojacek's laterometer, i.e., transmitting sound separately to each ear, Alekseenko and coworkers (1948, 1949) showed that the lateralization of sound is undisturbed in patients with complete unilateral destruction of the temporal lobe, including the auditory cortex, as the result of wounding.

These workers found that the lateralization of sound is disturbed in patients with a unilateral lesion of the temporo-parieto-occipital and inferior parietal region of the brain. These disturbances disappeared a few months after wounding. Similar results were obtained by Ageeva-Maikova and Sviridova (1951). Schankweiler (1961) investigated patients with pathological foci in the temporal lobe and likewise found no disturbance of localization of a source of sound.

Blagoveshchenskaya (1962) found a disturbance of the localization of sound in an acoustic field on the opposite side to the pathological focus in patients with lesions not confined to the temporal lobe, but in the parieto-temporal regions of the cortex.

After investigating the localization of sound in a free acoustic field, a number of investigators (Sanchez-Longo, Forster, and Auth, 1957; Sanchez-Longo and Forster, 1958; Jerger, 1960; Teuber and Diamond, 1956) found disturbances of the localization of sound in patients with unilateral lesions of the temporal lobe, in an acoustic field contralateral to the side of the temporal lobe lesion. These workers state that the sound was displaced toward the side opposite to the pathological focus.

The same method was used by Kaidanova, Meierson, and Tonkonogii (1965), who found disturbances of the localization of sound in patients with local lesions of the temporal and also of the parietal lobe when the sound was applied from the side of the healthy hemisphere, and discovered a tendency for the sound to shift toward the affected hemisphere.

Matzker (1957, 1958, 1959) applied a series of short pulses of sound to each ear separately, to one ear after a delay of 0.018-0.6 msec compared with the other. He showed that in healthy subjects the minimal difference in the times of arrival of the acoustic pulses in the right and left ear at which the sound was no longer heard in the midline was 0.018 msec. He confirmed the value of 0.684 msec, as determined by Hornbostel and Wertheimer (1920), as the minimum essential for displacement of the sound by 90° from the midline in healthy human subjects. Matzker (1959) used this test on 400 patients and found that in those with a lesion of the temporal lobes the midline zone was widened on the side contralateral to the focus, while in patients with a lesion of the brain stem it was widened on the side of the focus. In addition, in each concrete case care must be taken to ensure that the observed deviation is not due to unilateral peripheral damage.

Contrary to the results obtained by Sanchez-Longo and coworkers, Matzker (1959) showed that disturbances of the localization of sound do not necessarily mean injury to the temporal lobe. Unilateral foci of injury in the frontal, parietal and occipital lobes, and also in the brain stem can give rise to disturbances of the lateralization of sound.

The localization of sound in patients with temporal lesions was also investigated by Walsh (1957), Sedlaček (1960), and Norlund (1962). Walsh observed that in central auditory lesions the ability to localize sound in the vertical plane is affected, while the ability to localize sound in the horizontal plane remains intact.

Other types of binaural tests are those based on binaural summation or integration. They have been used in two forms: first, in summation facilitating the identification of signals through summation of their loudness or summation of two filtered, mutually complementary signals, and second, in the presence of noise applied to the opposite ear. Discrimination of speech or tonal thresholds was also investigated during the application of noise or of spoken announcements to the opposite ear.

The use of these tests showed that the discrimination of speech is impaired in the ear opposite to the pathological focus when any of these forms of interference are applied to the other ear.

If speech is applied alternately to the right and left ears (frequency 1-50/min) no reliable evidence can be obtained of a pathological focus in the temporal cortex, for identification is disturbed in old people and in patients with lesions of the auditory system in the brain stem (Bocca and Calearo, 1963; Hennebert, 1955). These results are attributed to difficulty in switching attention rapidly. A disturbance of attention in temporal lesions has also been described by Feldman (1960).

Tests based on binaural summation were suggested by Bocca (1961), Matzker (1959), and others. In Bocca's (1961) investigation normal speech of subthreshold intensity (level of intelligibility 25-45%) was applied to one ear, and the same text but after filtration to remove low frequencies (up to 500 Hz) was applied to the other ear at an intensity of 40 dB above threshold. When this text was applied monaurally, the level of intelligibility was 40%. On simultaneous application of these signals to both ears of healthy subjects binaural summation takes place and the mean level of intelligibility of the text for healthy subjects is 76%. In patients with lesions of the auditory cortex, no improvement of intelligibility follows binaural presentation of the text. Similar tests were used by Calearo (1957).

Matzker (1958, 1959), in his test of binaural summation, applied the same text to both ears but to one ear in the frequency band of 500-800 Hz and to the other ear in the band from 1815 to 2500 Hz. On simultaneous presentation of the filtered text to healthy subjects, 100% intelligibility resulted, while in patients with central lesions of the auditory system the level of intelligibility was very low.

Matzker regards this test as diagnostic of lesions of the auditory system in the brain stem, whereas Linden (1960, 1964) claims that it can detect foci in the temporal lobe.

In the investigations described above the intelligibility of speech was studied when signals were presented to the ear homolateral or contralateral to the pathological focus, i.e., attention was concentrated on the direct and crossed auditory pathways and the role of commissural connections was disregarded. This gives special interest to the description of an investigation of one patient (Sparks and Geschwind, 1968) in whom the commissural pathways connecting the left and right temporal lobes were divided for the treatment of temporal epilepsy. The use of audiometric tests revealed impairment of hearing in the right and left ears to high frequencies (4.6 and 8 kHz) on the average by 85-90%. If numbers consisting of 2 digits or monosyllabic words were presented to both ears the patient was quite unable to distinguish the signal (numbers and monosyllabic names of animals) when applied to the left ear, contralateral to the temporal lobe lesion, whereas 44% of the words applied to the right ear were repeated correctly. If the signal was presented to one ear and noise simultaneously presented to the other, 95-100% of correct responses were obtained, i.e., on account of division of the commissural connections the noise had no effect on perception of words by the other ear. Monaural speech tests revealed a 95-100% level of intelligibility of loud speech and a 23% level of intelligibility of filtered speech when applied to the left ear contralateral to the pathological focus, whereas the intellibility of the same signal when applied to the right ear was 66%.

Tests of binaural summation showed that when a weak signal was applied to the left ear and a filtered signal to the right no summation took place and the intelligibility of the signal was not improved by comparison with that of monaural presentation.

Complex excitatory and inhibitory relationships between the hemispheres were also demonstrated by the work of Chocholle (1957). For the diagnosis of temporal lobe lesions he investigated the smallest perceptible changes in intensity by the Lüscher – Zwislocki method by applying an amplitude-modulated tone to one ear and interference simultaneously to the other ear in the form of a continuous tone of the same or a different frequency, but of much lower intensity.

Chocholle found that when tones of equal frequency were applied to both ears of healthy subjects the smallest perceptible change in intensity (i.e., the differential threshold of intensity) is increased. If different tones are applied to the right and left ears the threshold of discrimination of intensity is reduced. In patients with lesions of the temporal cortex no integration is observed, and amplitude modulation is not suppressed by application of a tone of the same frequency to the opposite ear.

The same results were obtained by Maspétiol, Semette, and Mathieu (1960). However, these workers observed similar results also in patients with lesions of the auditory system in the brain stem.

Elevation of the thresholds of audibility only on the side contralateral to the lesion was also observed in patients with lesions of the temporal lobe and manifestations of sensory aphasia by Tonkonogii and Kaidanova (1963) when they tested the perception of tonal stimuli applied against the background of masking noise. Similar results were obtained by Sinha (1959).

However, Greiner and coworkers (1951) found no disturbance of hearing in patients with temporal lobe tumors during tonal audiometry against a background of noise.

The use of specialized speech tests, of binaural summation, and of the interpretation of stimuli against a background of noise or other interference applied to the opposite ear thus showed that disturbances of the recognition of mono- and bisyllabic words and of sentences composed of bisyllabic words always takes place on the side opposite to the side of extirpation, regardless of whether the pathological focus lies in the left or the right temporal lobe. These results indicate the role of the right temporal lobe in the recognition of speech under complex conditions (interference, interruption, compression), and at the same time they demonstrate the absence of asymmetry between the results of partial (unaccompanied by sensory aphasia) lesions of the left or right temporal lobe.

Nevertheless, after tests on patients with atrophic changes in the cortex of the left or right temporal lobes Milner (1962, 1967) found a clearly defined asymmetry of functions.

Damage confined to the left temporal lobe, where the speech center is located,* disturbs the perception of verbal material, and the defect is particularly clear after removal of the temporal lobe. However, no difference was found in these patients before and after operation as regards the number of mistakes made when solving problems on the differentiation of the duration, rhythm, pitch, and loudness of tonal stimuli. On the other hand, after removal of the right temporal lobe for the treatment of temporal epilepsy in patients with cortical atrophy, a statistically significant impairment of duration and timbre discrimination and of tonal memory was found although the perception of pitch and loudness remained intact. Although the volume of brain tissue removed from the right hemisphere was greater, on the average, than from the left, regardless of this difference none of these patients could distinguish the timbre of sounds after the operation. The difficulty of differentiation between these stimulus characteristics was also independent of the presence or absence of Heschl's gyrus.

Asymmetry in the functions of the left and right temporal lobes has also been demonstrated by tests on healthy persons (Kimura, 1961b).

---

*The localization of the speech center in all patients was based on the results of Wada's test (Wada and Rasmussen, 1960).

By comparing the assessments of perception of verbal material and tunes by the left and right ears during dichotic* presentation Kimura (1961b) showed that healthy subjects make fewer mistakes in the recognition of tunes presented to the left ear and fewer mistakes in the recognition of verbal material, including numbers, presented to the right ear.

Since it is generally accepted that the crossed auditory pathway is the more important, Kimura considers that his results confirm Milner's (1962) views of the localization of musical hearing in the right temporal lobe. Further support is given by the case of severe sensory aphasia resulting from an extensive lesion of the left temporal lobe in a well-known composer, whose musical ability remained completely unimpaired, described by Luria et al. (1968).

The great importance of the right temporal lobe in tune discrimination was also shown by the work of Schankweiler (1966). He examined 45 patients with atrophic changes in the right or left temporal lobes and demonstrated an impairment of the discrimination of tunes presented to the left ear, contralateral to the temporal lobe lesion. The disturbances increased in severity after removal of the right temporal lobe, leaving Heschl's gyrus intact.

Milner (1958) found disturbances of the discrimination of simple melodies consisting of 4 notes in patients after removal of the right temporal lobe. On repetition of the melody, one of the notes was replaced.

The appearance of amusia in patients with lesions of the right temporal lobe has also been described by Feuchtwanger (1930), Ustwedt (1937), and Krol' (1936).

It will be clear that in the study of disorders of musical hearing in patients with central lesions a change has occurred from the investigation of perception and discrimination of individual

*One form of testing binaural summation is the dichotic method of presenting stimuli suggested by Broadbent (1954), which tests "conflicting" hearing. For example, two numerals constituting a single number of 2 digits may be presented simultaneously to both ears. Usually when hearing is tested in this way the subject is given two series of digits, with six in each series, so that half the digits are received by the right and half by the left ear. The digits are grouped so that each two simultaneously presented to the different ears formed one bidigital number, i.e., each group of digits formed three bidigital numbers.

static acoustic signals to the investigation of discrimination of complex acoustic series and of stimuli changing with time. Stockert (1954), for instance, described the results of tests on a patient in whom, after an illness in childhood accompanied by hemiplegia, the differentiation of a single sound from a chord was disturbed; she could not recognize tunes, she could not distinguish simple rhythms, and could not tap out a rhythm she had just heard. She could not distinguish between an iamb and a trochee. Measurement of the differential thresholds of intensity by the Lüscher – Zwislocki method showed that she perceived an amplitude-modulated signal as continuous, whatever the depth of modulation. She did not understand speech in a noisy room, but could understand sentences in ordinary conversation. These disorders of hearing were combined with a disturbance of the localization of sound in space. The localization of the brain lesion in this patient was not determined.

Disturbance of the perception and reproduction of fast rhythms in patients with local lesions of the temporal lobe was described by Luria and Semernitskaya (1945). Similar observations were described by Richter (1957). The patient with a pathological focus in the temporal lobe, whom he investigated, could count rhythmic stimuli (clicks) correctly when presented slowly, but if presented rapidly (80/min) their perception was disturbed. Hearing disturbances of similar character in lesions of the thalamic portions of the auditory system were described by Arnold (1951), Pötzl (1946), and Stockert and Fresser (1954).

Two cases of auditory agnosia, i.e., disturbance of the recognition of sounds, in patients without manifestations of aphasia, which are described in the literature (Nielsen and Sult, 1939; Spreen, Benton, and Fincham, 1965), are of special interest.

The patient described by Nielsen and Sult (1939) could not recognize the splashing of water or the sound of metal when thrown about, but could recognize the striking of a clock. This patient also showed agnosia of other forms of sensory perception. For example, he insisted that it was dark when it was light, he could not recognize the smell of tobacco or the taste of an apple.

A case of isolated auditory agnosia was described by Spreen, Benton, and Fincham (1965). This was a man aged 65 who, after a cerebrovascular illness, was unable to understand familiar sounds such as coughing, the mewing of a cat, whistling, the crying of a child, the gurgling of water, and the ticking of a clock. He made many mistakes when asked to distinguish two pure tones of different pitch. However, the same patient could understand speech perfectly well. Audiometric tests showed slight impairment of hearing at high frequencies, but no worse than could be expected on account of his age. He had no difficulty in identifying the direction of a sound and could identify objects without mistakes by taste and smell. Postmortem examination showed an extensive lesion including the right frontal, temporal, and parietal regions and also the insula. There was no damage to the left hemisphere or the corpus callosum.

The possibility of isolated auditory agnosia had been suggested earlier (Kehrer, 1913; Kleist, 1934). However, the localization of the defect in such cases was considered by them to be bilateral and in the temporal lobe, with only minimal involvement of the dominant hemisphere.

Conditioned-Reflex Activity in Patients with Local Lesions of the Temporal Lobe

Great importance is attached to the investigation of neurodynamics, i.e., the relationship between excitation and inhibition, in patients with local lesions of the temporal lobe, using the conditioned-reflex method.

Traugott (1946, 1947) found that children with sensory alalia and aphasia had great difficulty in forming conditioned reflexes and differentiation to simple and combined acoustic stimuli. Yet the use of the same method revealed no difficulty in visual conditioning. Subsequent investigations confirmed the results of this original work. For example, Lubovskii (1952), Babenkova (1954), Shmidt and Sukhovskaya (1954), Kaidanova (1967), Kaidanova and Meierson (1961), and Stolyarova-Kabelyanskaya (1961) showed by a conditioned-reflex method that patients with sensory aphasia had difficulty in differentiating combined acoustic stimuli if their components were rearranged, whereas the same patients could still distinguish single acoustic stimuli. In patients with sensory aphasia a direct correlation was found between the degree of impairment of analysis and synthesis of conditioned acoustic stimuli and the severity of the sensory-aphasic syndrome (Traugott, Kaidanova, and Meierson, 1967).

Babenkova (1954) also found a direct correlation between disturbance of analysis and synthesis of simple and complex non-verbal acoustic stimuli and the severity of speech disorders.

Shmidt and Sukhovskaya (1954) demonstrated difficulty in the formation of conditioned reflexes to verbal stimuli and in their differentiation. They regard the disturbance or differentiation of oppositional phonemes as one of the main symptoms of sensory aphasia. Conditioned reflex formation in patients with various forms of temporal aphasia has also been investigated by Kryshova (1959), Tkachev (1955), and Dorofeeva (1965).

Pathological inertia of trace processes in the auditory system, manifested as a disturbance of the perception of sounds applied at a comparatively short interval after the preceding stimulus, was discovered in patients with local lesions of the temporal lobe (Golomshtok, 1952; Spirin, Fantalova, and Filippycheva, 1955; Korst and Fantalova, 1959).

Korst and Fantalova (1959) showed that patients with temporal lobe lesions often make mistakes when identifying single sounds applied soon after preceding sounds. The discrimination and identification of the stimuli were improved by spacing them more widely apart. These results confirmed Semernitskaya's observations that patients with sensory aphasia had difficulty in the auditory evaluation of repetitive structures applied in rapid succesion. Similar results were obtained by Richter (1957).

Prolongation of acoustic sensation was observed by Stockert (1954), who called it the "acoustic echo." However, he associated this disturbance of function with a pathological focus in the thalamic portion of the auditory system. The duration of the intervals between stimuli giving rise to a disturbance of discrimination of the subsequent stimulus in these investigations was 300-700 msec. On the other hand, Traugott, Kaidanova, and Meierson (1967) showed that the differentiation of two tonal stimuli was improved by bringing them closer together in time, and was impaired by increasing the interval between the positive and differential stimuli.*

An interesting method of assessing the state of the trace processes was used by Kaidanova (1967). In this investigation she

*Unfortunately, these workers do not state the duration of the interval between the stimuli in these investigations.

showed that discrimination of complex acoustic stimuli, which differ only in the duration of the pauses between the end of one component and the beginning of the next, is disturbed in children with sensory alalia. Discrimination of the pauses between the components of visual complexes was unimpaired in these children.

The investigation of conditioned-reflex activity in patients with sensory aphasia and alalia thus revealed a disturbance of the function of the auditory system (defects of analysis and synthesis of acoustic stimuli) and demonstrated a direct relationship between the degree of disturbance of auditory analysis and the severity of the sensory aphasia. However, since these studies involved application of the stimulus in an acoustic field, they have no bearing on lateralization.

Manifestations of Irritation of the Temporal Lobe

A focal lesion of the temporal lobe not only causes loss of functions, but also accompanying manifestations of irritation.

Noise, hyperacusia, and auditory hallucinations have been described as symptoms of cortical irritation.

In tumors of the temporal lobe noise resembling the ringing of a bell, whispering, or loud noises localized in both ears are observed. According to Rapoport (1948), they are due mainly to increased intracranial pressure and associated secondary changes in the nervous apparatus of the cochlea (of the "congested ear" type). They are of no importance in localization for they can be observed in lesions of the ascending auditory pathway at any level. The same view is held by Blagoveshchenskaya (1962).

According to Rapoport (1948), auditory hallucinations are observed in one-fifth of all cases of temporal lobe lesions, and they have the character of voices, music, or singing. Sensations of whistling, noises, and other elementary acoustic sensations are regarded by Rapoport as characteristic of stimulation of peripheral portions of the auditory system. However, these views are not supported by the observations of Penfield and Erickson (1945), who described auditory hallucinations, in the form of elementary sounds (noise, rustling, whistling) during direct electrical stimulation of the temporal cortex in man.

Shmar'yan (1937, 1949) distinguishes 3 types of auditory disturbances in temporal lobe tumors. The first group consists of acoustico-vestibular disorders, the second of a syndrome of disturbance of the tonal quality of auditory perception with features of hyperpathia and depersonalization of speech, found most typically in patients with lesions of the right temporal lobe. The third group consists of auditory and verbal hallucinations. According to Shmar'yan's observations auditory psychosensory disorders are a feature predominantly of the first stage of the illness in patients with temporal lobe tumors, when signs of irritation are predominant.

Rapoport found that auditory hallucinations are usually associated with intracerebral tumors of the temporal lobe.

Karaseva (1967) observed auditory hallucinations in only 2 of 37 patients with temporal lobe lesions, and the lesion in these patients was extensive and affected not only the temporal cortex, but also the subjacent white matter and neighboring brain structures. In both cases the auditory hallucinations resembled the noise of the sea or whistling of the wind in the ears.

Bender and Diamond (1965) found no strict relationship between the presence and character of auditory hallucinations and the localization of the pathological focus. They consider that auditory hallucinations and illusions usually arise in patients with lesions of the auditory nerve or medulla, but they may also be of cortical origin. In that case they are projected to the side contralateral to the affected hemisphere. The frequency of auditory hallucinations in temporal tumors, according to cases reported in the literature, did not exceed 4%.

Auditory hyperpathia (hyperacusia) may also be a symptom of irritation of the temporal cortex. It is characterized by the perception of speech with altered tonal qualities, so that it becomes strangely loud and unpleasant, and in the depersonalization of the speaker's voice (Rapoport, 1948). These phenomena were observed in very few patients, and as a rule they were combined with auditory hallucinations and epileptic fits. The disturbances described above corresponded to the localization of the pathological focus (usually a tumor) in the region of the sylvian fissure and in areas of the cortex bordering on Heschl's gyrus.

The importance of central psychosensory disorders (tinnitus, hallucinations, and hyperacusia) in the localization of lesions has not been adequately investigated.

Perception of Acoustic Stimuli of Different Durations

This review of the literature makes it clear that lesions of the auditory cortex in man do not disturb the detection of stationary acoustic stimuli, such as are used in ordinary audiometric tests, or their discrimination by frequency and intensity.

Similar results have been obtained after extirpation of the auditory cortex in animals. In most investigations a disturbance of the identification and discrimination of fragments of speech or music was detected, especially if presented in a form in which their information content was limited, or when tests based on binaural interaction were used. However, the use of these tests has certain limitations, first, because of their complexity, and, second, because speech tests have language restrictions* for they naturally can only be used to investigate persons who speak a certain language. The results of these tests depend on the subject's intellectual level and their use is restricted to patients with manifestations of sensory aphasia. Consequently, the search for new methods of investigation for use in the diagnosis of central lesions still remains an urgent problem.

Changes in auditory perception depending on the time of action of the stimuli have recently been extensively used in psychophysical experiments on healthy subjects (see the surveys by Zwislocki, 1960; Doughty and Garner, 1947). The purpose of these investigations was to study the relationship between stimulus intensity and duration (within certain limits), characterized by the phenomenon of temporal summation or integration well known in the physiology of the central nervous system.

One method of studying temporal summation is by measuring it at the threshold level, i.e., by determining the range of durations

*All speech tests suggested by Bocca and his collaborators (Bocca, 1961-1965) are designed specifically for the Italian language.

within which the threshold of detection or discrimination of the stimulus depends on its duration.

Psychophysical investigations on healthy persons showed that 200 msec is the critical period during which the auditory system can integrate a stimulus (Garner, 1947; Miscolczy-Fodor, 1953; Plomp and Bouman, 1959; Zwislocki, 1960).

Quantitative studies showed that the change in threshold intensities as a function of duration is linear within the range 5-200 msec and has a slope of 9-10 dB per decade (tenfold increase in stimulus duration) at a frequency of 1000 Hz. For white noise and low-frequency tones the slope of the curves of threshold intensity versus stimulus duration is significantly reduced* (Garner, 1947; Miscolczy-Fodor, 1953).

According to Garner's (1947) observations, with a decrease in the duration of series of tonal stimuli at 1000 Hz from 1000 to 1 msec the threshold intensities of the series are increased by 30 dB, while according to Miscolczy-Fodor (1953), they are increased by 27 dB. This shortening of bursts of white noise causes an increase of 24-26 dB in the threshold intensities. In these investigations on healthy subjects no differences were found between the results of measurements on the right and left ears.

Investigation of hearing by acoustic stimuli of different duration is now used to study patients with peripheral lesions of the auditory system and it has enabled lesions of the sound-receiving portion of the cochlea and auditory nerve to be detected much more precisely than the methods used previously (Miscolczy-Fodor, 1953; Harris, Haines, and Myers, 1958; Elliott, 1963; Kishonas, 1966, 1967; Wright, 1967, 1968). These investigations showed that the slope of the temporal summation curves in patients with a disturbance of the sound-conducting system of the middle ear is indistinguishable from the slope in healthy subjects, but the curves themselves are shifted in accordance with the impairment of hearing at the frequency tested. In lesions of the sound-receiving portion of the cochlea, on the other hand, the slope of the threshold intensity versus stimulus-duration curves is significantly reduced. Whereas in healthy subjects, in response to a tenfold decrease in

*Some investigators have found that the change in threshold with a decrease in stimulus duration is independent of frequency (Plomp and Bouman, 1959).

stimulus duration (a series of tones at 2-4 kHz) the increase in threshold was 9-10 dB, in patients with disturbances of sound perception the increase in threshold was 3-6 dB for the same decrease in stimulus duration.

For several years a systematic investigation of the role of the temporal parameters of stimuli and the temporal characteristics of responses of various parts of the auditory system in sound discrimination has been undertaken in the Laboratory of the Physiology of Hearing, directed by G. V. Gershuni, at the I. P. Pavlov Institute of Physiology. One part of this investigation is the study of the relationship between the thresholds of detection of acoustic stimuli and their duration in animals, using both electrophysiological and behavioral methods. The investigation has shown that the stimulus duration factor has an essential role in the assessment of function of the auditory cortex in the analysis of acoustic stimuli. Results of electrophysiological investigations published in the literature indicate the spatial projection of frequencies on the surface of the auditory cortex (Tunturi, 1946). However, total bilateral extirpation of the auditory cortex does not disturb the thresholds of detection of stationary acoustic stimuli or of their discrimination by frequency and intensity (Mering, 1962; Neff, 1961).

The reasons for the disagreement between the results of the electrophysiological and behavioral experiments were examined by Gershuni (1963). He postulated that the discrepancy between the results can be explained by the very great difference in duration of the stimuli used in the electrophysiological and behavioral experiments. This suggestion was confirmed by subsequent work.

By using measurements of threshold as functions of stimulus duration after extirpation of different parts of the auditory cortex in behavioral experiments on animals (dogs) it was shown that the thresholds of detection of acoustic stimuli are increased only in response to the action of sounds whose duration is limited to 10-16 msec (Baru, 1964, 1966).

Unilateral extirpation of the temporal cortex (areas AI, AII, Ep, and SS, and in some animals AIV and IT also), followed by retrograde degeneration of the medial geniculate body, caused an increase in the thresholds of detection of acoustic stimuli shorter than 16 msec in all dogs undergoing the operation if the sound was applied to the ear contralateral to the side of extirpation. If the sounds were applied to the homolateral ear relative to the operation the threshold intensities were unchanged by comparison with those before the operation.

After extirpation of the auditory cortex of the opposite hemisphere in these animals, similar changes in threshold intensities of short stimuli were observed when the sounds were applied to the ear contralateral to the side of the second operation. After the first operation, as well as after the second, the threshold intensities of longer acoustic stimuli were unchanged by comparison with their preoperative level.

The increase in the threshold intensities of series of tones at 1000 Hz, 1-2 msec in duration, immediately after the operation was 20-25 dB. The difference 8-10 months after the operation was 10-14 dB, compared with 8.7 ± 0.4 dB for bursts of white noise of the same duration. More complete compensation was not achieved after 1-2 years.

Similar results were observed after isolated unilateral and bilateral extirpation of part of the cortex of the middle ectosylvian gyrus or area AI (the primary projection area of the auditory pathway). The increase in thresholds to short stimuli ($t < 10$ msec) in these animals during the first 1-1.5 months after the operation was 20-22 dB, i.e., 3-5 dB less than in the animals after extensive extirpations of the auditory cortex including areas AI, AII, Ep, and SS. The range of durations within which the increase in thresholds was statistically significant was slightly narrowed to values of the order of 10 msec. The difference between the threshold intensities of short stimuli of 1-2 msec before and 2-4 months after extirpation of the auditory cortex averaged 10 dB in these dogs, i.e., it was not significantly different from the increase in threshold intensities in dogs with extensive extirpation of the auditory cortex.

The threshold intensities of short acoustic stimuli were not restored to the characteristic values for intact animals after small or more extensive extirpations, despite long periods of observation after the operation (1-3 years).

An increase in the thresholds of detection of short acoustic stimuli was also found on the investigation of threshold intensities of acoustic stimuli of different duration in patients with vascular lesions of the temporal lobe (Baru, Gershuni, and Tonkonogii, 1964). In patients with a lesion of the temporal lobe the thresholds of detection of short acoustic stimuli ($t < 7$ msec) were increased in the ear opposite to the pathological focus. The actual magnitude of the increase in thresholds was 8 dB for stimuli 3.6 msec in duration and 9 dB for stimuli of 1.2 msec (limit of variation 6-23 dB). The threshold intensities of stimuli of longer duration, measured in the same ear (contralateral to the focus) and stimuli of all durations in the ear on the same side as the lesion were indistinguishable from the corresponding values in a control group of 5 patients with a lesion in other parts of the cerabral hemispheres and in a group of healthy subjects. The results of investigation of a group of patients with brain lesions in different situations thus demonstrate that selective impairment of the discrimination of short sounds is present in patients with a temporal lobe lesion. The increase in thresholds for these sounds is observed when the sound is applied to the ear contralateral to the pathological focus. However, no variation in the 8 thresholds in response to shortening of the stimuli could be detected in patients with sensory-acoustic, sensory-amnestic, and conduction aphasia, i.e., with differences in the precise localization of the focus in the left temporal lobe.

Changes in the threshold intensities of long and short stimuli were found after administration of pharmacological agents with a selective action on nuclei of the posterior hypothalamus and reticular formation or on cortical neurons and thalamic structures (Baru, 1967; Traugott et al., 1968). The reduction in the threshold intensities of short stimuli is evidence of the activating effect of the nonspecific systems on the auditory projection area.

On the basis of the results already obtained by the workers cited above it seemed possible that this method could be used to establish the localization of pathological foci in the temporal lobe. However, quite apart from the fact that further investigations on large groups of patients were necessary to verify this hypothesis, the work of Baru, Gershuni, and Tonkonogii still left unsolved the problem of the relationship between the effect of detection of short acoustic stimuli and hemispheric dominance. There are no clinical–anatomical comparisons to provide an answer to the question of how perception of acoustic stimuli of different duration is connected with injury to particular brain structures. Nevertheless, an elucidation of these problems is absolutely essential before the method of testing hearing with acoustic stimuli of different duration can be used for topical diagnosis.

Because of the difficulty of reaching a decision on the dominant role of individual structures of the temporal lobe from the results of investigation of patients with cerebrovascular lesions, it was decided to made a clinical neurosurgical study of the character of perception of acoustic stimuli of different durations so that advantage could be taken of the more precise methods available for localizing the pathological focus and of the opportunity of seeing the affected region during operation.

CHAPTER 2

Characteristics of the Patients and Methods of Investigation

Patients with local lesions of the temporal cortex of vascular origin or resulting from intracerebral and extracerebral tumors or traumatic and inflammatory foci were investigated.

The main group consisted of 96 patients admitted for treatment to the N. N. Burdenko Institute of Neurosurgery (Karaseva, 1966, 1967). Besides this main group, another 36 patients admitted for treatment to the V. M. Bekhterev Leningrad Psychoneurological Research Institute were studied (Baru, Gershuni, and Tonkonogii, 1964; Vasserman, 1969).

The character of the pathological process differed in the 96 patients studied. The diagnosis in 68% of cases was a brain tumor, in 12% vascular diseases, in 11% the sequelae of brain trauma, and in 9% inflammatory diseases.

The age of the patients ranged from 8 to 62 years. With respect to localization of the focus, the main group consisted of patients with lesions of the temporal lobe (52 patients). The control group consisted of patients with lesions of the cerebral hemispheres outside the temporal lobe (27 cases), patients with lesions of the brain stem at various levels (9 cases), and patients with a syndrome of intracranial hypertension with hydrocephalus, with no clearly defined focal lesions. Eight healthy adult subjects aged from 19 to 65 years also were investigated.

Irrespective of the nature of the disease, a clearly defined local brain lesion was present in the 88 patients observed.

Analysis of the clinical picture was based on the results of a combined examination of the patient using neurological, x-ray contrast, electrophysiological, and other methods of investigation. The state of the higher cortical functions was judged from the results of a neuropsychological examination. The state of the patients' hearing was assessed by otoneurological investigation. In 68 cases the lesion was verified at operation, and in 6 cases at autopsy.

The main purpose of the investigation was to assess the patients' hearing quantitatively. Besides the usual otoneurological methods of examination, the patients were subjected to a special investigation, including measurement of the threshold intensities of acoustic stimuli of different duration. The technique of the otoneurological investigation is fully described in textbooks of special otoneurology (Blagoveshchenskaya, 1962, 1965; Zhukovich, 1966).

The acuity of hearing of all patients was assessed by a set of tuning forks with resonance frequencies C128-C2048, and also by pure-tone audiometry, using the type AA-01 automatic audiometer. The threshold sensitivity was measured for both air and bone conduction. Lateralization of the sound was determined by Weber's test. The intelligibility of loud and whispered speech and the state of vestibular function of all patients also were investigated.

The relationship between the threshold intensity of acoustic stimuli and their duration was studied as follows. Threshold intensities of bursts of white noise and of tones of 1000 Hz with durations of 1200, 120, 45, 4, 2, and 1 msec were measured. The acoustic stimuli were produced by a type ZG-2A audiofrequency generator and a type G-2-12 wide-band noise generator.

Signals from the generator output were led to the input of an electronic switch which gave the stimulus its correct duration. From the output of the switch the signals were led through attenuators, graduated in decibels, to a type TD-6 electrodynamic telephone. The telephone was calibrated against a type IU-3 standard "artifical ear" apparatus. The amplitude characteristic curve of the acoustic system was linear within the working range of intensities. The time constant of the telephone was 0.6 msec at 1000 Hz.

Square signals with minimal build-up time were used. The duration of the stimulus was verified during each test by means of a type S1-19 oscilloscope.

A high-value electronic switch was used for part of the investigation, because the spectrum of the short stimuli employed in the tests formed a frequency band with maximum corresponding to the frequency applied. The energy diminished on either side of the maximum within limits determined by the formula $f_0 \pm 1/t$ (where f_0 is the frequency of the oscillations applied, in Hz, and t the duration of the tone, in sec).

As a result of the random phase of stimulus application and removal and the consequent random limits of the spectrum of each individual stimulus, the energy of the short stimuli equal in duration to that emitted by the telephone was too unstable. Because of this, an electronic switch with a low interference level and allowing smooth phase regulation was developed (Lebedev, 1966) and used in the greater part of the work. Stimuli were applied in the zero phase, at which transient distortions were least marked.

Special attention was paid to reducing the click level when switching on the stimuli. In the apparatus used the "on" stimulus–noise level was 50 dB, i.e., during measurement at the threshold level the click was never heard.

Bursts of white noise were used as acoustic stimuli because white noise is an acoustic stimulus with uniform spectral density at all frequencies. If the bursts were shortened the changes in spectral composition were less marked than those produced by shortening the bursts of tonal stimuli. However, the use of white noise has disadvantages of its own, because the level of intensity is unstable as the result of stimulus fluctuation when the bursts are shortened. In order to detect the character of the change in threshold intensities during a decrease in stimulus duration it is therefore necessary to use two types of stimuli: tonal and noise. Threshold measurements were carried out at 1000 Hz, a frequency lying in the region of maximum sensitivity of the human ear. The absolute thresholds at this frequency are not, as a rule, reduced by age changes in hearing or in diseases of the cochlea. For this reason, with a decrease in stimulus duration as the result of widening of their spectrum, bursts with a basic frequency of 1000

Hz lost their tonal color,* and the subjects were warned that they had to report any sound which they heard.

Thresholds were measured monaurally by the limit method. The stimulus intensity was changed initially by 5 dB, and nearer to the threshold by 1 dB. The measurements began with long stimuli, and these were gradually replaced by shorter. A voluntary movement (pressing on a button, as a result of which the control lamp in front of the experimenter lit up) served as the subject's response. The threshold was taken as the lowest stimulus intensity which the subject could detect with a probability of 0.5.

The threshold intensity of the acoustic stimulus at each duration studied was determined for all patients at least 5-10 times and the mean value of the measurements was taken as the threshold of audibility.

When measuring the threshold intensities of acoustic stimuli of different duration the examiner's object was to assess the degree of increase in the threshold for a short stimulus (1 msec) compared with a long stimulus (1200 msec) on the ipsilateral and contralateral sides relative to the lesion. The solution of this problem would be simple if in all patients the thresholds of long stimuli were equal and differed only slightly from the thresholds in healthy subjects. However, absolute values could not be used for this purpose because the threshold intensities of long acoustic stimuli in the patients examined were variable. Auditory sensitivity can be reduced as the result of previous diseases of the middle or inner ear, or though the action of a pathological process on auditory structures in the brain stem. As characteristics of the degree of the defect of auditory perception it was therefore decided to use the difference between thresholds measured to short ($t = 1$ msec) and long ($t = 1200$ msec) acoustic stimuli, described by Gershuni and Kishonas (see Kishonas, 1966) as the duration effect. The magnitude of the duration effect on the side ipsi- and contralateral to the lesion was compared in different patients and the deviation of this characteristic from its value in healthy subjects was also taken into account.

*The relationship between the sensation of pitch (tonality), the duration, and the intensity of a sound has been fully investigated by Doughty and Garner (1947).

Besides the study of the relationship between the threshold intensities of acoustic stimuli and their duration, some additional tests also were carried out. The integrity of spatial hearing was determined with the aid of Vojacek's laterometer (the technique of this test is described by Blagoveshchenskaya, 1962, in her textbook of otoneurology).

To assess musical hearing, because of the great variability between people's musical abilities very simple tests were used, which made allowance for the patient's level of musical education. The patient was asked to recognize a popular tune played on the xylophone. Two musical fragments were presented and the patient was asked to state whether they were identical or different. The patient had also to distinguish two notes separated by an interval of a half or complete tone.

Ability to assess rhythmic structures by ear also was studied. Simple rhythmic groups of 2, 3, or 4 individual beats, each about 20 msec in duration, and complex accentuated rhythms were presented.

The beats were presented in slow (interval 0.8-1 sec) and quick (interval 20-40 msec) time by tapping a pencil on the table or from a tape recorder. The subject had either to count the number of beats or to reproduce them by tapping with his finger or a pencil on the table.

CHAPTER 3

Threshold Intensity of Acoustic Stimuli as a Function of Duration in Healthy Subjects

Before the character and degree of disturbance of acoustic perception could be estimated in patients with local brain lesions, measurements of threshold intensities had to be made on healthy subjects under the same circumstances, one of which was that the measurements were made not in a soundproof room, but in an ordinary quiet room. Threshold intensities of series of tones at 1000 Hz were measured in 7 individuals aged from 19 to 65 years. The results of measurements of such series of varied duration are given in Table 1.

TABLE 1. Changes in Threshold Intensities of Series of Tones at 1000 Hz (in dB) as a Function of Their Duration in Healthy Individuals

Subjects	Duration of stimulus in msec						
	1200	120	45	14	4.5	2	1
P-va	0*	3.0±0.2	6.0±0.5	11.5±1.0	18.0±1.0	23.5±1.5	26.5±1.3
S-zh	0	5.5±1.0	9.5±1.2	14.5±1.5	18.0±0.5	23.0±1.0	25.0±1.0
Ya-v.	0	3.2±0.3	9.7±0.5	12.5±1.0	18.0±0.7	22.8±1.0	25.5±0.8
K-v.	0	3.2±1.2	5.5±0.5	11.7±0.7	17.5±1.0	22.7±1.0	26.0±0.4
K-v.	0	4.5±1.0	6.9±0.7	13.0±1.0	17.7±0.8	22.5±1.0	25.5±0.8
R-aya	0	3.6±0.6	5.0±0.3	13.1±0.8	16.0±0.5	22.6±1.0	25.6±1.3
M-va	0	3.5±1.0	6.3±1.0	12.3±1.0	14.8±1.0	21.5±1.2	25.3±0.9
Mean	0	3.7±0.7	7.0±0.7	12.0±1.0	17.0±0.8	22.4±0.8	25.6±0.8

*Threshold intensity of series of tones at 1000 Hz and 1200 msec in duration taken as zero level. Change in thresholds on shortening of stimulus from 1200 to 1 msec is defined as the duration effect.

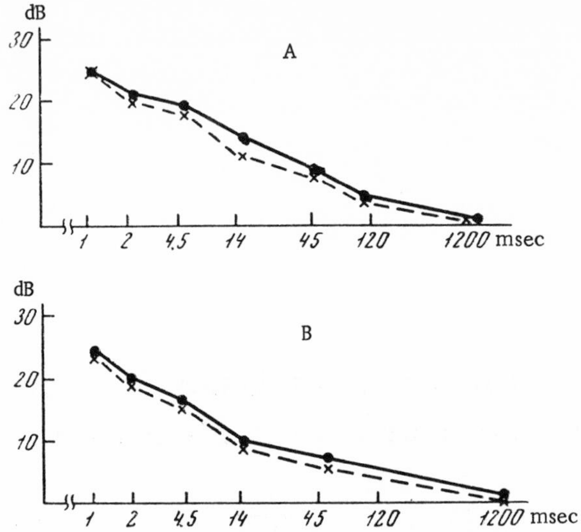

Fig. 2. Thresholds of detection of series of tones at 1000 Hz (A) and bursts of white noise (B) as functions of their duration in healthy subjects (mean results for 7 subjects). Continuous line shows results of measurements of thresholds in left ear, broken line corresponding results for the right ear. Abscissa, stimulus duration in msec; ordinate, thresholds in dB from conventional level. Threshold for stimuli with duration of 1200 msec taken as zero level for counting decibels.

TABLE 2. Changes in Threshold Intensities of Bursts of White Noise (in dB) as a Function of Their Duration in Healthy Subjects

Subjects	Stimulus duration in msec						
	1200	120	45	14	4,5	2	1
S-zh	0*	1.3±1.0	2.5±0.2	10.5±1.0	16,8±0.5	18.8±0.5	25.0±0.5
Ya-v	0	2.0±0,8	3,5±1.0	11,5±0.5	18.3±1.0	19.0±1,0	26,0±0.6
K-v.	0	2.0±0.3	4.0±0.5	10.0±1.2	17.0±0.7	17.9±0.4	24,0±0.8
P-va	0	1.5±0.7	4,8±1.2	8.8±0.5	16.4±1,2	17.6±0,3	26.5±1,0
M-va	0	2.0±0.1	4.6±0.6	12,2±0.3	17,5±0,4	19,9±0.1	25.7±1.0
Mean	0	1.8±0,6	3,9±0.7	10.6±0.5	17,4±0.8	18.3±0.5	25,0±0.7

*Threshold intensity of bursts of white noise 1200 msec in duration taken as zero level for counting decibels.

The mean duration effect for 7 healthy adults was thus 25.6 ± 0.8 dB. Curves showing threshold intensities as a function of the duration of series of tones at 1000 Hz (also the mean values of 7 subjects) are given in Fig. 2A. They show that the results of measurements on the right and left ears are identical. Similar results were obtained in tests of threshold intensities of bursts of white noise of different durations (Table 2; Fig. 2B).

As Table 2 and Fig. 2B show, the change in thresholds in response to shortening the intensity of bursts of white noise from 1200 to 1 msec averaged 25.0 dB. Variations in the results of individual measurements did not exceed ±1 dB.

The duration effect in healthy subjects thus shows no significant difference when measured in the right and left ears, and for series of tones at 1000 Hz its value is 25.6 ± 0.8 dB, and for bursts of white noise 25.0 ± 0.7 dB.

CHAPTER 4

Effect of Stimulus Duration on Thresholds of Detection of Acoustic Stimuli of Patients with Local Lesions of the Temporal Lobe

The investigations revealed differences in the character of perception of acoustic stimuli of short duration in patients with pathological lesions of the superior zone of the temporal lobe and those with lesions in its other (basal and polar) zones. The results of the measurements in these two groups of patients will thus be examined separately.

LOCAL LESIONS OF THE SUPERIOR ZONE OF THE TEMPORAL LOBE

Threshold intensities were studied in 37 patients with a pathological focus in the superior zone of the temporal lobe. The character of the lesion was as follows: intracerebral tumors – 18 patients, extracerebral tumors – 8, sequelae of head injuries – 7, scarring and atrophic changes after arachnoencephalitis – 2, aneurysm of a branch of the middle cerebral artery – 1, and brain abscess – 1 patient.

Despite the difference in nature of the pathological process, a common feature of all the patients of the group was the presence of clearly defined focal injury to the superior zone of the temporal lobe (the superior temporal gyrus, Heschl's gyrus, and their pathways) although their general condition at the time of the test was satisfactory.

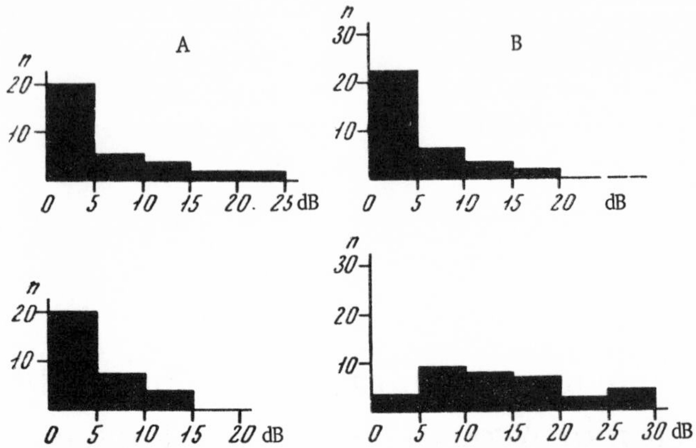

Fig. 3. Absolute thresholds (in dB) in patients with local lesions of the temporal lobe compared with corresponding values for healthy subjects to series of tones at 1000 Hz and with durations of 1200 msec (A) and 1 msec (B). Mean results for 7 healthy subjects taken as zero level for counting decibels. Above – difference between thresholds, i.e., loss of hearing measured in ear homolateral to the pathological focus; below – measured in the ear contralateral to the focus. Abscissa, difference between thresholds (dB); ordinate, number of patients.

The results of measurements of the threshold intensities of series of tones at 1000 Hz and with durations of 1200 and 1 msec are given in Fig. 3A and B and compared with the results of the tests on the healthy subjects.

It is clear from Fig. 3A that the threshold intensities of series of tones at 1000 Hz and with a duration of 1200 msec show no significant difference when measured in the right and left ears. The threshold intensities of these stimuli in 26 patients (84%), when measured in the ear homolateral to the pathological focus, and in 27 patients (87%) when measured in the contralateral ear, were not more than 10 dB higher than the mean value of the thresholds in the healthy subjects.

Measurement of the threshold intensities to series of tones at 1000 Hz and 1 msec in duration (Fig. 3B) gave considerably different results. In the first place, the results of measurements of threshold intensities in the homolateral ear differed significantly from those in the ear contralateral to the lesion. Whereas in most patients (28, or 89%) the thresholds measured in the ear homolateral to the focus did not differ from the threshold intensities in healthy subjects by more than 10 dB, in measurements on the ear contralateral to the affected temporal lobe, in 24 patients (66%) the threshold intensities to series of tones at 1000 Hz and 1 msec in duration were more than 15 dB higher than the corresponding values in healthy subjects.

Measurements of threshold intensities of bursts of white noise of different duration also gave analogous results.

Just as when tonal stimuli were used, the threshold intensities of bursts of white noise 1200 msec in duration were identical whether measured in the ear homolateral or contralateral to the pathological focus. In neither case were they more than 10-15 dB higher than the thresholds of audibility measured in healthy subjects. For stimuli of short duration (1 msec) the threshold intensities measured in the ear homolateral to the focus in 77% of patients likewise were not more than 15 dB higher than the mean thresholds in healthy subjects, whereas the threshold intensities measured in the contralateral ear were not more than 15 dB higher than normal in only 46% of patients, and in the other 54% the thresholds of bursts of white noise 1 msec in duration were 15-25 dB above the mean thresholds in healthy subjects.

Measurement of the thresholds to long acoustic stimuli thus revealed no difference in the character of the thresholds on the sides homolateral and contralateral to the focus. When thresholds to short stimuli were measured, patients with lesions in the superior zone of the temporal lobe showed a tendency for the thresholds to increase more when measured in the ear opposite to the pathological focus.

As an example the results of measurement of the threshold intensities of series of 1000-Hz tones and of different durations in the case of patient K-v can be considered. This patient had undergone resection of part of the superior and middle gyri of the right temporal lobe for suspected tumor. Table 3 gives results showing the character of the increase in thresholds relative to a conventional zero line taken as the threshold intensity of series of tones at 1000 Hz and with a duration of 1200 msec, in response

Table 3. Threshold Intensities of Series of Tones at 1000 Hz as a Function of Their Duration in Patient K-v after Resection of the Right Temporal Lobe

Stimulus duration, msec	Changes in threshold intensity in dB relative to conventional zero level*		Difference between thresholds for right and left ears
	Right ear	Left ear	
1200	0	0	
120	+4	+4	0
45	+6	+5	1 (R > L)
14	+15	+14	1 (R > L)
4.5	+18	+25	7 (L > R)
2	+22	+40	18 (L > R)
1	+24	+47	23 (L > R)

*Threshold intensity of series of tones at 1000 Hz and with a duration of 1200 msec taken as the zero level for counting decibels.

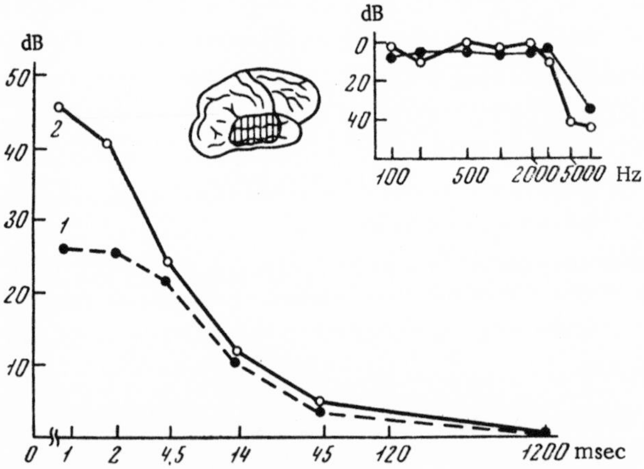

Fig. 4. Thresholds of detection of series of tones at 1000 Hz as a function of duration. Patient K-v after resection of superior and middle temporal gyri on the right side for tumor: 1) measurements on right ear, on side homolateral to pathological focus; 2) on left ear, contralateral to lesion. Diagram on the right shows this patient's audiogram. Shaded area on diagram of brain shows area of resection. Legend as in Fig. 2.

to shortening the stimulus duration. From the results of this table the curves of temporal summation shown in Fig. 4 are plotted.

The increases in threshold intensities in response to stimuli less than 14 msec in duration, when measured in the ear contralateral to the affected temporal lobe, are shown in Table 3 and Fig. 4. The difference between the threshold intensities of series of tones at 1000 Hz and with durations of 1 sec and 1200 msec (the duration effect) was 24 dB in the right ear, homolateral to the focus, i.e., almost the same as in healthy subjects, while in the left ear, contralateral to the focus, the duration effect was 47 dB.

Consequently, the duration effect in patient K-v when measured in the ear contralateral to the side of operation was 23 dB higher than the duration effect in the ear homolateral to the side of the focus. Changes of this nature, in the form of an increase in the duration effect as a result of an increase in the thresholds of audibility of sounds less than 14 msec in duration when measured on the side opposite to the focus in the temporal lobe, were found in all 37 patients in whom the pathological process involves the superior zone of the temporal lobe (Fig. 5). It will be clear from Fig. 5 that before the operation the duration effect on application of series of tones at 1000 Hz to the ear on the same side as the temporal lobe lesion varied between 21 and 28 dB. In 13 patients the effect was 24-26 dB, in agreement with the results of the measurements from the healthy subjects. After operation the duration effect on the side of the focus varied from 18 to 31 dB. In 7 patients the duration effect was 24-27 dB, i.e., it differed by not more than 2 dB from the results of measurements of the duration effect in the healthy subjects.

When the sound was applied to the ear contralateral to the lesion, before the operation the duration effect varied from 24 to 39 dB, while after operation it varied from 23 to 47 dB, with a mean of 35 dB. The duration effects in the patients were independent of the degree of impairment of hearing due to factors unconnected with the lesion of the auditory cortex (the relationship between the duration effect and degree of impairment of hearing will be examined in more detail in a special section).

In all patients, irrespective of the degree of loss of hearing, the duration effects measured in the ear contralateral to the focus

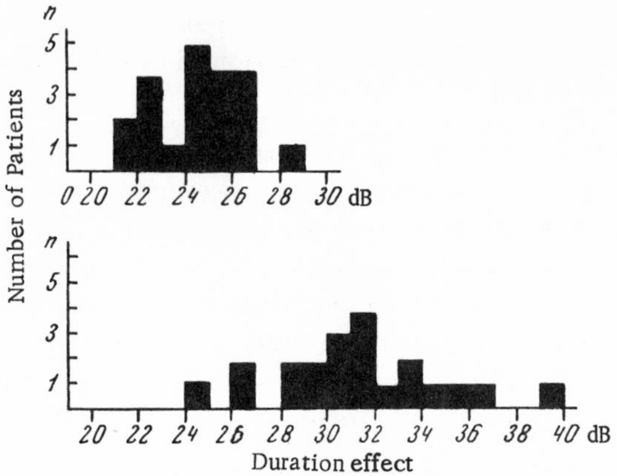

Fig. 5. Distribution of duration effects (in dB) measured to series of tones at 1000 Hz in patients with lesions of the superior zone of the temporal lobe. Above – duration effect on side homolateral to lesion; below – on contralateral side. Abscissa, difference in dB between threshold intensities of stimuli with durations of 1200 and 1 msec; ordinate, number of patients.

were much greater than those measured in the ear on the side of the focus and greater than the duration effects obtained as a result of measurements on healthy subjects.

The duration effects measured on the ear homolateral to the lesion were not significantly different from those measured in healthy subjects.

Analysis of these 37 cases, in 2 of which the diagnosis was confirmed at autopsy or at subsequent histological examination, in 28 at operation, and in 8 by means of contrast methods (arteriography and ventriculography), showed that in every case the pathological focus involved Heschl's gyrus, the superior temporal gyrus, or their pathways.

The case described below, verified at autopsy, will serve as an example.

Patient B-ov, a man aged 56 years (case No. 41851), was admitted to the Burdenko Neurosurgical Institute on February 23.

He complained of a swelling on the right side of the head which had appeared about 5 months previously, and was accompanied by headache.

On examination: a swelling slightly tender on palpation could be felt in the right parieto-occipital region. Pupils R > L. Left-sided homonymous hemianopia. Marked papilledema. Central paresis of the left facial nerve. In Barre's position the left arm drops. Astereognosis of the left hand. Bilateral positive Babinski's sign.

Examination by the otologist revealed no defect of hearing.

EEG: against the background of interhemispheric asymmetry a focus of pathological activity is present in the right parieto-temporo-occipital region.

Lumbar puncture: pressure 500 mm water, protein 0.9‰, cells 30/3.

Roentgenograms of the skull: marked changes of increased intracranial pressure.

Right-sided carotid angiography: vessels of a tumor can be seen in the temporo-parieto-occipital region.

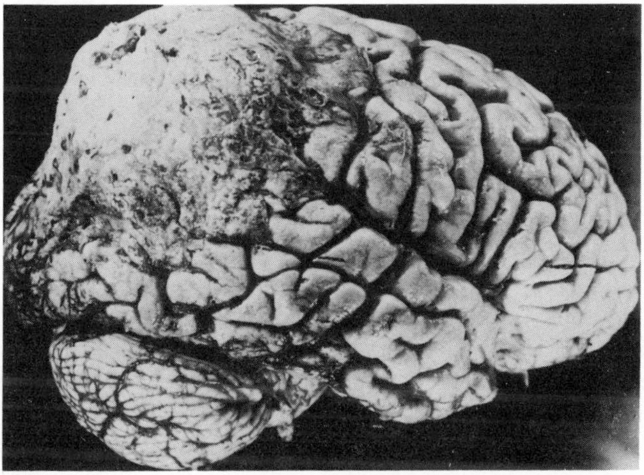

Fig. 6. Photograph of the brain. The tumor occupies the whole of the parietal lobe and the boundary between the superior temporal gyrus and supramarginal gyrus (patient B-ov).

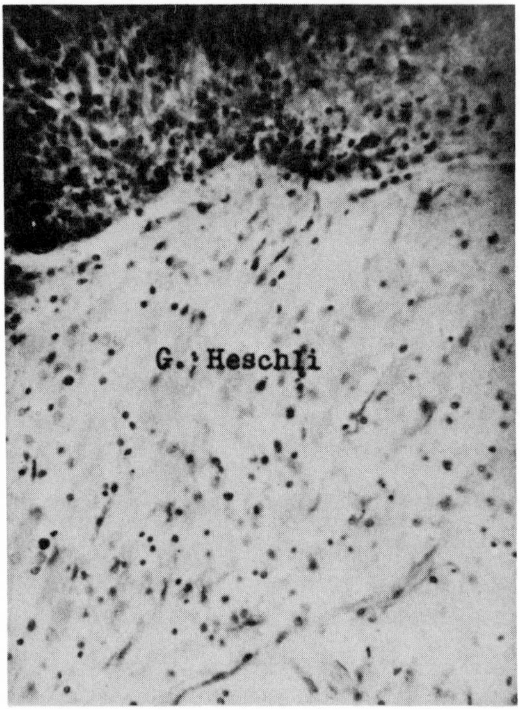

Fig. 7. Photomicrograph of section through cortex of Heschl's gyrus, stained by Nissl's method (patient B-ov). Masses of tumor cells filled the sylvian fissure. Structure of the cortex of Heschl's gyrus is completely destroyed. No intact nerve cells can be seen in the section.

On March 25, operation: resection of the affected bone tissue in the right parieto-occipital region and biopsy of the tumor.

April 10: the patient died.

At autopsy a carcinoma of the right lung with multiple metastases in the liver was found. A solitary metastatic nodule was present in the posterior part of the right cerebral hemisphere. The nodule occupied the parietal lobe and the junction between the superior temporal gyrus and the supramarginal gyrus (Fig. 6).

Frontal sections showed that the tumor had invaded the hemisphere and extended as far as the lateral wall of the ventricular triangle.

In sections stained by Spielmeyer's and Nissl's methods the tumor was seen to fill the subarachnoid space of the sylvian fissure between the adjacent gyri of the temporal and parietal lobes, to invade the posterior part of the sylvian fissure, and to spread to the operculum parietale et temporale, in the latter case as far as the posterior part of Heschl's gyrus.

In sections stained by Nissl's method masses of tumor cells could be seen to fill the subarachnoid space of the sylvian fissure. The cortical structure in that region was totally destroyed (Fig. 7). No intact nerve cells whatsoever could be seen. Areas of necrosis and hemorrhage were visible in the tumor tissue. Necrosis was observed in the walls of the blood vessels and the small vessels were infiltrated by tumor cells. A clear line of demarcation was present on the outer surface of the superior temporal gyrus between the zone of gross pathological changes in the cortex and the rest of the cortex with its perfectly normal structure.

In sections stained by Spielmeyer's method the intensity of staining of the fibers was considerably reduced in the white matter of the temporal lobe and where the central auditory pathway leaves the medial geniculate body.

In series of sections through the medial geniculate body the cells were heavily laden with pigment. On the side of the tumor the nerve cells were considerably reduced in number, while the glial cells were more numerous and formed a massive band running along the medial border of the medial geniculate body where, according to Peele (1954), the central auditory pathway leaves that structure (Fig. 8).

The density of the cells in the medial geniculate body on the side of the tumor and on the opposite side is given in Table 4.

TABLE 4. Cell Density in Medial Geniculate Body

Region of measurement	Number of cells per mm^3				Glial index	
	Glial		Nerve			
	Healthy subject	Patient	Healthy subject	Patient	Healthy subject	Patient
Rostral part						
Medial part	90 633	152 172	8099	181	10.8	841
Lateral part	87 740	108 009	7647	181	10.8	596.8
Caudal part	87 784	180 271	2876	220	30.4	620

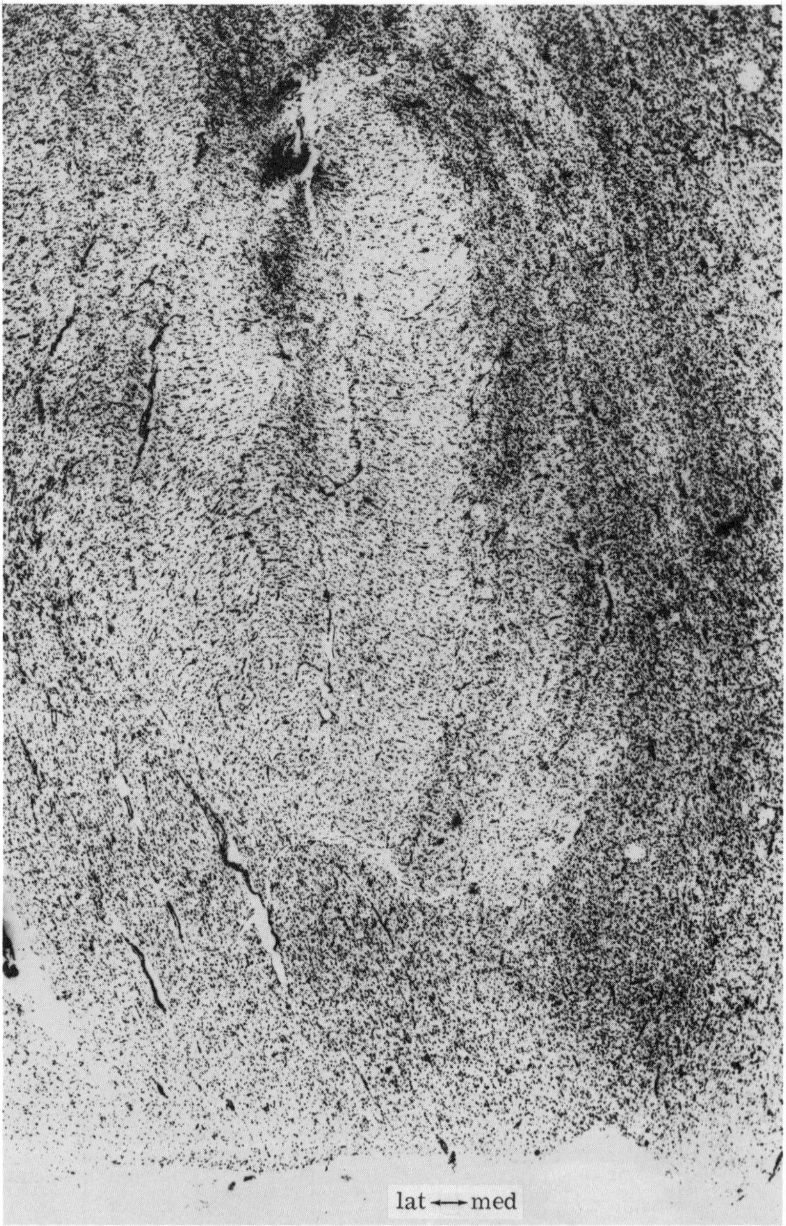

Fig. 8. Photomicrograph of brain section through medial geniculate body at point of exit of central auditory pathway (patient B-ov). Explanation in text. Stained by Nissl's method.

The cells which remained intact were very palely stained and exhibited neuronophagy. Vascular changes were minimal. Infiltration of the vessel walls was absent. Dilation of the vessels and slight perivascular edema were visible. Changes in the medial geniculate body can be interpreted as the final phase of retrograde degeneration. On the left side the nerve tissue was unchanged, and although the cells were rather palely stained, the nucleus and nucleolus were clearly visible.

After the patient's admission to the clinic, the threshold intensities of acoustic stimuli of different durations were measured twice. The two measurements of threshold intensities of series of tones at 1000 Hz, but of different duration, showed that the thresholds in the right ear were almost indistinguishable from normal. In the left ear the threshold to tones 1200 msec in duration was 3 dB above normal, but to tones 1 msec in duration it was 11 dB above normal. The duration effect on the right side was 25 dB and on the left side 38 dB, i.e., 13 dB higher on the left than on the right.

In this patient with metastasis of a carcinoma in the right cerebral hemisphere a lesion of the posterior part of Heschl's gyrus was caused by growth of the tumor into the posterior part of the sylvian fissure and the adjacent portion of the parietal and temporal lobes. Degeneration of the central auditory pathway and cells of the medial geniculate body also was seen.

Measurement of the thresholds of audibility revealed an increase in the threshold intensity of short acoustic stimuli in the ear contralateral to the focus.

What determines the degree of the increase in threshold values to short acoustic stimuli?

The observations show that the volume of the affected brain tissue influences the degree of elevation of the threshold. In the case described below the whole temporal lobe was removed because of invasion by a tumor.

Patient S-ev, a youth aged 19 years (case No. 41241), was admitted to the Burdenko Neurosurgical Institute on February 22, 1965. His illness dated from 1958 when he began to have spasms of the right hand with deviation of the mouth to the right and disturbance of speech. In 1960 he underwent an operation at the Burdenko Neurosurgical Institute, when part of a tumor (a ganglio-astrocytoma) was removed from the middle portions of the temporal lobe. His condition remained satisfactory until 1965 when he began to have severe headaches and attacks of *petit mal*. Examination in 1965 showed papilledema, central paresis of the right facial nerve, and signs of pyramidal insufficiency on the right side.

Otological investigation: whispered speech is heard on the right side at 3 m and on the left at 6 m. No disturbance of hearing was detected by tuning fork tests or tonal audiometry.

Speech audiometry: 100% intelligibility at 40 dB on the right and 35 dB on the left. The EEG showed a focus of pathological activity in the left temporal lobe. Bilateral carotid angiography revealed medial displacement of the intracavernous and supraclinoid segment of the internal carotid artery and the initial part of the middle meningeal artery. The anterior cerebral artery was displaced to the right and medially.

At operation on December 7, 1965 the whole left temporal lobe was found to be invaded by a tumor. The whole of this lobe was removed. After removal of the tumor the wing of the sphenoid bone, anterior cranial fossa, tentorium cerebelli and the tentorial notch, and the pyramid of the temporal bone could be seen.

Histological examination of the tumor after its removal showed that it was a ganglio-astrocytoma.

On examination 3 weeks after the operation the papilledema was slightly reduced, but total right-sided hemianopia had developed. The headache had disappeared. Otoneurological examination showed no change compared with the preoperative condition. Measurement of the threshold intensities of series of tones at 1000 Hz, of different duration, gave the results which are shown in Table 5.

Investigation before the operation showed an almost uniform increase in the thresholds in the left ear to stimuli of all durations tested, amounting on the average to 4-5 dB. The duration effect was almost indistinguishable from that measured in healthy subjects. Measurements on the right ear showed that the threshold intensity of series of tones at 1000 Hz, 1 msec in duration, was 11

TABLE 5. Threshold Intensities of Series of Tones at 1000 Hz as a Function of Their Duration in Patient S-ev before and after Removal of the Left Temporal Lobe in Healthy Subjects

Stimulus duration, msec	Change in threshold intensity from conventional level, in dB*			
	Before operation		After operation	
	Left ear	Right ear	Left ear	Right ear
1200	0	0	0	0
4.5	19.5±1.0	24.0±1.0	20.0±0.4	36.0±0.8
2.0	21.5±1.0	26.0±1.0	23.0±0.6	38.0±0.2
1.0	24.5±1.0	31.0±2.7	26.0±0.5	43.0±3.0
Duration effect	25 dB	31 dB	26 dB	43 dB

*Threshold intensity of series of tones at 1000 Hz, 1200 msec in duration, taken as the zero level for counting decibels.

dB above normal, but the threshold intensity of series 1200 msec in duration was raised by only 5 dB, so that the duration effect was greater than in healthy persons by 5 dB.

After the operation, when stimulation was applied to the left ear, homolateral relative to the operation, the thresholds to a series of tones at 1000 Hz and with durations of 1200 and 1 msec and, consequently, the duration effect, were all indistinguishable from those measured in healthy subjects. In measurements on the right ear, on the side contralateral to the operation, the threshold intensity of series of tones 1200 msec in duration was only 4 dB above normal. The threshold to tones 1 msec in duration was increased still further, and was now 21 dB higher than that measured in healthy subjects. As a result, the duration effect determined in the right ear of patient S-ev was 43 dB and 17 dB higher than normal and than that measured in the left ear respectively (Fig. 9).

In this patient with a tumor occupying the whole of the left temporal lobe, against the background of a marked rise of intracranial pressure before the operation a slight increase in thresholds by 10 dB to long acoustic stimuli measured in both ears and a greater increase (by 15 dB) in the threshold to short tones 1 msec in duration in the right ear were thus observed. Three weeks after operation at which the whole temporal lobe invaded by the

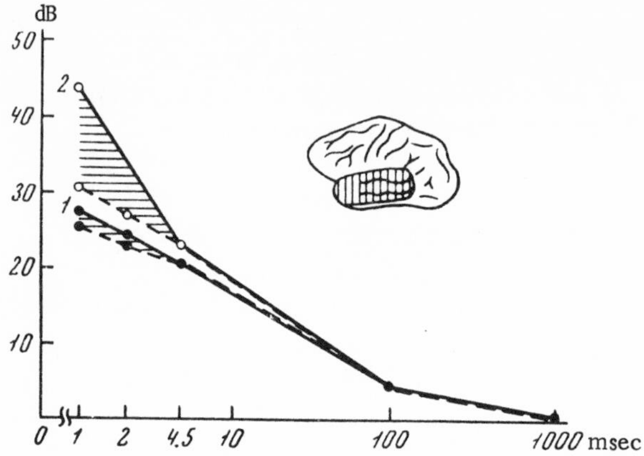

Fig. 9. Threshold intensities of series of tones at 1000 Hz and of different duration in patient S-ev with a lesion of the superior zone of the left temporal lobe: 1) measurements on left ear homolateral relative to the focus; 2) on right ear contralateral to the focus. Shaded area on graph shows change of threshold after removal of left temporal lobe invaded by tumor. Shaded area on diagrams of brain represents area of resection. Remainder of legend as in Fig. 4.

tumor was removed, against the background of a general improvement in the patient's subjective state and normalization of hearing, as shown by the results of audiometric tests, there was an even greater increase in the threshold to short tones (by 21 dB) than before the operation in the ear on the side contralateral to the pathological lesion.

Total removal of the temporal lobe thus did not cause deafness in the ear contralateral to the focus, but merely led to a substantial increase in the threshold intensities of short acoustic stimuli.

A larger increase in thresholds to short stimuli was observed as a rule in patients with an intracerebral lesion than in patients with extracerebral tumors. This can be attributed to the anatomical relations of the auditory cortex and its connections. Pathways to the auditory cortex run through the isthmus of the temporal lobe in a narrow bundle, and in the white matter of the temporal lobe they are also compactly arranged. For this reason, even a small focus in the white matter of the superior or middle temporal gyrus can disturb the functional state of many fibers simultaneously.

Extracerebral tumors can disturb the functions of the auditory cortex if they are situated on the lateral surface of the temporal lobe and compress the superior temporal gyrus, or if they are situated in the sylvian fissure and compress predominantly the transverse gyri. Simultaneous damage to the entire auditory cortex by an extracerebral tumor is therefore improbable. The slight severity of the defect before operation on extracerebral tumors can be attributed to the fact that these tumors cause little disturbance to the blood supply of the underlying cortex, for although they may grow around the blood vessels they rarely obliterate them completely (Arutyunova, 1959).

The smallest degree of elevation of the thresholds to acoustic stimuli of short duration was found in patients examined a long time after the operation. In 5 cases the thresholds were measured at times ranging between 2 and 24 years after the operation. The results of measurement of the threshold intensities in these patients are shown in Table 6.

The results in Table 6 show that in all patients the increase in the duration effect in measurements on the ear contralateral to the pathological focus compared with the corresponding value on the homolateral side and with the results of measurements on healthy subjects still persisted even 20-24 years after removal of the temporal lobe. The fact that the defect of hearing persisted for such a long time is evidence that it is not fully compensated by the activity of other brain regions.

Is there a direct link between disturbances of the perception of short sounds and disturbances of verbal acoustic gnosis?

The observations provide a negative answer to this question. Of the 37 patients showing elevation of the thresholds to short stimuli, in 22 the pathological focus was located in the left temporal lobe, and in the other 15 it was in the right temporal lobe. Of the 22 patients with a left-sided lesion, gross sensory aphasia was found in 10 patients and elements of sensory aphasia in the form of defects of phonemic hearing during special tests in 7 patients. No symptoms of sensory aphasia were present in 2 left-handed patients and in 2 patients with a pathological focus in the interior of the temporal lobe.

TABLE 6. Threshold Intensities of Series of Tones at 1000 Hz and Bursts of White Noise as a Function of Their Duration in Patients Examined a Long Time after Operation

Patient's name	Character and location of pathological focus	Time after operation	Duration effect: On side of lesion, 1000 Hz	Duration effect: On side of lesion, White noise	Duration effect: On opposite side, 1000 Hz	Duration effect: On opposite side, White noise	Difference between sides
D-ov	Meningioma of left sylvian fissure	14 years	25.0	–	28.6	–	+3.6
	Penetrating wound of left parieto-temporal region	21 years	26.0	27.0	31.7	30.0	+5.7
	Removal of intracerebral scar with cyst and metallic splinter from interior of temporal lobe	18 years					
E-ov	Penetrating wound of left temporal lobe	20 years	20.8	–	30.0	–	+9.2
	Excision of scar from meninges and brain tissue	8 years					
B-ov	Penetrating wound of left temporo-parietal region	24 years	30.0	–	36.0		+6.0
N-kii	Meningioma of right temporo-parietal region	6 months	–	18.8	–	31.0	+12.2
		1.6 years	–	19.0	–	27.0	+8.0

An increase in the thresholds to acoustic stimuli of short duration in 15 patients with a lesion of the right temporal lobe and in patients with a left-sided lesion in whom the syndrome of sensory aphasia was slight or absent suggests that this defect of hearing is independent of hemispheric dominance and of the severity of the speech disorders.

Conclusions

In patients with a local lesion of the superior zone of the temporal lobe (37 persons) the duration effect on the side contralateral to the focus is 3-23 dB greater than the corresponding effect on the homolateral side (mean difference 10 dB). The increase in the duration effect is the result of a higher increase in the threshold to short acoustic stimuli.

A greater increase in thresholds in the ear contralateral to the focus than in the homolateral ear is found to stimuli shorter than 14 msec in duration. Elevation of the thresholds to short stimuli is observed in lesions of both the dominant and the nondominant hemisphere.

The severest defect is observed in patients with an intracerebral lesion. The increase in the duration effect observed on the side contralateral to the lesion compared with the value obtained on the homolateral side in patients 20-24 years after injury to the temporal lobe is evidence that complete compensation of this defect by the activity of other parts of the brain does not take place.

LOCAL LESIONS IN THE BASAL PORTION AND POLE OF THE TEMPORAL LOBE

The second group of patients with pathological lesions of the temporal lobe consisted of 15 persons with lesions of the basal and polar zones: the lesion was intracerebral in 9 cases and extracerebral in 6. All patients had clearly defined signs and symptoms of a local brain lesion.

The distribution of the increases in threshold intensities of series of tones at 1000 Hz, with durations of 1200 and 1 msec, in

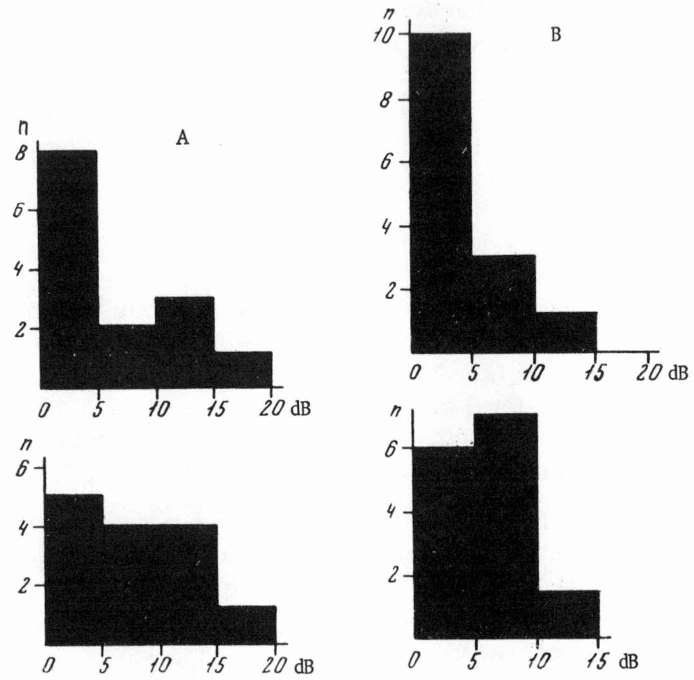

Fig. 10. Absolute thresholds (dB) in patients with local lesions of the basal portion and pole of the temporal lobe compared with corresponding values in healthy subjects to series of tones at 1000 Hz and with durations of 1200 msec (A) and 1 msec (B). Mean results for 7 healthy subjects taken as the zero level for counting decibels. Above – difference in thresholds measured in the ear homologous to the lesion; below – in the ear contralateral to the focus. Abscissa, difference in thresholds (dB); ordinate, number of patients.

14 patients of this group, compared with the results obtained in healthy subjects, is shown in the histogram in Fig. 10.

It is clear from Fig. 10 that the threshold intensities of tonal series with durations of 1200 and 1 msec, measured in the ears homolateral and contralateral to the lesion, do not differ significantly in the patients of this group. Measurements in the ear homolateral to the lesion in 10 patients and in the contralateral ear in 9 patients showed that the increase in threshold intensities of series of tones 1200 msec in duration did not exceed 10 dB. To stimuli 1 msec in duration an increase in the threshold intensities by less than 10 dB was found in 13 of 14 patients tested when the stimuli were applied similarly to the right and left ears.

A graph of threshold intensities of series of tones at 1000 Hz as a function of their duration in patient K-ov with an intracerebral tumor of the polar zone of the right temporal lobe, is shown in Fig. 11.

Patient K-ov, a man aged 27 years, was admitted to the Burdenko Neurosurgical Institute on October 16, 1965 (case No. 41034). His illness began a year ago with attacks of unconsciousness lasting 1-2 min, before which he saw bright pictures before his eyes. Later he developed headaches and his visual acuity was impaired.

Examination revealed moderate signs of increased intracranial pressure and evidence of a local lesion of the right hemisphere: anosmia on the right side and central paresis of the left facial nerve. The EEG showed a focus in the anterior zones of the right temporal region. Carotid angiography on the right side revealed displacement of the middle cerebral artery and anterior choroid artery upward and medially.

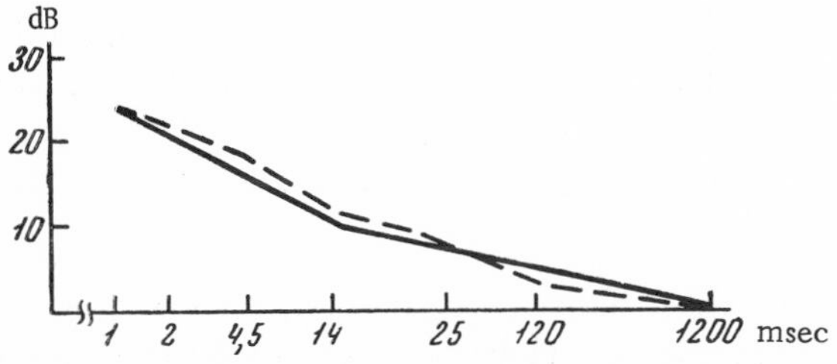

Fig. 11. Thresholds of detection of series of tones at 1000 Hz as a function of their duration. Patient K-ov with a tumor of the polar zone of the right temporal lobe. Continuous line shows results of measurements on left ear contralateral to tumor; broken line measurements on right ear homolateral to tumor. Threshold for series of tones at 1000 Hz, 1200 msec in duration, taken as zero level for counting decibels. Abscissa, stimulus duration in msec; ordinate, thresholds in dB.

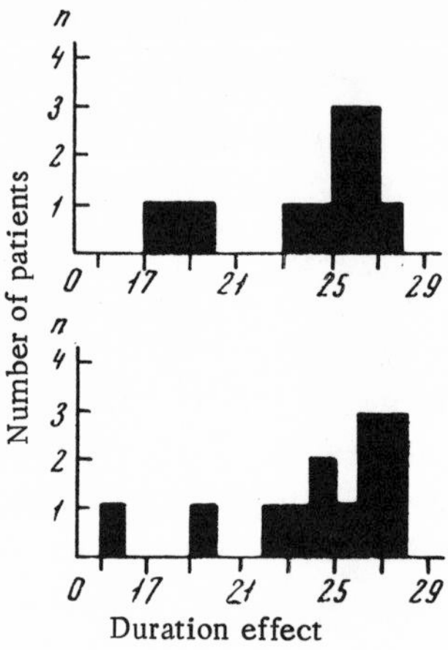

Fig. 12. Distribution of duration effect (in dB) measured to series of tones at 1000 Hz in patients with focal lesions of the basal and polar zones of the temporal lobe. Above – duration effect on side homolateral to lesion; below – on side contralateral to lesion. Abscissa, difference between threshold intensities of stimuli with durations of 1200 and 1 msec, in dB; ordinate, number of patients.

On October 25, 1965 an intracerebral tumor (astrocytoma) of the right temporal lobe, occupying its pole, was removed.

The curves of threshold intensities as a function of stimulus duration for patient K-ov, measured during acoustic stimulation of the right and left ears coincide completely (Fig. 11). On both sides the duration effect was 23 dB. Similar results were obtained in the remaining patients of this group.

The distribution of the duration effect among this group of patients on the sides homolateral and contralateral to the focus is shown in Fig. 12. In no patient did the duration effect exceed 28 dB, i.e., in no patient did it differ by more than 2 dB from the corresponding value in healthy subjects.

The results of these measurements show also that the difference between the duration effect on the side of the lesion and on the contralateral side did not exceed ± 2 dB in all patients of this group, and in 10 of the 14 patients it did not exceed ± 1 dB.

No increase in threshold intensities to stimuli of any duration was thus found in the patients of this group. There was likewise no difference between the results of measurements of threshold intensities on the side of the lesion or the contralateral side, whether long or short acoustic stimuli were used.

The reason for the absence of an increase in threshold intensities of short acoustic stimuli in the patients of this group is evidently that although the pathological focus lay within the temporal lobe, it had not spread to the auditory projection cortex or to the ascending auditory pathway.

An extracerebral lesion compressing the basal zone of the temporal lobe was present in 6 patients. An intracerebral tumor of the polar zone of the temporal lobe was found in 2 patients, and in the remaining 7 patients the pathological focus was in the interior of the temporal lobe, involving mainly the basal zone. The following case is very demonstrative.

Patient K-ii, a man aged 26 years (case No. 41634), right-handed, was admitted to the Burdenko Neurosurgical Institute on January 22, 1966, where he died on February 27, 1966. On admission he complained of headaches with nausea and vomiting and loss of the right half of the visual field. He suffered from olfactory hallucinations.

On examination: right-sided hemianopia. Outlines of the optic disks indistinct. Central paresis of right facial nerves. Right-sided hemihypoesthesia. Positive Gordon's and Oppenheim's signs on the right side.

Otoneurological examination showed no disturbance of hearing. The EEG showed a well-marked focus of pathological activity in the left temporo-occipital region against the background of distinct interhemispheric asymmetry.

Roentgenograms of the skull showed changes due to increased intracranial pressure. Pineal gland displaced to the right.

Lumbar puncture: CSF pressure 340 mm water, protein 0.87‰, cells 34/3.

Neuropsychological tests showed gross disturbances of audio-verbal memory.

Left-sided carotid angiography: displacement of the middle cerebral artery upward and medially.

On February 27 the patient had a sudden attack of severe headache and vomiting, with a rigor, and respiratory and cardiac arrest.

Autopsy: a large unilocular hydatid cyst was found in the interior of the left temporal lobe.

A

B

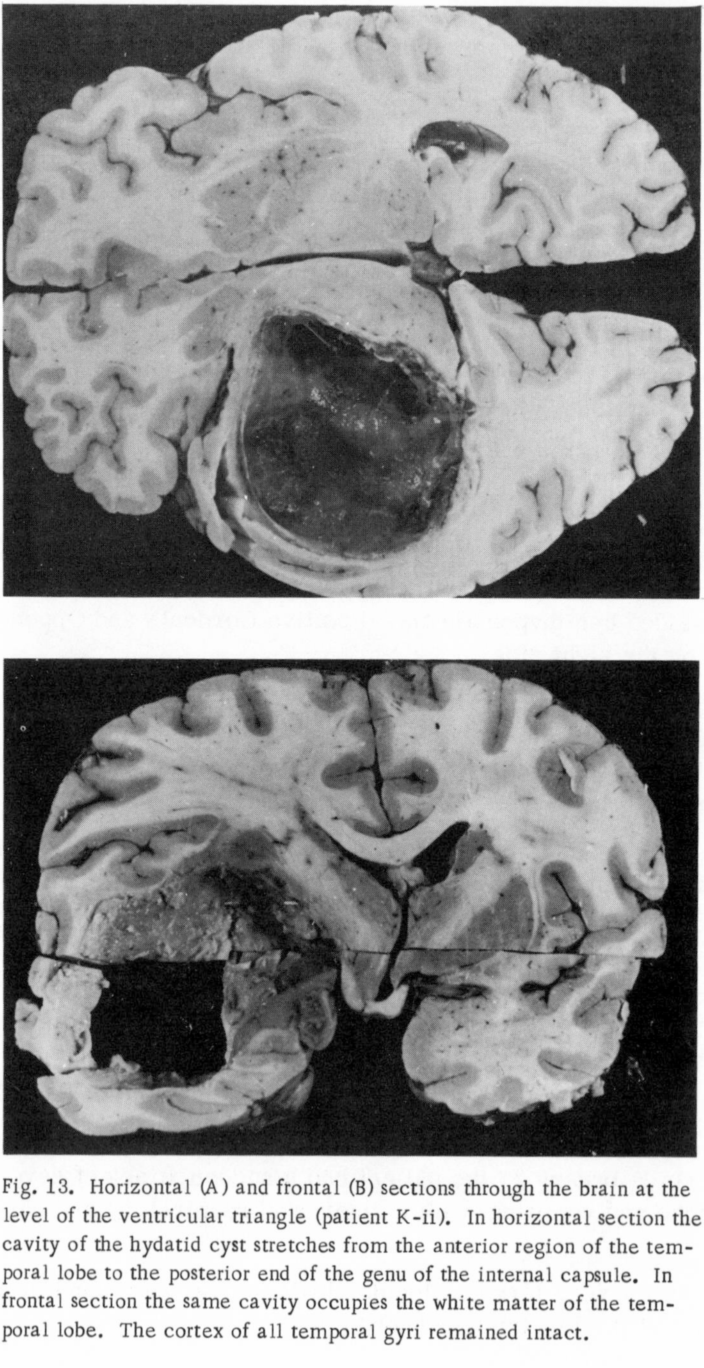

Fig. 13. Horizontal (A) and frontal (B) sections through the brain at the level of the ventricular triangle (patient K-ii). In horizontal section the cavity of the hydatid cyst stretches from the anterior region of the temporal lobe to the posterior end of the genu of the internal capsule. In frontal section the same cavity occupies the white matter of the temporal lobe. The cortex of all temporal gyri remained intact.

In horizontal sections the cavity of the hydatid cyst extends from the anterior region of the temporal lobe to the posterior end of the genu of the internal capsule, compressing the posterior genu and pulvinar of the thalamus modially (Fig. 13A).

In frontal sections at the level of the ventricular triangle the cyst occupies the white matter of the temporal lobe. The cortex of all temporal gyri is preserved. In a section at the level of Heschl's gyrus, the cavity 5 cm in diameter occupies the white matter in the region of the middle and inferior temporal gyri, the lower part of the capsular externa et extrema, and the cortex of the hippocampal gyrus. The temporal gyri are displaced to the periphery (Fig. 13B).

The central gray matter of the temporal lobe, the hippocampus, and the amygdala were thus destroyed. The whole of the internal capsule, including its posterior portion, was intact.

Series of sections stained by Spielmeyer's method showed that the fibers in the superior temporal gyrus were well stained. In sections stained by Nissl's method the cytoarchitectonic structure of the cortex of Heschl's gyrus remained intact and no vascular changes were seen.

The medial geniculate body was intact on both sides. Slight degeneration was observed in the dorsal layers of the left lateral geniculate body. No gliosis was visible in the region of the central auditory pathway. Slight infiltration of the blood vessel walls was visible on the affected side. Counting the number of satellite cells in the medial geniculate bodies showed no significant differences. No difference likewise was found in the shape of the nerve cells.

Measurements on the right ear showed an increase in the thresholds of audibility of series of tones at 1000 Hz, 1200 msec in duration by 4.5 dB over normal, and of series 1 msec in duration by 5 dB.

In measurements on the left ear the threshold for stimuli 1200 msec in duration was normal, while that to stimuli of 1 msec in duration was 1.5 dB above normal.

The duration effect was 27 dB for stimuli applied both to the left and right ear.

Consequently, in this patient with a large hydatid cyst in the interior of the temporal lobe the superior and middle zones of the temporal lobe were compressed by the large, space-occupying lesion but not destroyed. The medial geniculate body – central auditory pathway – cortex of Heschl's gyrus system was unchanged. Investigation of the threshold intensities of acoustic stimuli of different duration showed no selective disturbances of the detection of short duration sounds on either side.

Conclusions

In patients with local lesions of the basal and polar zones of the temporal lobe (15 cases) the duration effect on the side of the focus and on the opposite side do not differ by more than 2 dB. No definite predominance was found on either side.

In two-thirds of the patients of this group who were tested, the duration effects do not differ by more than 1 dB from the results of the corresponding measurements on healthy subjects.

COMBINED LESIONS OF THE TEMPORAL LOBE AND PERIPHERAL PORTION OF THE AUDITORY SYSTEM

Threshold intensities of acoustic stimuli of different durations have been investigated in patients with lesions of the peripheral portion of the auditory system by a number of workers (Miscolczy-Fodor, 1953; Harris, Haines, and Myers, 1958; Elliott, 1963; Kishonas, 1967). They found that in diseases of the middle ear a disturbance of sound conduction does not alter the slope of the curves of threshold intensity versus stimulus duration. In lesions of the organ of Corti the slope of the curves of threshold intensity versus duration is significantly reduced. Whereas under normal conditions in response to a tenfold decrease in stimulus duration the threshold intensities increased by 9-10 dB, in patients with lesions of the organ of Corti the mean increase in thresholds is 3-5 dB for a tenfold decrease in duration (this reduced steepness of the curves of temporal summation is particularly marked at frequencies of 2000 and 4000 Hz or more). Consequently, in diseases of the organ of Corti the character of the change in the temporal summation curve is opposite to that observed in central cortical lesions of the auditory system. A substantial decrease in the duration effect would therefore be expected in patients with lesions of the superior zones of the temporal lobe associated with Menière's disease or neuritis of the auditory nerve.

Accordingly, during the investigation of patients with combined lesions of the temporal lobe and the peripheral portion of the auditory system, as attempt was made to determine how the hearing defect due to the peripheral lesion affected the duration effect in patients with a local lesion in the superior zones of the temporal lobe and, consequently, to ascertain whether disturbances of function of the auditory cortex can be detected in the presence of a concurrent lesion of the peripheral part of the auditory system.

Of the 96 patients undergoing otoscopic examination 10 showed signs of previous otitis (dullness and indrawing of the tympanic membranes). The results of pure-tone audiometry on all the patients of this group showed a slight impairment of hearing in the region of low and middle frequencies (in 9 patients the loss of hearing did not exceed 10 dB, while in 1 patient it was 15 dB).

In 7 of these patients, in whom the pathological process was outside the superior zone of the temporal lobe, an almost uniform elevation of the thresholds to short and long acoustic stimuli was found by comparison with measurements on healthy subjects. The duration effect in these patients was the same as in healthy persons. In 3 patients with a local lesion of the superior temporal subregion, against the background of raised thresholds to long acoustic stimuli, there was an even greater increase in the thresholds to short acoustic stimuli when applied to the ear on the side contralateral to the focus. The duration effect on the side contralateral to the focus was, correspondingly, 9-10 dB higher on the average than the duration effect of the homolateral side, i.e., a previous attack of otitis did not interfere with the diagnosis of the localization of the pathological focus in the superior zone of the temporal lobe by means of the test now under consideration.

In 10 of the total group of patients investigated by pure-tone audiometry, a bilateral impairment of hearing within the range of high frequencies (4000 Hz and higher) with respect to both air and bone conduction was found. In 4 of these patients, with no local lesion of the temporal lobe, the increase in thresholds was greater to long acoustic stimuli and was particularly marked when white noise was used as the stimulus. As a result, the duration effect in these patients was 17.0–27.0 dB, or 5–8 dB below normal.* In 6 patients with combined lesions (a focus in the superior zone of the temporal lobe and neuritis of the auditory nerves) the same pattern was found on the side of the focus. On the contralateral side in these patients the increase in thresholds to short stimuli was greater and the duration effect was 8–13 dB greater than when measured in the ear homolateral to the lesion.

The results of measurements of the threshold in patient Ch–v (case No. 41624), with a meningioma of the left temporal lobe and bilateral neuritis of the auditory nerve, will serve as an example.

Measurements on the ear homolateral to the focus revealed an increase in the threshold intensities of series of tones at 1000 Hz and 1200 msec in duration by 18 dB compared with normal and by 14 dB compared with sounds 1 msec in duration. As a result of the greater increase in threshold to long acoustic stimuli the duration effect was 22.0 dB (4 dB less than normal).

In the right ear the threshold to acoustic stimulation 1200 msec in duration was 16.5 dB above normal, and to stimuli 1 msec in duration 24 dB above normal. As a result of the greater increase in the threshold to the short acoustic stimulus the duration effect was 7.5 dB above normal, with an absolute value of 33.5 dB.

This case shows, first, the greater degree of increase in threshold to long acoustic stimuli in the presence of neuritis of the auditory nerve, so that the duration effect is less than normal.

In measurements on the right ear, opposite to the focus in the temporal lobe, a marked increase in the threshold to the long acoustic stimulus is also found. However, the increase in threshold to the short acoustic stimulus due to the cortical defect of

*The value of the duration effect to series of tones at 1000 Hz thus obtained is in agreement with the results (Kishonas, 1966), of measurements on patients with neuritis of the auditory nerve. In response to series of tones at 2000 and 4000 Hz, Kishonas found a smaller duration effect (9-12 dB).

hearing is even more marked in this ear, so that there is a net increase in the duration effect, as is characteristic of all patients with a pathological focus in the superior zones of the temporal lobe.

A loss of auditory sensation can be produced not only by a lesion of the peripheral part of the auditory system, but also by increased intracranial pressure which was found in most of the patients investigated. For this reason, the effect of differences in the degree of loss of hearing due to factors unconnected with the lesion of the auditory cortex on the duration effect in patients with temporal lesions deserves special examination.

The distribution of duration effect measured to series of tones at 1000 Hz (A) and white noise (B) in relation to the degree of impairment of hearing of these stimuli in 37 patients with a lesion of the superior temporal zones is shown in Fig. 14.

It is clear that the duration effect in these patients is independent of the degree of impairment of hearing. In all patients, regardless of the degree of loss of hearing, the duration effects measured in the ear contralateral to the lesion are much greater than those measured in the ear homolateral to the lesion and than the values obtained with healthy subjects.

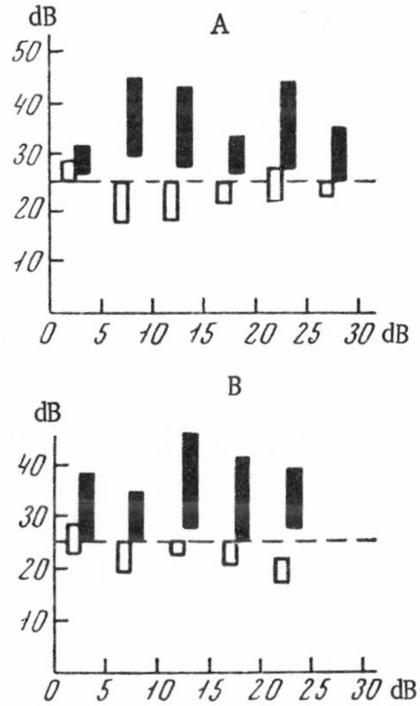

Fig. 14. Distribution of values of duration effect plotted with respect to loss of hearing to tones at 1000 Hz (A) and white noise stimuli (B) in patients with lesions of the superior temporal zone. Columns show range of distribution of duration effect for a loss of hearing indicated on abscissa (filled columns denote side contralateral to lesion, empty columns side homolateral to lesion). Broken line shows duration effect in healthy persons. Abscissa, loss of hearing in dB (below threshold of normal hearing, taken as zero); ordinate, duration effect (dB).

A combination of lesions of the peripheral and cortical portions of the auditory system thus does not prevent the detection of a defect of hearing short stimuli due to a lesion of the auditory cortex.

Conclusions

In patients with a lesion of the superior zone of the temporal lobe the duration effect on the side contralateral to the focus is 2-3 dB greater than the corresponding effect measured on the same side as the focus. The increase in duration effect is the result of a greater increase in the threshold to short acoustic stimuli.

An increase in the thresholds to short acoustic stimuli is observed in lesions of both dominant and nondominant hemispheres.

In patients with a local lesion of the basal and polar zones of the temporal lobe there is no predominant increase in thresholds to acoustic stimuli of any particular duration.

A combined lesion of the cortical and peripheral portions of the auditory system does not prevent the detection of a defect due to a cortical lesion.

CHAPTER 5

Thresholds of Detection of Acoustic Stimuli as a Function of Duration in Patients with Local Brain Lesions Outside the Temporal Lobe

LOCAL BRAIN LESIONS OUTSIDE THE TEMPORAL LOBE

Altogether, 27 patients with a local lesion of the brain outside the temporal lobe were investigated. Depending on the character of the disease, this group contained 18 patients with tumors (10 extracerebral and 8 intracerebral), 7 patients with sequelae of head injuries, 1 patient with cystic arachnoiditis, and 1 patient with thrombosis of the internal carotid artery. All patients had clearly defined focal symptoms.

The patients were subdivided as follows depending on the location of the lesion: in 2 patients the lesion was in the parieto-occipital region, in 4 in the parietal lobe, in 8 in the fronto-parietal region, and in 8 in the frontal lobe. In 5 more patients, although the lesion lay outside the temporal lobe, it also affected the region of the temporal lobe to some extent. One patient had a penetrating wound of the basal fronto-temporal region. In the patient with a diagnosis of thrombosis of the internal carotid artery, the clinical features indicated that the functions of the frontal and parietal lobes were most severely affected. There were also indications of a disturbance of the functions of the deep zones of the temporal lobe (disturbance of auditory memory). In these two cases, because of the character of the clinical picture it was difficult to decide whether the lesion extended to the superior zone of the temporal lobe. Three other cases are of particular interest, for the pathological focus lay in the posterior zone of the temporal

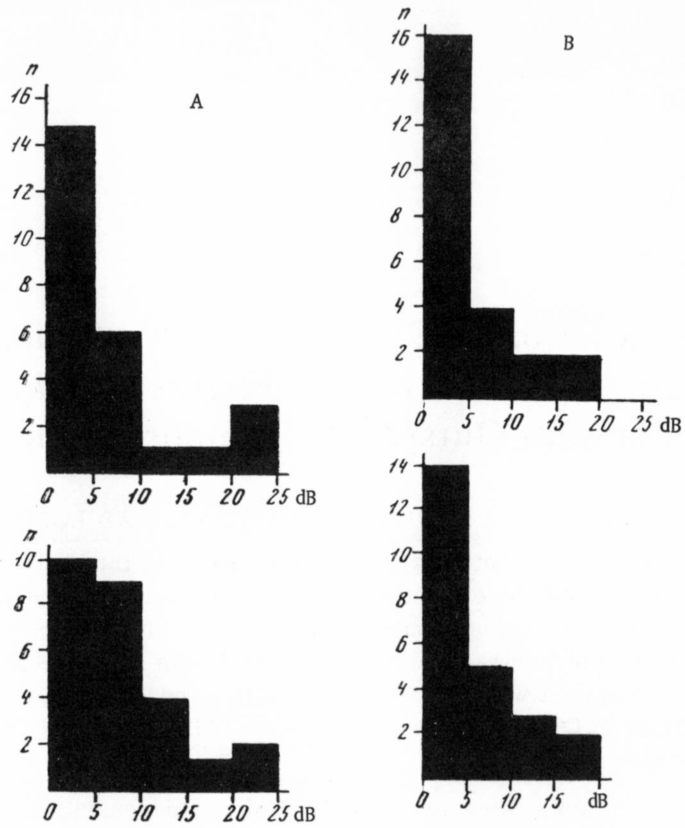

Fig. 15. Absolute thresholds (in dB) in patients with local lesions of the brain outside the temporal lobe compared with the corresponding values for healthy subjects to series of tones at 1000 Hz and with durations of 1200 msec (A) and 1 msec (B). Mean results for 7 healthy subjects taken as zero level for counting decibels. Above: difference between thresholds in ear homolateral to the lesion; below, difference in thresholds in ear contralateral to the lesion. Abscissa, difference in thresholds (in dB); ordinate, number of patients.

lobe, at its junction with the inferior parietal and occipital regions, i.e., close to the auditory cortex, but without affecting it.

The results of measurement of the threshold intensities (dB) in 22 patients with a lesion outside the temporal lobe are compared in Fig. 15 with those measured in healthy subjects to a tonal stimulus at 1000 Hz and 1200 msec and 1 msec in duration. Clearly the thresholds on the sides homolateral and contralateral to the focus do not differ significantly. To stimuli with a duration of 1200 msec the threshold intensities were not more than 10 dB higher than those measured in healthy subjects, when tested in the ear homolateral to the focus in 21 patients and in the ear contralateral to the focus in 19 patients. Similar results were obtained when the threshold intensities to stimuli 1 msec in duration were measured.

Curves showing threshold intensities of series of tones at 1000 Hz as a function of their duration in patient M-v with the sequelae of an injury to the right parieto-occipital region are shown in Fig. 16. The curves reflecting the shift in thresholds in response to shortening the duration of the stimuli, when measured in the ears homolateral and contralateral to the focus, clearly coincide. On both sides the duration effect is 26 dB, i.e., it is indistinguishable from the results of measurements made on healthy subjects.

The duration effects in this group of patients, when measured in the ears both homolateral and contralateral to the focus, are shown in Fig. 17. In the great majority of patients the duration effect both before and after the operation does not differ by more than 2 dB from the corresponding value measured in healthy subjects. In 13 patients the duration effect was greater on the side contralateral to the lesion, in 7 patients it was greater on the

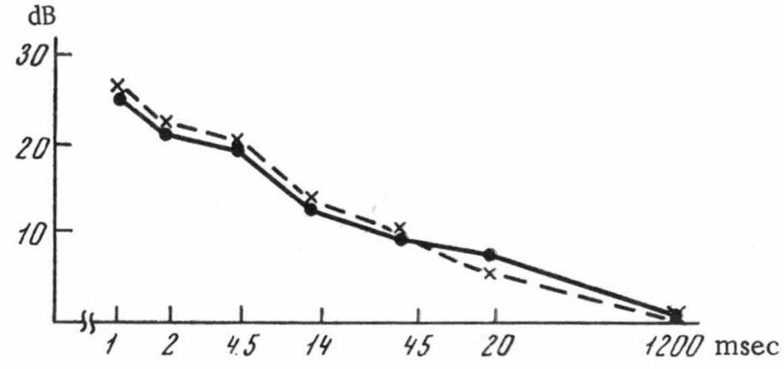

Fig. 16. Thresholds of detection of series of tones at 1000 Hz as a function of duration. Patient M-v with sequelae of an injury to the right parieto-occipital region. Continuous line shows results of measurement in left ear, contralateral to the focus; broken line results in the right ear homolateral to the focus. Abscissa, stimulus duration; ordinate, thresholds, in dB. Threshold for series of tones at 1000 Hz, 1200 msec in duration, taken as zero level for counting decibels.

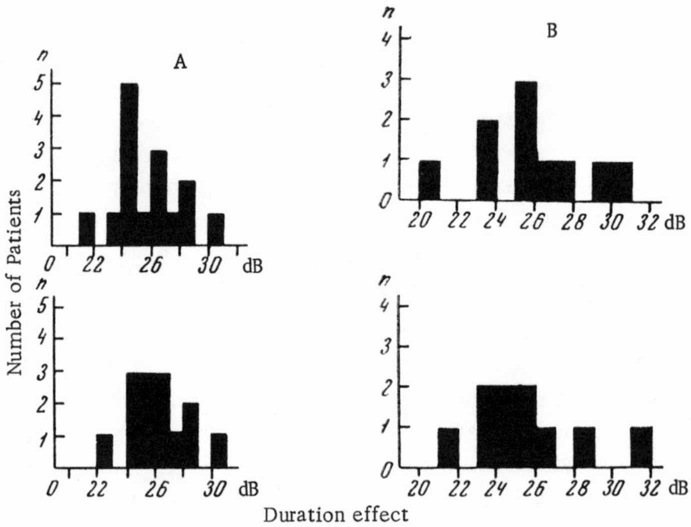

Fig. 17. Distribution of duration effect (in dB) measured to series of tones at 1000 Hz in patients with local lesions of the brain outside the temporal lobe, before (A) and after operation (B). Above: duration effect on side homolateral to lesion; below: effect on side contralateral to lesion. Abscissa, difference in dB between threshold intensities of stimuli 1200 msec and 1 msec in duration; ordinate, number of patients.

same side as the lesion, and in 4 patients the results of the measurements were the same on both sides.

In all cases the difference between the duration effect measured on the two sides did not exceed 2.5 dB.

Conclusions

In patients with a local lesion of the brain outside the temporal lobe the duration effects on the side of the focus and on the opposite side differ by not more than 2.5 dB, with no clearly defined predominance on either side. In most patients of this group the duration effects do not differ by more than 2 dB from those measured in healthy subjects. No predominant increase in thresholds to acoustic stimuli of any particular duration is found.

LESIONS OF THE BRAIN STEM

Nine patients with lesions of the brain stem were investigated: 8 with tumors and 1 with an arachnoid cyst. Depending on

TABLE 7. **Duration Effects in Patients with Local Lesions of the Brain Stem**

Name	Location of lesion	Duration effect (in dB)				Difference between two sides (in dB)	
		In left ear		In right ear			
		Before operation	After operation	Before operation	After operation	Before operation	After operation
	A. Tone of 1000 Hz						
R-ov	Pons (destruction of corpora quadrigemina)	23.2	–	21.6	–	−1.6	–
K-va	Third ventricle	24.0	26.0	24.0	26.0	0	0
P-ov	Mesencephalon	25.3	–	23.5	–	−1.8	–
V-va	Fourth ventricle	–	16.0	–	21.3	–	+5.3
F-in	Fourth ventricle	23.7	25.0	22.9	26.0	−0.8	+1.0
L-ev	Pons	21.0	–	22.0	–	+1.0	–
R-ev	Posterior cranial fossa	26.0	–	26.5	–	+0.5	–
P-va	Posterior cranial fossa	25.0	–	25.7	–	−0.7	–
E-va	Cerebellum	23.5	–	25.0	–	+0.5	–
	B. White noise						
R-ov	Pons (destruction of corpora quadrigemina)	22.0	–	21.3	–	−0.7	–
P-ov	Mesencephalon	24.5	–	22.0	–	−2.5	–

+ denotes that duration effect is greater when measured in right ear, - denotes effect is greater in left ear.

the location of the lesion the patients were distributed as follows: 3 patients had a lesion mainly in the region of the mesencephalon and pons, 1 patient in the region of the pons, 2 in the region of the floor of the fourth ventricle, and 1 in a cerebellar hemisphere. In 2 patients the precise location of the lesion in the posterior cranial fossa could not be determined.

In most patients of this group (7 cases) only a slight decrease in hearing was observed at a frequency of 1000 Hz (5-10 dB), equally whether the measurements were made on the right or left ears. Only in 1 patient, with a tumor in the floor of the fourth ventricle and destruction of the cochlear nuclei, was the loss of hearing found to be different when measured in the right ear (21 dB) and in the left (35 dB). The results of measurement of the duration effect in these patients are shown in Table 7.

It will be clear from Table 7 that the magnitude of the duration effect in all the patients of this group did not exceed 26 dB, and that its mean value was 24 ± 0.5 dB. Consequently, in the patients of this group a tendency was observed for the duration effect to be reduced compared with its value measured in healthy subjects.

Two cases in which the auditory structures of the brain stem were directly involved in the pathological process may now be examined.

Patient R-ov, a man 24 years (case No. 41419), was admitted to the Burdenko Neurosurgical Institute on December 20, 1965 and remained there until January 26, 1966. He complained of increasing headaches.

On examination: corneal reflexes diminished on both sides. Anisocoria R > L. Pupils do not respond to light. Convergence disturbed. Paresis of upward movement of eyes. Nystagmus on looking upward, downward, and straight ahead. Marked disturbances of standing, walking, and coordination on both sides.

Optic disks pale, outlines indistinct, veins wide.

Otological investigation: whispered speech heard at 5 m on both sides. Tests with tuning fork show hearing 90% at all frequencies. Pure-tone audiometry: loss of hearing of 10-20 dB in both ears in zone of middle frequencies and 20-30 dB in zone of high frequencies.

Ventriculography: marked hydrocephalus, posterior and inferior portions of third ventricle not filled.

On account of the occlusion at the level of the aqueduct of Sylvius an operation was performed on January 7, 1966, when the lamina terminalis was perforated. On January 26, however, the patient died.

At autopsy a tumor of the tegmentum of the pons was found. The tumor was 3.5 cm in diameter and it invaded the lamina quadrigemina, more especially on the left side, and the left cerebral peduncle, and it obstructed the lumen of the aqueduct of Sylvius (Fig. 18).

Microscopic study of a series of sections through the pons and mesencephalon showed that the tumor was an astrocytoma

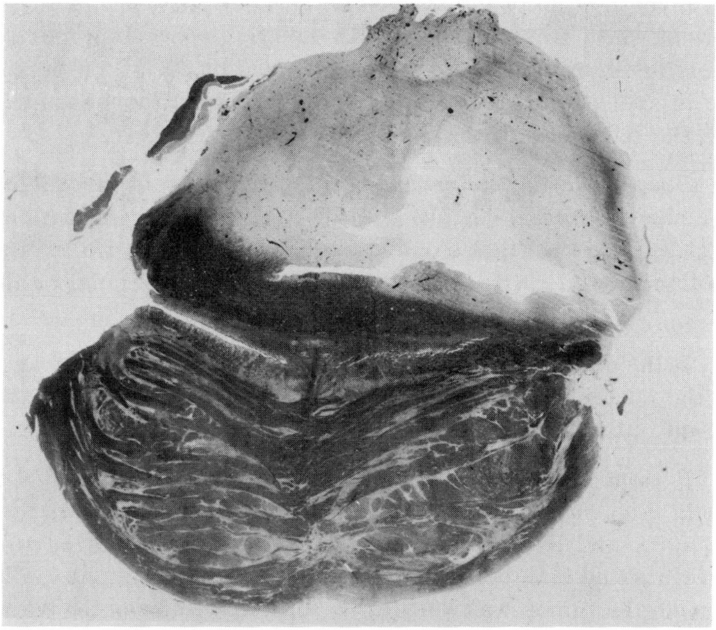

Fig. 18. Section through pons stained by Spielmeyer's method (patient R-ov). The tumor invades a large part of the tegmentum of the pons. Transverse fibers were preserved at the border between the base and tegmentum, as well as the medial lemniscus on both sides. The lateral lemniscus on the right side is surrounded by tumor tissue and completely degenerated, while on the left side it is better preserved.

invading the tegmentum of the pons and the tegmentum and tectum mesencephali. The lateral lemniscus was ill-defined, especially on the right. No cellular structures remained intact in the left inferior colliculus; in the right inferior colliculus, more or less degenerated nerve cells could be seen here and there among the tumor cells.

Measurement of the threshold intensities of series of tones at 1000 Hz and 1200 msec in duration revealed an increase of 10 dB in their level on the right side and of 9 dB on the left. In response to tones 1 msec in duration the threshold was raised by 6 dB on both sides. As a result of the somewhat greater increase in thresholds to long acoustic stimuli (by 3-4 dB), the duration effect was 21.6 dB (in the right ear) and 23.2 dB (in the left ear), i.e., 2.8 dB below normal on the left and 4.4 dB below normal on the right.

Investigation of the thresholds of audibility of this patient to bursts of white noise 1200 msec in duration showed an increase in their level by 6 dB on the left side and by 10 dB on the right, while to acoustic stimuli 1 msec in duration the increases were 3 dB on the left and 6 dB on the right.

Because of the somewhat greater increase in thresholds to long acoustic stimuli (by 3-4 dB) the duration effect in patient R-ov was 21.3 dB in the right ear and 22.0 dB in the left, i.e., it was 3 dB below normal on the left side and 4 dB below normal on the right.

In the next case, in which the diagnosis was verified at operation, the cochlear nuclei in the floor on the fourth ventricle were involved in the pathological process.

Patient V-va, a woman aged 26 years (case No. 42193) underwent 3 operations at the Burdenko Neurosurgical Institute in 1951, 1952, and 1960, for the partial removal of an astrocytoma of the vermis and both hemispheres of the cerebellum. At the last operation the tumor was seen to be intimately connected with the floor of the fourth ventricle, especially in the lateral zones.

On examination in 1960: corneal reflexes absent; peripheral paresis of the left facial nerve; coordination and maintenance of the static posture disturbed; bulbar dysarthria, dysphonia. Whispered speech heard on the right and left at a distance of 1 m. Tuning-fork tests: on the right C 40%, C_1 43%, C_2 45%, C_3 50%; C_4 50%, on the left C 33%, C_1 35%, C_2 40%, C_3 43%, C_4 45%. Pure-tone audiometry: hearing reduced by 40 dB to all frequencies on both sides.

The threshold intensities of series of tones at 1000 Hz and 1200 msec in duration were increased in patient V-va by comparison with those measured in healthy subjects, by 21 dB in the right ear and by 35 dB in the left. The duration effect was 21.3 dB when measured in the right ear and 15.2 dB when measured in the left ear.

Consequently, in patient V-va, with a tumor of the cochlear nuclei of the floor of the fourth ventricle, the duration effect was 5 dB less than in healthy subjects on the right side and 10 dB less on the left.

In patients with tumors of the brain stem, in whom the pathological process directly involved the cochlear nuclei and auditory pathways, disturbances of hearing, of varied severity, were thus observed. If the cochlear nuclei in the floor of the fourth ventricle were involved in the pathological process, the disturbances of hearing were more severe than in lesions of the inferior colliculi. The thresholds to long acoustic stimuli were increased more in these patients than those to short stimuli.

Conclusions

Investigation of the relationship between threshold intensities and duration of the stimulus showed that in patients with local brain lesions outside the temporal lobe the increase in thresholds was not more marked for acoustic stimuli of any particular duration.

The magnitude of the duration effect is identical with the results of measurements in healthy subjects and not significantly different when measured in the ears homolateral and contralateral relative to the pathological focus. In patients in whom auditory structures in the brain stem are involved in the pathological process, the duration effect is reduced on account of the greater increase in threshold intensities to long acoustic stimuli than to short.

CHAPTER 6

Results of Additional Investigations

As was mentioned above, besides the main method of investigation (a study of the relationship between threshold intensities and duration of acoustic stimuli in 8 healthy subjects and 96 patients with lesions in different parts of the brain) some aspects of the activity of the auditory system also were examined.

1. An investigation of three-dimensional hearing, using an instrument of the Vojacek's laterometer type, showed that the ability to locate a source of sound was unimpaired in all 37 patients with lesions of the superior zone of the temporal lobe.

The ability to localize sound was also unimpaired in patients with lesions in the frontal lobe. Only in patients with lesions in the parieto-temporo-occipital region was the localization of the source of a sound grossly impaired. Localization of a sound was particularly severely disturbed on the side contralateral to the lesion.

2. The evaluation of rhythms, whether in slow or quick time, gave rise to no difficulty in healthy subjects.

Most patients with a lesion in any part of the brain could correctly reproduce rhythmic structures if presented in slow time, whereas patients with lesions of the temporal zones (both the superior temporal and basal zones) and patients with lesions of the frontal and parietal lobes made many mistakes when evaluating rhythmic structures applied in quick time. However, the mistakes in patients with lesions of the superior temporal zone were always in the form of an underestimation of the number of beats, whereas patients with lesions in other parts of the brain made mistakes of random character (they were just as likely to overestimate as to underestimate the number of beats).

If the attention of patients with lesions outside the temporal lobe was mobilized, this often prevented them from making mistakes when evaluating rhythms.

It is interesting to note that patients with lesions of the superior temporal zones as a rule could easily reproduce the accentuations of rhythmic structures.

3. Healthy subjects had no difficulty in discriminating between two musical fragments or two notes differing by a complete or half tone. Consequently, all the tests which were used to study musical hearing were sufficiently easy for healthy subjects.

Investigations showed that patients with pathological lesions in the temporal lobe distinguish musical fragments or series of tones differing by a complete or half tone, i.e., in terms of the criteria used they showed no evidence of amusia.

General Conclusions

The survey of the literature shows that classical methods of testing hearing, such as pure-tone audiometry, tuning-fork tests, measurement of differential thresholds of frequency and intensity, speech audiometry, suprathreshold equalization of loudness, and also the tests of Weber and Schwabach, as a rule do not enable a pathological focus in the central portions of the auditory system to be localized.

By the use of new methods in conjunction with the classical methods of investigation the localization of the pathological process can be determined more precisely. Tests based on binaural interaction reveal deviations from normal in lesions at any level of the auditory system above the first decussation of the central auditory pathway. On the basis of deviation of the acoustic image, the localization of a pathological process can be placed with an equal measure of probability in the brain stem on the side to which the acoustic image is displaced or in the contralateral temporal lobe.

Tests of the recognition of fragments of speech or music presented monaurally and binaurally under conditions when the excess of information which they contain is reduced (by filtration, compression, or periodic interruption of the fragments, by introduction of noise or irrelevant speech conducted to the same ear as that receiving the test fragment, or to the opposite ear) are of great importance for the diagnosis of pathological lesions in the temporal lobe. By the use of these methods it is possible to locate a lesion in the right or left temporal lobes on the basis of the disturbance of discrimination of a text or fragment if presented to the ear contralateral to the side of the affected temporal lobe. However, tonal tests for the diagnosis of central lesions have definite advantages over speech tests, because they are independent of the subject's native tongue or of the level of his intelligence and they can be used on patients with various forms of aphasia. Consequently, the large group of patients with diseases of the brain accompanied by marked disturbances of speech are not excluded from investigation by these tests.

The use of monaural tests for the diagnosis of central lesions is preferable to the use of binaural tests, for they allow definite conclusions to be drawn from comparison of the results of measurements when the stimulus is applied to the right and left ears. With tests of this type some of the factors which have a marked effect on the results of the measurements can be equalized (or neutralized): the level of education, the intellectual state, or attention of the patient, as well as general cerebral symptoms such as drowsiness, ease of fatigue, and so on.

In the investigation described above the use of acoustic stimuli of different durations for the investigation of hearing has been examined as a possible method for use in the diagnosis of temporal lesions. This method fully satisfies the requirements examined above, for it is a tonal monaural threshold test.

The results show that destruction of the superior temporal subregion, or even of the entire temporal lobe, by a pathological process or its surgical removal does not significantly raise the thresholds of detection of stationary acoustic stimuli. Audiometric tests, as Fig. 5 shows, revealed a very slight impairment of hearing at a frequency of 1000 Hz by 5-10 dB in most patients by comparison with measurements made on healthy subjects.* Meanwhile, in all these patients the thresholds of intensity of acoustic stimuli under 10 msec in duration were found to be increased when measured in the ear contralateral to the affected temporal lobe. No such increase in the thresholds of detection of short acoustic stimuli could be found in patients with lesions in the basal and polar zones of the temporal lobe, in other parts of the cerebral hemispheres, or in the brain stem.

*Elevation of the threshold by 5-10 dB was also observed in other patients with tumors in the basal and polar zones of the temporal lobe and also in other zones of the cerebral hemispheres.

As a result of the increase in the thresholds of audibility of short acoustic stimuli and the absence of changes in long acoustic stimuli in patients with pathological foci in the superior temporal zone, the duration effect is considerably greater than that measured in healthy subjects or in patients with lesions elsewhere. These results, obtained in the investigations just described, confirm those obtained by Baru, Gershuni, and Tonkonogii (1964), who found an increase in the thresholds of detection of short acoustic stimuli in patients with local lesions of the temporal cortex of vascular origin. However, the authors cited investigated predominantly patients with lesions in the left temporal lobe. It was not clear whether the defect of detection of short acoustic stimuli was connected with hemispheric dominance. In the present investigation, an increase in the thresholds of detection of short acoustic stimuli was found in all 37 patients with lesions of the superior zone of the temporal lobe tested, regardless of the fact that in 17 patients the lesion was in the nondominant hemisphere (in the right hemisphere of 15 right-handed patients and the left hemisphere of 2 left-handed patients), while in the remaining 20 (right-handed) patients it was in the left temporal lobe, i.e., in the dominant hemisphere. The increase in threshold intensities was independent of whether the lesion was in the dominant or nondominent hemisphere.

In the patients K-ov and S-ev, with lesions in the temporal lobe of the right (nondominant) and left (dominant) hemisphere respectively, resulting from removal of about equal volumes of brain tissue invaded by a tumor of the temporal lobe, an increase of identical magnitude in the threshold intensities of short acoustic stimuli was observed after the operation. In these patients the threshold intensities of series of tones at 100 Hz and 4, 5, 2, and 1 msec in duration, when measured in the ear contralateral to the side of the operation, were 16-17 dB higher than the corresponding values measured in the ear homolateral to the side of the operation. Consequently, the results of this investigation afford convincing evidence that the thresholds of detection of short acoustic stimuli are raised equally by lesions of the superior zones of the temporal lobe of the dominant and nondominant hemispheres.

One problem which arose was to determine the role of particular brain structures in the perception of acoustic stimuli of different durations. An investigation of the threshold intensities of acoustic stimuli of different durations detectable by patients with local lesions of the auditory system at different levels (cortex, inferior colliculi and lateral lemniscus, cochlear nuclei, receptors of the cochlea, sound-conducting system of the middle ear) showed an increase in the thresholds of detection of short acoustic stimuli only in patients with lesions of the superior temporal zone, in whom the thresholds of detection of long acoustic stimuli remain unaffected, so that the duration effect in these patients is increased.*

The duration effect measured in the ear contralateral to the lesion in patients with a pathological focus in the temporal lobe was considerably higher than the duration effect measured in healthy subjects.

In patients with lesions of the auditory system at other levels (inferior colliculi and lateral lemniscus, cochlear nuclei, receptor system of the cochlea) the duration effect was much smaller than in healthy subjects. The results of tests on patients with lesions of the auditory system at its various levels are given in Fig. 19. They also show that the magnitude of the duration effect is independent of the impairment of hearing, for in patients with greatly reduced hearing as the result of disease or injury to the receptor and nervous apparatus of the cochlea, the duration effect was 10-14 dB, while in patients with equal or even greater impairment of hearing as the result of injury to the sound-conducting system of the middle ear the duration effect was indistinguishable from that measured in healthy subjects.

The degree of increased threshold intensities of short acoustic stimuli depended on the location of the pathological focus and the volume of affected brain tissue. The most important factor was integrity of the central auditory pathway and cortical projection area. In patient B-ov, for example, a disturbance of the thresholds of detection of short stimuli applied to the left ear was found, indicating a local lesion of the auditory cortex in the right hemisphere. Macroscopic examination of the brain at autopsy gave the impression that the principal tumor nodule was located in the parietal lobe at a considerable distance from the auditory cortex.

*As already mentioned, the duration effect is the term applied to the difference between threshold intensities of acoustic stimuli 1200 msec and 1 msec in duration.

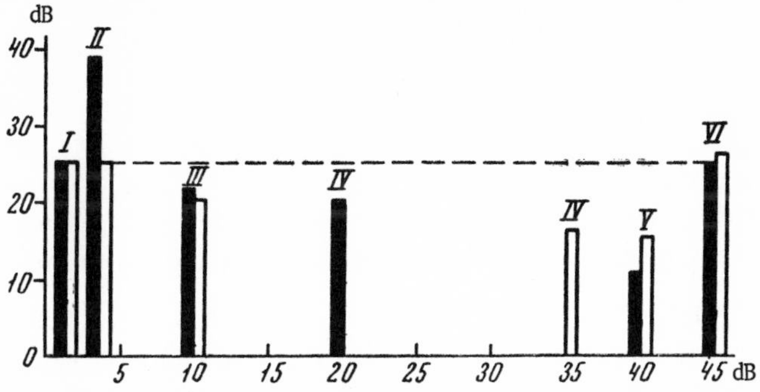

Fig. 19. Effect of duration of series of tones at 1000 Hz, 1200 and 1.2 msec in duration, in healthy subjects and patients with lesions of the auditory system at various levels, in relation to degree of impairment of hearing in dB, obtained from the results of audiometric tests: I) healthy subjects; II) patients with lesions of the auditory cortex; III) patient with lesion of the inferior colliculi and lateral lemniscus; IV) patient with lesion of the cochlear nuclei; V) patient with lesion of the receptor system of the cochlea; VI) patient with disturbance of sound conduction. Abscissa, degree of impairment of hearing, in dB; ordinate, difference between threshold intensities, in dB. Unshaded column represents results of measurement on the side of the lesion, shaded column — on the side contralateral to the lesion.

Microscopic study of a series of brain sections showed considerable pathological changes in the cortex of Heschl's gyrus and the central auditory pathway and secondary degeneration of cells in the medial geniculate body.

By contrast to this, no increase in threshold intensities of long or short acoustic stimuli was found in patient K-ii. At autopsy the whole of the central part of the temporal lobe was found to be occupied by a large hydatid cyst, and it could be assumed that the central auditory pathway was involved in the pathological process. A microscopic study of a series of brain sections showed that cells of the auditory cortex and medial geniculate body remained completely intact.

It can be concluded from a comparison of these results that the disturbance of perception of short acoustic stimuli is associated with a lesion of the auditory cortex and central auditory pathway. The increase in threshold intensities of short acoustic stimuli was more marked in patients with intracerebral lesions than in those in whom the brain tissue was damaged by a pathological process arising from extracerebral structures (the meninges or blood vessels, for example).

The greater disturbance of functions resulting from an intracerebral pathological process can evidently be explained by the topographical features of the auditory cortex and its connections.

Pathways to the auditory cortex run in a narrow bundle in the isthmus of the temporal lobe, and their arrangement is also compact in the white matter of the temporal lobe. Even a small focus in the white matter of the superior or middle temporal gyrus can thus simultaneously disturb the functional state of a large number of fibers.

Extracerebral tumors can cause disturbance of the functions of the auditory cortex on the lateral surface of the temporal lobe, either by compressing the superior temporal gyrus or, if they are located in the Sylvian fissure, by compressing mainly the transverse gyri. Simultaneous damage to the whole of the auditory cortex by an extracerebral tumor is thus unlikely.

The slight severity of the defect before operation for extracerebral tumors can also be explained by the fact that these tumors cause little disturbance to the blood supply of the subjacent cortex, for although they grow around the blood vessels they rarely obliterate them completely (Arutyunova, 1959).

The increase in threshold intensities of acoustic stimuli discovered in this investigation is reasonably stable. In 3 patients with intracerebral lesions resulting from a penetrating wound of the left superior temporal region, investigated 20-24 h after wounding and 14-18 years after operation for the excision of scars affecting the meninges and brain tissues, the increase in threshold to short acoustic stimuli on the side contralateral to the injury was 6-9 dB compared with the results of measurements in the ear homolateral to the pathological focus.

The results of tests on a series of patients with considerable impairment of hearing as the result of previous diseases of the middle ear and also on patients with lesions of the nervous apparatus of the cochlea show that lesions of the peripheral portions of the auditory system do not prevent the appearance of an increase in threshold intensities of short stimuli, which is a characteristic phenomenon of lesions of the superior and middle zones of the temporal lobe.

An increase in the threshold intensities of acoustic stimuli under 10 msec in duration when measured in the ear contralateral to a temporal lesion was thus recorded surprisingly constantly in all patients with lesions of either the right or the left temporal lobe tested. The precise nature of the results and their stability over a period of time, the relative simplicity of the measurements, and the possibility of detecting a pathological process in the temporal cortex even against the background of diseases of the peripheral portion of the auditory system are features such that the method of testing hearing by the use of acoustic stimuli of different duration can be recommended for the diagnosis of a pathological focus in the superior temporal subregion in either the left or the right hemisphere.

The increase in differential thresholds of intensity with a decrease in duration of acoustic stimuli observed recently in patients with lesions of the superior zones of the temporal lobe (Baru and Vasserman, 1968), indicate that the perception of short acoustic stimuli is disturbed not only at threshold, but also at suprathreshold levels.

Similar results have been obtained in model experiments on animals. For example, after extensive ablation of the temporal cortex in dogs (the superior zones of the anterior and posterior sylvian gyrus, anterior, middle, and posterior ectosylvian, and middle and posterior suprasylvian gyri – areas AI, AII, εP, IT, and SS, and in some animals AIII and AIV also), or simply of area AI, an increase in the thresholds of detection of acoustic stimuli shorter than 10-16 msec is observed.

An increase in the differential thresholds of frequency and intensity of short acoustic stimuli has also been found after extensive ablation of the auditory cortex.

The similarity between the results of investigations on patients with destruction of the temporal cortex by a pathological process or surgical ablation and the results of experimental studies on animals indicates that in the present writers' investigation the mechanism of analysis of acoustic stimuli which is common to both man and animals is injured.

Electrophysiological findings explain why the detection and discrimination of short acoustic stimuli are disturbed in lesions of the auditory cortex.

To begin with, the time scale within which the detection of short acoustic stimuli is disturbed in lesions of the auditory cortex coincides with the critical summation time calculated from the thresholds of evoked responses recorded from the auditory area (Gershuni, Gasanov, Zaboeva, and Lebedinskii, 1964; Gershuni, Shevelev, and Likhnitskii, 1964).

The present investigation also showed that the initial time of action of the stimulus is recorded in the primary response.

Electrophysiological studies (Gershuni, 1967; Radionova, 1967; Marueseva, 1967) revealed two types of responses to acoustic stimuli, differing in a number of very important features, at different levels of the auditory system. On the whole, it can be considered that the responses of one type are produced by a system working with a low time constant (fast-summating, phasic neurons), while those of the other type are produced by a system with high time constant (slowly summating tonic neurons). The role of the fast and slow neurons in the transmission of information in the auditory system has been examined by Gershuni (1967). He suggests that information on short acoustic stimuli or on the initial portion of a long stimulus, within the range of 10-20 msec, can be transmitted by fast neurons or by the initial short-latency spikes of slow neurons. These flows of information evidently converge on neurons of the auditory cortex whose initial response develops during the first 10-20 msec after the beginning of action of the acoustic stimulus. If these neurons of the auditory cortex with whose activity the primary response of the auditory area is connected are injured, the cause of the disturbance of discrimination of short acoustic stimuli will be obvious.

Gershuni also assumes that fast neurons are associated at the periphery predominantly with the inner hair cells, whose particular sensitivity to the transitional qualities of the stimulus has been asserted by Neubert (1960).

A channel of transmission of information concerning the start of action of a stimulus and of transitional processes can thus be distinguished in the auditory system, in which it may play an essential role in stimulus segmentation. The differentiation of the beginning of a stimulus is also very important in all operations requiring the counting of time. Furthermore, the ability of some neurons of the auditory cortex to generate prolonged afterdischarges when the action of short acoustic stimuli has ceased is regarded as one mechanism of short-term memory. Gershuni (1963, 1966) has put forward a hypothesis to explain the mode of operation of the mechanism for distinguishing short acoustic stimuli involving the use of "reproduction" phenomena (short-term memory).

As a result of the activity of this "reproducing" mechanism, a slowly responding discriminatory system is formed which is capable of prolonging the effect of a short stimulus to the necessary values.

Injury to cells of the auditory cortex must naturally also disturb the activity of neurons analyzing information about a stimulus during the short period of time after its application and it must disturb the mechanism of short-term memory essential to the discrimination of short stimuli.

It is thus neither the complexity nor the simplicity of an acoustic stimulus which predetermines the role of the auditory cortex in its identification, but the character of those operations of information analysis which must be carried out to distinguish and identify the useful features of the stimulus. If the useful features require the selection of information originating from segments with marked transitional phenomena, discrimination of the stimulus will be disturbed, regardless of its simplicity or complexity, in lesions of the auditory cortex.

It can be concluded from the results of electrophysiological and behavioral investigations that auditory cortical projection is not just the spatial, but also the temporal projection of the process taking place on the receptor surface of the cochlea.

The method of investigating auditory thresholds as a function of stimulus duration is an essential part of the analysis of auditory cortical function because it enables disturbances of the temporo-spatial organization of the auditory function to be detected.

Bibliography

Ageeva-Maikova, O. G., and Sviridova, A. E., 1951, "The topical importance of disturbances of binaural hearing after head injuries," in: Problems in Neurosurgery, Moscow, Medgiz, pp. 68-73.

Alajouanine, T., Aubry, M., and Pialoux, P., 1955, "Note préliminaire sur l'atteinte auditive dans l'aphasie," in: Les Grandes Activités du Lobe Temporal, Paris, pp. 203-210.

Alekseenko, N. Yu., Blinkov, S. M., Gershuni, G. V., Klaas, Yu. A., and Maruseva, A. M., 1948, "Symptomatology of injury to the temporoparieto-occipital region (Brodmann's Area 37) and the anterior zone of the inferior parietal region (Brodmann's Area 40)," Zh. Nevropat. i Psikhiat., No. 17, pp. 9-13.

Alekseenko, N. Yu., Blinkov, S. M. and Gershuni, G. V., 1949, "Disturbance of perception of the direction of sound as a symptom of a local lesion of the human brain," Problems in Physiological Acoustics, No. 1, Moscow–Leningrad, Izd. AN SSSR, p. 43.

Allen, W. F., 1945, "Effect of destroying 3 localized cerebral cortical areas for sound on correct conditioned differential responses of the dog's foreleg," Amer. J. Physiol., 144:415-428.

Appaix, A., Roche, R., Pech, A., Henin, J., and Aymard, J., 1957, "L'otologiste devant les affections de l'angle pontocérébelleux," Soc. d'Oto-Rhino-Laryngol., No. 6, pp. 77-99.

Arnold, G., 1946, "Thalamische Hörstörung mit Paramusie nach Fleckfieber," Mschr. f. Ohrenheilk., 79/80:11-27.

Arnold, G., 1951, "Die Untersuchung zentraler Hörstörungen mit neuen Hörprüfungsmethoden," Arch. Ohr. Heilk und Z. Hals. Heilk., No. 157, pp. 521-542.

Arutyunova, A. S., 1954, The Superior Temporal Gyrus and Medial Geniculate Body in Man, Candidate's Dissertation, Moscow, Acad. Med. Sci. USSR.

Arutyunova, A. S., 1959, "Changes in brain tissue in arachnoid-endotheliomas receiving an additional blood supply from the pial arteries," in: Current Problems in Neurosurgery, Moscow, Medgiz, pp. 363-378.

Avakyan, R. V., Baru, A. V. Gershuni, G. V., and Tonkonogii, I. M., 1963, "The role of higher levels of the auditory system in the detection and discrimination of acoustic stimuli," Abstracts of Proceedings of the 20th Conference on Problems in Higher Nervous Activity, Moscow–Leningrad, Izd. AN SSSR, p. 6.

Babenkova, S. V. 1954, "Features distinguishing the interaction between central brain systems during recovery of speech in various forms of aphasia," Abstracts of Proceedings of the 7th Session of the Institute of Neurology, Moscow, Izd. AMN SSSR.

Babkin, B. P., 1911, "Further investigations of the normal and injured central auditory system of the dog," Trudy Obshchestva Russkikh Vrachei (SPb), No. 77, pp. 249-288.

Baru, A. V., 1964, "Role of the cerebral cortex in the detection of acoustic stimuli of different duration," Abstracts of Proceedings of the 10th Congress of the All-Union Physiological Society, No. 2, Moscow—Leningrad, Nauka, pp. 79-80.

Baru, A. V., 1966, "Role of the temporal cortex in the detection of acoustic stimuli of different duration," Zh. Vyssh. Nervn. Deyat., No. 16, pp. 655-665.

Baru, A. V., 1967a, "Effect of some pharmacological agents on the detection of acoustic stimuli of different duration," Zh. Vyssh. Nervn. Deyat., No. 17, pp. 107-115.

Baru, A. V., 1967b, "Differential thresholds of frequency in relation to duration of tonal series in animals after ablation of the auditory cortex," in: Mechanisms of Hearing, Leningrad, Nauka, pp. 121-135.

Baru, A. V., Gershuni, G. V., and Tonkonogii, I. M., 1964, "The importance of detection of acoustic stimuli of different duration in the diagnosis of temporal brain lesions," Zh. Nevropat. i Psikhiat., 64(4):481:485.

Baru, A. V., and Vasserman, L. I., 1968, "Discrimination of the intensity of acoustic stimuli of different duration by patients with local lesions of the temporal lobe," Abstracts of Proceedings of the 3rd All-Union Congress of the Society of Psychologists, Kiev.

Bein, É. S. 1948, The Psychological Analysis of Temporal Aphasia, Candidate's Dissertation, Moscow, Akad. Med. Sci. USSR.

Bein, É. S. 1964, Aphasia and Ways of Overcoming It, Leningrad, Meditsina.

Bekhterev, V. M., 1905, Fundamentals in the Science of Brain Function [in Russian], No. 5, St. Petersburg, pp. 407-460.

Bekhterev, V. M., 1907, Fundamentals in the Sciences of Brain Function, No. 7, pp. 1264-1317.

Belenkov, N. Yu., 1965, The Conditioned Reflex and Subcortical Brain Structures, Moscow, Meditsina.

Bender, M. B., and Diamond, S. P., 1965, "An analysis of auditory perceptual defects with observations on the localization of disfunction," Brain, 88:675-685.

Bittrich, K., 1956, "Otologisches bei Hirntumoren im Kindes und Jugendlichen Alter," Z. Laryng., 36:287-298.

Blagoveshchenskaya, N. S., 1962, The Topical Importance of Disturbances of Hearing, Vestibular Function, Olfaction, and Taste in Brain Lesions, Moscow, Medgiz.

Blagoveshchenskaya, N. S., 1965, Otoneurological Symptoms in the Clinical Picture of Brain Tumors, Moscow, Medgiz, p. 255.

Blinkov, S. M., 1955, Structural Features of the Human Brain, Moscow, Medgiz.

Blinkov, S. M., and Brazovskaya, F. A., 1957, Current Problems in Neurosurgery, No. 1, Moscow, Medgiz, p. 41.

Blinkov, S. M., and Zvorykin, V. P., 1950, "Size of the auditory cortex and medial geniculate body in man and monkeys," Dokl. Akad. Nauk SSSR, 74(1):123-126.

Bocca, E., 1951, "Interrupted masking as a differential test of auditory function." Acta Oto-Laryngol. (Stockholm), 39:452-463.

Bocca, E., 1961, "Factors influencing binaural integration of periodically switched messages," Acta Oto-Laryngol. (Stockholm), 53:142-144.

Bocca, E., and Calearo, C., 1963, "Central hearing processes," in: Modern Developments in Audiology, New York and London, pp. 337-370.

Bocca, E., Calearo, C., and Cassinari, V., 1954, "A new method for testing hearing in temporal lobe tumors (preliminary report)," Acta Oto-Laryngol. (Stockholm), 44:219-221.

Boiko, Z. S., 1966, "Changes in the differential threshold of perception of strength of acoustic stimuli in patients with sensory aphasia," in: Transactions of Leningrad Research Institute of Diseases of the Ear, Throat, Nose, and Speech, No. 14, Leningrad, p. 74.

Bozzi, R., 1929, "Contributo clinico e anatomopatologico allo studio dei tumori del lobo temporale," Rev. Ot. Nerv. Ment., 34:349.

Bremer, F., 1943, "Etude oscillographique des réponses sensorielles de l'aire acoustique corticale chez le chat." Arch. Internat. Physiol., pp. 53-103.

Bremer, F., and Dow, R. S., 1939, "The cerebral acoustic area of the cat. A combined oscillographic and cytoarchitectonic study," J. Neurophysiol., 2:308-318.

Broadbent, D. E., 1954, "The role of auditory localization in attention and memory span," J. Exp. Psychol., 47:191-196.

Broca, P., 1861, "Remarques sur le siège de la faculté du langage articulé," Bull. Soc. Anthropol. (Paris), No. 6.

Brower, B., cited by Bumke and Foerster, 1936.

Brunetti, F., 1961, "Modifications de l'adaptation auditive d'origine centrale par interférences sensorielles," Acta Oto-Laryngol. (Stockholm), 53:145-150.

Bumke, O., and Foerster, O., 1936, Handbuch der Neurologie, Berlin, pp. 459-482.

Butler, R. A., Diamond, J. T., and Neff, W. D., 1957, "Role of auditory cortex in discrimination of changes in frequency," J. Neurophysiol., 20:108-120.

Calearo, C., 1957, "Binaural summation in lessions of the temporal lobe," Acta Oto-Laryngol. (Stockholm), 47:392-395.

Calearo, C., and Antonelli, A. R., 1963, "Cortical hearing tests and cerebral dominance," Acta Oto-Laryngol., (Stockholm), 56:17-26.

Chocholle, R., 1957, "La sensibilité auditive différentielle d'intensité en présence d'un son contrelatéral de même fréquence," Acustica, 7:75-83.

Citron, L., Dix, M.R., Hallpike, C.S., and Hood, J.D. 1963, "A recent clinocopathological study of cochlear degeneration resulting from tumor pressure and disseminated sclerosis with particular reference to the finding of normal threshold sensitivity from pure tone," Acta Oto-Laryngol. (Stockholm), 56:330.

Clark, W., LeGros, E. and Russell, W. Ritchie, 1938, "Cortical deafness without aphasia," Brain, 61:375.

Crosby, E., Humphrey, T., and Lauer, W. E., 1962, Correlative Anatomy of the Nervous System, New York.

Cushing, H., 1921, "The field defects produced by temporal lobe lesions," Brain, 44:341-346.

Dandy, W. E., 1933, "Physiological studies following extirpation of the right cerebral hemisphere in man," Bull. Johns Hopkins Hosp., 53:31-51.
Dorofeeva, S. A., 1965, "Disturbances of auditory function and methods of restoring speech in sensory aphasias of vascular genesis," in: Rehabilitative Treatment and Social and Occupational Readaptation of Patients with Nervous and Mental Diseases, Leningrad, pp. 216-218.
Doughty, J. M., and Garner, W. R., 1947, "Pitch characteristics of short tones," J. Exp. Psychol., 37:351-365.
Efron, R., 1963, "Temporal perception, aphasia, and déjà vu," Brain, 86:403-423.
Elliott, L. L., 1963, "Tonal thresholds for short duration stimuli as related to subject hearing level," J. Acoust. Soc. Amer., 35:578-580.
El'yasson, M. N., 1908, Investigation of the Hearing Ability of Dogs Under Normal Conditions and After Partial Bilateral Extirpation of the Cortical Hearing Center, Candidate's Dissertation, St. Petersburg.
Feldmann, H., 1960, "Untersuchungen zur Discrimination differenter Schallbilder bei simultaner, monauraler und binauraler Darbeitung," Arch. Ohr. Heilk. und Z. Hals Heilk., 176:601-605.
Ferrier, D., 1876, The Function of the Brain, London.
Feuchtwanger, E., 1930, Amusie, Berlin.
Flechsig, P., 1920, Anatomie des menschlichen Gehirn und Rückenmarks auf myelogenetischer Grundlage, Leipzig.
Garner, W. R., 1947, "The effect of frequency spectrum on temporal integration of energy in the ear," J. Acoust. Soc. Amer., 19:808-810.
Gershuni, G. V., 1959, "Methods of Investigation of the Function of the Central Auditory System," in: Physiological Methods in Clinical Practice [in Russian], Leningrad, Medgiz, pp. 349-406.
Gershuni, G. V., 1963, "Evoked potentials and the mechanism of discrimination of an external stimulus," Zh. Vyssh. Nervn. Deyat., 13:882-890.
Gershuni, G. V., 1966, "The temporo-spatial organization of the auditory system," Proceedings of the 18th International Psychological Congress, Symposium 15, Moscow, Nauka, pp. 105-119-128.
Gershuni, G. V., 1967, "The mechanisms of hearing (in connection with investigation of temporal and temporal-frequency characteristics of the auditory system)," in: Mechanisms of Hearing, Leningrad, Nauka, pp. 3-32.
Gershuni, G. V., Shevelev, I. A., and Likhnitskii, A. M., 1964, "Dependence of the primary response of the cat auditory cortex on temporal parameters of the stimulus under waking conditions," Zh. Vyssh. Nervn. Deyat., 14:489.
Gershuni, G. V., Gasanov, U. G., Zaboeva, N. V., and Lebedinskii, M. M., 1964, "The electrical primary response of the cortical projection zone and temporal parameters of the external stimulus," Biofizika, 9:597.
Goldberg, J. M., and Neff, W. D., 1961, "Frequency discrimination after bilateral ablation of cortical auditory areas," J. Neurophysiol., 24:119.
Gol'din, S. Ya., 1951, Otoneurological Symptoms and Syndromes, Moscow, Medgiz.
Goldstein, K., 1948, Language and Language Disorders, New York, Grune and Stratton.
Goodman, A. C., 1957, "Some relations between auditory functions and intracranial lesions with particular reference to lesions of the cerebellopontine angle," Laryngoscope, 67:987-1010.

Grahe, K., 1932, Hirn und Ohr, Leipzig.

Greiner, G., Kantzer, L., and Rohmer, F., 1951, "Résultats de tests audiométriques nouveaux après ablation d'un lobe temporal," Rev. d'Oto-Neuro-Ophtalm., 23: 249-256.

Greiner, G., Rohmer, F., Mengus, M., and Eissen, F., 1957, "Surdité unilatérale avec recrutement accompagnant une lesion du tronc cérébral," Rev. d'Oto-Neuro-Ophtalm., 29:422-424.

Greiner, G., Rohmer, F., Mengus, M., and Isch, F., 1956, "Considérations sur les surdités et bulbi-protubérantielles," Rev. d'Oto-Neuro-Ophtalm., 28:391-396.

Grinberg, G. E., 1962, "Classification of lesions of the central acoustic system and their differential diagnosis," Zh. Ushn., Nos., i Gorl. Bol., 22(4):3.

Guild, S. R., 1932, "Correlations of histologic observations and the acuity of hearing," Acta Oto-Laryngol., 17:207-249.

Hansen, C. C., and Reske-Nielsen, A., 1963, "Cortical hearing loss in a patient with glioblastoma," Arch. Otolaryngol., 77:461-473.

Harris, J., Haines, H., and Myers, G., 1958, "Brief-time audiometry (temporal integration in the hypacuses)," Arch. Otolaryngol., 67:699-713.

Harris, J., Haines, H., and Myers, G., 1960, "The importance of hearing at 3 kc for understanding speeded speech," Laryngoscope, 70:131.

Harrison, J. M., and Irving, R., 1965, "The anterior ventral cochlear nucleus," Comp. Neurol., 124:15-42.

Harrison, J. M., and Warr, W. B., 1962, "A study of the cochlear nuclei and ascending auditory pathways of the medulla," Comp. Neurol., 119:3.

Head, H., 1926, Aphasia and Kindred Disorders of Speech, Cambridge, p. 2.

Heilbronner, K., 1910, "Die aphasischen, apraktischen und agnostischen Störungen," Handbuch der Neurologie, Berlin, pp. 982-1093.

Hennebert, D., 1955, "L'intégration de la perception auditive et de l'audition alternante," Acta Otol. Belg., 9:344-346.

Henschen, S. E., 1918, "Über Hörsphäre," J. Psychol. Neurol., 22:319-472.

Henschen, S. E., 1920, Klinische und anatomische Beiträge zur Pathologie des Gehirns, Part 5, Stockholm.

Hirsch, I. J., 1952, The Measurement of Hearing, New York.

Hornbostel, E. M., and Wertheimer, M., 1920, "Über die Wahrnehmung der Schallrichtung," Stizungsber. Preuss. Akad. der Wissenschaft. (Berlin), p. 388.

Jatho, K., 1954, "Beitrag zue audiometrischen Diagnostik der zentralen Hörstörung," Arch. Ohr. Heilk. Z. Hals. Heilk., 165:331-336.

Jerger, J., 1960a, Audiological Manifestations of Lesions in the Auditory Nervous System, Laryngoscope, 70:417-425.

Jerger, J., 1960b, "Observations on auditory behavior in lesions of the central auditory pathways," Arch. Oto-Laryngol., 71:797-806.

Jerger, J., 1964, "Auditory tests for disorders of the central auditory mechanism," in: Neurological Aspects of Auditory and Vestibular Disorders, Springfield, pp. 77-86.

Kabelyanskaya, L. G., 1957, "The state of the auditory system in sensory aphasia," Zh. Nevropat. Psikhiat. im. Korsakova, 57(6):712-716.

Kachuro, M. N., 1964, Frequency Localization in the Auditory Cortex and Medial Geniculate Body Under Conditions of Waking, Anesthesia, and Local Strychninization of the Cortex, Candidate's Dissertion.

Kaidanova, S. I., 1967, "Differentiation of pauses between components of rhythmic stimuli by children with sensory alalia," in: Physiological Mechanisms of Speech Disturbances, Leningrad, Nauka, pp. 54-62.

Kaidanova, S. I., and Meierson, Ya. A., 1961, "Activity of the central auditory system in aphasia," Zh. Vyssh. Nervn. Deyat., 11:602.

Kaidanova, S.I., Meierson, A. Ya., and Tonkonogii, I. M., 1965, "Disturbance of localization of sound in space in local brain lesions," Vestn. Otorinolaring., No. 2, pp. 39-42.

Kalinina, T. E., 1962, "Effect of ablation of the auditory and adjacent areas of the cortex on acoustic conditioned reflexes," Zh. Vyssh. Nervn. Deyat., 12:720-725.

Karaseva, T. A., 1966, "The role of the temporal cortex in detection of acoustic stimuli of short duration in man," Proceedings of the 18th International Psychological Congress, Symposium 15, Moscow, Nauka, pp. 142-147.

Karaseva, T. A., 1967, "Detection of acoustic stimuli fo short duration in local lesions of the temporal lobe," in: Mechanisms of Hearing, Leningrad, Nauka, pp. 135-143.

Khananashvili, M. M., 1965, "Differentiation of acoustic conditional stimuli by time of rise of intensity and the role of the temporal cortex in this function," Zh. Vyssh. Nervn. Deyat., No. 15, p. 5.

Kimura, D., 1961a, "Some effects of temporal lobe damage on auditory perception," Canad. J. Psychol., 15:156-165.

Kimura, D., 1961b, "Cerebral dominance and the perception of verbal stimuli," Canad. J. Psychol., 15:166-171.

Kimura, D., 1963, "Right temporal-lobe damage," Arch. Neurol. (Chicago), 8:264.

Kimura, D., 1964, "Left-right differences in the perception of melodies," Quart J. Exp. Psychol., 16:355-358.

Kishonas, A. P., 1966, "The use of short acoustic stimuli (the duration effect under normal and pathological conditions)," Vestn. Otorinolaring., No. 2, pp. 25-29.

Kishonas, A. P., 1967, "Relationship between threshold of audibility and duration of acoustic stimuli in diseases of the organ of hearing," in: Mechanisms of Hearing, Leningrad, Nauka, pp. 144-150.

Kleist, K., 1934, "Kriegsverletzungen des Gehirns in ihrer Bedeutung für die Hirnlokalisation und Hirnpathologie," in: Geistes und Nervenkrankheiten, No. 5, Leipzig, pp. 643, 645, and 797.

Kolodny, A., 1928, "Symptomatology of tumors of the temporal lobe," Brain, 51:385.

Kornyanskii, G. P., 1950, "Clinical syndromes of tumors of the floor of the fourth ventricle," Voprosy Neirokhir., No. 1, pp. 34-35.

Korst, L. O., and Fantalova, V. L., 1959, "Characteristics of disorders of some cortical functions in patients with tumors of the temporal and occipital lobes of the brain," in: Current Problems in Neurosurgery, No. 3, Moscow, Medgiz, pp. 153-164.

Krassing, M., 1950, "Das klinische Bild der Hirnstammschwerhörigkeit," Arch. Ohr. Heilk. Z. Hals. Heilk., 158:449-453.

Krol', N. M., 1946, "Acoustic allesthesia and acoustic disorientation with reversal of acoustic perception through 180°: a syndrome of right temporal lobe lesions," in: Transactions of Evacuation Hospitals of Voronezh Military District, Moscow, Medgiz, pp. 204-209.

Kryshova, N. A., and Shteingart, K. M. 19--, "A study of the activity of the articulatory system in aphasia," Scientific report of the I. P. Pavlov Institute of Physiology, Academy of Sciences of the USSR, Leningrad, Nauka, pp. 72-75.

Kryter, K. D., and Ades, H. W., 1943, "Studies of the function of the higher acoustic nervious centers in the cat," Amer. J. Psychol., 56:501-536.

Kryzhanovskii, N. N., 1909, Conditioned Acoustic Reflexes After Ablation of the Temporal Areas of the Brain in Dogs, Candidate's Dissertation, St. Petersburg.

Ladyzhenskaya, E. A., 1960, "Hearing disorders and deafness in midbrain lesions," Vestn. Otorinolaring., 22:240-247.

Larsell, O., 1951, Anatomy of the Nervous System, New York.

Lebedev, A. P., 1966, "An electronic switch with a low intereference level permitting smooth phase regulation," Zh. Vyssh. Nervn. Deyat., 16:742-748.

Lebedinskii, M. S., 1941, Aphasia, Agnosia, and Apraxia, Khar'kov.

Lemoyne, J., and Mahoudea, D., 1959, "A propos d'un cas d'agnosie auditive pure avec surdité corticale associée avec une dysphonie fonctionelle. Observation anatomoclinique," Ann. Oto-Laryngol., 76:293-310.

Levin, G. Z., 1959, "Basic features of evolution of the medial geniculate body," Arkh. Anat. Gistol. i Embriol., No. 6, pp. 23-32.

Levin, G. Z., 1961, "Evolution of the inferior colliculi," Arkh. Anat. Gistol. i Émbriol., 47:21-27.

Lhermitte, J., 1937, Système Nerveux Central, Paris, p. 422.

Linden, A., 1960, Talaudiometri med Frekvensdistorsion och Binauralt Hörselsyntesprov, Göteborg.

Linden, A., 1964, "Distorted speech and binaural speech resynthesis tests," Acta Oto-Laryngol., 58:32-47.

Lorente de Nô, R., 1933, "Anatomy of the 8th Nerve. General plan of structure of the primary cochlear nuclei," Laryngoscope, 43:327-350.

Luciani and Sepilli, 1866, Cited by Bekhterev, V. M., 1905-1907.

Luria, A. R., 1947, Traumatic Aphasia, Moscow, Izd. AMN SSSR.

Luria, A. R., 1952, "Fundamental clinical problems of local brain lesions in the light of I. P. Pavlov's ideas," Zh. Vyssh. Nervn. Deyat., 2:668-690.

Luria, A. R., 1962, Higher Cortical Functions in Man, Moscow University Press, Moscow. English translation, New York, 1966.

Luria, A. R., 1967, "Factor and forms of aphasia," in: Physiological Mechanisms of Speech Disturbances, Leningrad, Nauka, pp. 109-123.

Luria, A. R., Tsvetkova, L. S., and Futer, D. S., 1968, "Aphasia in a composer," in: Problems in Dynamic Localization of Brain Functions, Moscow, Meditsina, p. 328.

Marie, P., 1906, "Revision de la question de l'aphasie," Semaine Médicale.

Maruseva, A. M., 1967, "Temporal characteristics of neurons of the inferior colliculi in rats with different types of response to acoustic stimuli," in: Mechanisms of Hearing, Leningrad, Nauka, pp. 50-62.

Maspétiol, R., Semette, D., and Mathieu, C., 1960, "Introduction à l'étude des troubles auditifs corticaux," Ann. Oto-Laryngol. (Paris), 77:287-295.

Massopust, L. C., Wolin, L. R., Jr., Meder, R., and Frost, V., 1967, "Changes in auditory frequency discrimination thresholds after temporal cortex ablation," Exp. Neurol., 19:245.

Matzker, J., 1957, "Ein neuer Weg zur otologischen Diagnostik cerebraler Erkrankungen," Z. Laryngol., 36:177-189.

Matzker, J., 1958, Ein binauraler Hörsynthese-Test zum Nachweis zerebraler Hörstörungen, Stuttgart.

Matzker, J., 1959, "Two new methods for the assessment of central auditory function in cases of brain disease," Ann. Otol. (St. Louis), 68:1185-1197.

Matzker, J., 1965, "Die zentralen Hörstörungen und ihre Diagnostik," Studium Generale, 11:682-700.

Mering, T. A., 1952, "Conditioned reflexes in dogs after ablation of the auditory cortex," Zh. Vyssh. Nervn. Deyat., 2:894.

Mering, T. A., 1962, "Morpho-physiological investigation of conditioning to acoustic stimuli," in: Structure and Function of the Nervous System, Moscow, Medgiz, pp. 178-185.

Meyer, D. R., and Woolsey, C. N., 1952, "Effects of localized cortical destruction on auditory discriminative conditioning in cat," J. Neurophysiol., 15:149-162.

Milner, B., 1962, "Laterality effects in audition," in: Interhemispheric Relations and Cerebral Dominance, Baltimore, pp. 177-195.

Milner, B., 1967, "Brain mechanisms suggested by studies of temporal lobes," in: Brain Mechanisms Underlying Speech and Language, Baltimore, pp. 122-145.

Misch. W., 1928, "Über corticale Taubheit," Z. Ges. Neurol. Psychiat., 115:567-573.

Miscolczy-Fodor, F., 1953, "Monaural loudness-balance test and determination of recruitment degree with short sound impulses," Acta Oto-Laryngol. (Stockholm), 43:573-595.

Monakow, C. von, 1914, Die Lokalisation im Grosshirn und der Abbau der Funktion durch corticale Herde, Wiesbaden.

Morrell, F., 1935, "L'audition dans l'aphasie sensorielle," Encephale, 2:533-553.

Morest, D. K., 1964, "The neuronal architecture of the medial geniculate body of the cat," J. Anat. (London), 98:611-630.

Morest, D. K., 1965, "The laminar structure of the medial geniculate body of the cat," J. Anat. (London), 99:143-160.

Mosidze, V. M. 1965, Role of the Auditory Cortex in Conditioned-reflex Activity [in Russian], Tbilisi.

Mounier-Kuhn, P., and Lafon, J., 1962, "De quelques particularités phonétiques de l'audition de la parole," Acta Oto-Laryngol. (Stockholm), 53:155-167.

Munk, H., 1881, Über die Funktionen der Grosshirnrinde, Berlin.

Neff, W. D., 1961, "Neural mechanisms of auditory discrimination," in: Sensory Communication, New York, pp. 259-278.

Neubert, K., 1960, "Innere Haarzellen des cortischen Organs und Schallanalyse," Naturwissenschaften, 47:526.

Nielsen, J. M., 1946, "Agnosia, apraxia, aphasia. Their value in cerebral localization," in: Clinical Neurology, Vol. 1, New York.

Nielsen, J. W., and Sult, C. W., 1939, "Agnosias and body schema," Bull. Los Angeles Neurol. Sco., 4:69.

Norlund, B., 1962, "Angular localization, a clinical test for investigation of ability to localize airborne sound," Acta Oto-Laryngol. (Stockholm), 55:405-423.

Orfinskaya, V. K., 1958, "Classification of the forms of aphasia and principles of speech therapy with aphasics," Proceedings of the Leningrad Zonal Psychological Conference, Leningrad, pp. 85-86.

Peele, T. L., 1954, The Neuroanatomical Basis for Clinical Neurology, New York.

Penfield, W., and Erickson, T. C., 1945, Epilepsy and Cerebral Localization, Springfield.

Penfield, W., and Roberts, L., 1959, Speech and Brain Mechanisms, Princeton, New Jersey.

Pfaltz, R., 1963, Cited by Matzker, J., 1965.

Pfeifer, R. A., 1936, "Pathologie der Hörstrahlung und der corticalen Hörsphäre," in: Bumke, O., and Foerster, O. (Editors), 1936.

Philippides, M., and Greiner, G., 1950, "Troubles cochléares après ablation du lobe temporal gauche," Rev. Oto-Neuro-Ophtalm., 22:19-22.

Pialoux, P., 1962, Cited by Bocca, E., and Calearo, C., 1963.

Plomp, R., and Bouman, M. A., 1959, "Relation between hearing thresholds and duration of tone pulses," J. Acoust. Soc. Amer., 31:749-758.

Poljak, U. S., 1932, The Main Afferent Fiber Systems of the Cerebral Cortex in Primates, California.

Popov, N. A., 1959, "The clinical picture of temporal lobe tumors (difficulties and methods of diagnosis)," Voprosy Neirokhir., No. 5, pp. 38-43.

Pötzl, O., 1946a, "Die Pathophysiologie der thalamisch bedingten Hörstörung," Mschr. f. Ohrenheilk., 79/80:28-38.

Pötzl, O., 1946b, "Weiteres über die zerebralen Störungen der Tonperzeption," Mschr. f. Ohrenheilk., 79/80:471-481.

Quist-Hanssen, S., and Strömsnes, A., 1960, "Speech audiometry in persons with brain damage," Acta Oto-Laryngol. (Stockholm), 51:272-278.

Raab, D. H. and Ades, H. W., 1946, "Cortical and midbrain mediation of a conditioned discrimination of acoustic intensities," Amer. J. Psychol., 59:59-83.

Rabending, G., 1959, "Sprachtaubheit und acustischer Funktions Wandel," Arch. Psychiat. Nervenkrank., 198:633-642.

Radionova, E. A., 1967, "The role of temporal characteristics of unit responses in the cochlear nucleus to acoustic stimuli," in: Mechanisms of Hearing, Leningrad, Nauka, pp. 32-50.

Ramon y Cajal, S., 1909, Histologie du Système Nerveux de l'Homme et des Vertébrés, Paris.

Ranson, S. W., and Clark, S. L., 1959, The Anatomy of the Nervous System, Philadelphia, p. 371.

Rapoport, M. Yu., 1948, The Neurological Diagnosis of Temporal Lobe Tumors, Moscow, Medgiz.

Rasmussen, G. L., 1964, "Anatomical relationships of the ascending and descending auditory systems," in: Neurological Aspects of Auditory and Vestibular Disorders, Springfield, pp. 5-23.

Ratnikova, G. I., 1967, "The structure of the cochlear nuclei in the cat," in: Mechanisms of Hearing, Leningrad, Nauka, pp. 182-195.

Richter, 1957, Cited by Rabending, G., 1959.

Rosenzweig, M. R., 1946, "Discrimination of auditory intensities in the cat," Amer. J. Psychol., 59:127-136.

Rosenzweig, M. R., 1951, "Representation of the two ears at the auditory cortex," Amer. J. Physiol., 167:147-158.

Sa, G. de, 1958, "Audiologic findings in central nerve deafness," Laryngoscope, 68:308.

Saltzman, M., 1952, "Audiometric studies following mesencephalotomy and thalamotomy," Z. Hals.-Nas.-Ohrenheilk., 46:368.

Sanchez-Longo, L. P., and Forster, T. M., 1958, "Clinical significance of impairment of sound localization," Neurology, 8:119-126.

Sanchez-Longo, L. P., Forster, T. M., and Auth, T. L., 1957, "A clinical test for sound localization and its application," Neurology, 7:655-663.

Santos, P. S., and Corrée, A., 1957, "Fonction cochléo-vestibulaire après hémisphérectomie," Rev. Oto-Neuro-Ophtalm., 29:257-266.

Schubert, K., and Panse, F., 1953, "Audiologische Befunde bei sensorischer Aphasie," Arch. Ohr.-, Nas., Kehlk. Heilk., 164:23-40.

Sedlaček, K., 1960, "A new method for examination of principal factors of directional hearing in clinical praxis," Csl. Otolaryngol., 9:324-332.

Semernitskaya, S. M., 1945, Rhythm and Its Disturbance in Various Brain Lesions, Candidate's Dissertation, Moscow.

Schankweiler, D. P., 1961, 'Performance of brain-damage in patients on two test of sound localization," J. Comp. Physiol. Psychol., 54:375-381.

Schankweiler, D. P., 1966, "Effects of temporal-lobe damage on perception of dichotically presented melodies," J. Comp. Physiol. Psychol., 62:115-119.

Shileiko, Z. I., 1940, "Changes in hearing and in labyrinthine and olfactory function in temporal lobe tumors," Voprosy Neirokhir., No. 4, pp. 68-79.

Shmar'yan, A. S., 1937, "Auditory psychosensory disorders in temporal lobe lesions," Zh. Nevropat. i Psikhiat. im Korsakova, No. 6, p. 110-124.

Shmar'yan, A. S., 1949, Brain Pathology and Psychiatry, Moscow, Medgiz.

Shmidt, E. V., and Sukhovskaya, I. A., 1954, "The pathophysiology of sensory aphasia," Zh. Nevropat. i Psikhiat. im. Korsakova, 54:987.

Sinha, Cited by Milner, B., 1962.

Sosenkov, V. A., 1963, "Preservation of conditioned reflexes in cats after removal of the cerebral cortex," in: Proceedings of the 20th Conferences on Problems in Higher Nervous Activity, Leningrad, Izd. AN SSSR, p. 224.

Sparks, R., and Geschwind, N., 1968, "Dichotic listening in man after section of neurocortical commissures," Cortex, 4:3-16.

Spirin, B. G., Fantalova, V. L., and Filippycheva, N. A., 1955, "Investigation of the inertia of trace processes in the auditory system in patients with local brain lesions," Annotations of Scientific Works of the Academy of Medical Sciences of the USSR, Moscow, pp. 325-326.

Spoendlin, H., 1968, "Ultrastructure and peripheral inervation pattern of the receptor in relation to the first coding of the acoustic message," Ciba Foundation Symposium of Hearing in Vertebrates, London, pp. 89-119.

Spreen, O., Benton, A. L., and Fincham, R. W., 1965, "Auditory agnosia without aphasia," Arch. Neurol., 13:84-92.

Stockert, F. C., 1951, "Ein Fall von thalamischer Hörstörung," Arch. Psychiat. Neurol., 187:45-68.

Stockert, F. C., 1954, "Zentrale Hörstörungen," Fortschr. Neurol. Psychiat., 22:457-472.

Stockert, F. C., and Fresser, E., 1954, "Melodientaubheit bei akustischen Funktionswandel," Arch. Psychol. Z. Neurol., 192:174-184.

Stolyarova-Kabelyanskaya, L. G., 1961, "Clinical and pathophysiological differences between cortical and transcortical aphasia," in: Clinical and Pathophysiological Problems in Aphasia, Moscow, Medgiz, p. 24.

Street, B. C., 1957, "Hearing loss in aphasia," J. Speech Hearing Disord., 22:60-67.

Stroughton, G. S., and Neff, W. D., 1950, "Function of auditory cortex: the effects of one-stage versus two-stage ablation," Amer. Psychol., 5:747.

Swischer, L.P., 1967, "Auditory intensity discrimination in patients with temporal-lobe damage," Cortex, 2:179-193.

Sychowa, B., 1962, "Medial geniculate body of the dog," Comp. Neurol., 118:3.

Tato, J., and de Quiros, J. J., 1960, "Die sensibilisierte Sprachaudiometrie," Acta Oto-Laryngol. (Stockholm), 51:593-614.

Terr, M. A., Goetzinger, C. P., and Rousey, C. L., 1958, "A study of hearing acuity in adult aphasic and cerebral palsied subjects," Arch. Oto-Laryngol., 67:447.

Teuber, H. L., and Diamond, S., 1956, "Effects of brain injury in man on binaural localization of sounds," Cited by Milner, B., 1962.

Thiebaut, F., Greiner, G. F., and Mengus, M., 1956, "Lésions des voies auditives centrales s'accompagnant de recruitment," Ann. Oto-Laryngol. (Paris), 73:257-261.

Thompson, R. F., 1960, "Function of auditory cortex of cat in frequency discrimination," J. Neurophysiol., 23:321-334.

Tkachev, R. A., 1955, "Problems in the pathophysiology of aphasic disorders accompanying vascular diseases of the brain," Zh. Nevropat. i Psikhiat. im. Korsakova, Vol. 15, p. 422.

Tonkonogii, I. M., 1968, Strokes and Aphasia, Leningrad, Meditsina.

Tonkonogii, I. M., and Kaidanova, S. I., 1963, "Detection of acoustic stimuli against a noise background by patients with local brain lesions," Zh. Nevropat. i Psikhiat. im. Korsakova, No. 11, p. 1614-1619.

Traugott, N. N., 1947, "Sensory alalia and aphasia in children," Abstracts of Scientific Research of the Academy of Medical Sciences of the USSR.

Traugott, N. N., 1959, "Special features of auditory function in disturbances of the activity of the auditory cortex in children," Problems in Physiological Acoustics, No. 4, Moscow–Leningrad, Izd. AN SSSR, pp. 201-207.

Traugott, N. N., Kaidanova, S. I., and Meierson, Ya. A., 1967, "Activity of the auditory and motor systems in aphasia," in: Physiological Mechanisms of Speech Disturbances, Leningrad, Nauka, pp. 157-164.

Traugott, N. N., Bagrov, Ya. Yu., Balonov, L. Ya., Deglin, V. L., Kaufman, D. A., and Lichko, A. E., 1968, Outlines of Human Psychopharmacology, Leningrad, Nauka.

Tsimmerman, G. S., 1967, The Ear and the Brain, Moscow, Meditsina.

Tunturi, A. R., 1952, "A difference in the representation of auditory signals for the left and right ears in the iso-frequency contour of the right middle ectosylvian auditory cortex of the dog," Amer. J. Physiol., 168:712-727.

Tunturi, A. R., 1955, "Effects of lesions of the auditory and adjacent cortex on conditioned reflexes," Amer. J. Physiol., 181:225-229.

Tunturi, A. R., 1960, "Neural mechanisms of the auditory and vestibular systems," Chapter 13 in: Anatomy and Physiology of the Auditory Cortex, Springfield.

Undrits, V. F., 1963, "Topical diagnosis of lesions of the central auditory system," Proceedings of the 1st All-Union Congress of Otolaryngologists, Moscow, pp. 335-344.

Ustwedt, H. J., 1937, "Über die Untersuchung der musikalischen Funktionen bei Patienten mit Gerhirnleiden, besonders bei Patienten mit Aphasie," Acta Med. Scand., 86:737.

Vardapetyan, G. A., 1966, "Electrophysiological investigation of temporal summation in different parts of the cat's auditory system," Zh. Vyssh. Nervn. Deyat., 16:470.

Vardapetyan, G. A., 1967, "Characteristics of single-unit responses in the cat's auditory cortex," in: Mechanisms of Hearing, Leningrad, Nauka, pp. 74-90.

Vasserman, L. I., "Investigation of absolute thresholds as a function of duration of acoustic stimuli in patients with temporal lobe lesions," in: Experimental Psychology in Psychiatric and Neurological Clinics (Proceedings of the V. M. Bekhterev Leningrad Psychoneurological Institute), Vol. 46, Leningrad, pp. 77-89.

Venderovich, E. A., 1916, New Facts on the Course of the Sensory Auditory and Visual Systems in the Hemisphere and the Need for Surgical Investigation and Intervention on the Intrafissural Cortex During Operation on Cortical Projection Zones, St. Petersburg.

Wada, J., and Rasmussen, T., 1960, "Intracarotid injection of sodium amytal for the lateralization of cerebral speech dominance. Experimental and clinical observations," J. Neurosurg., 17:266-282.

Walsh, E. G. 1957, "An investigation of sound localization in patients with neurological abnormalities," Brain, 80:222-250.

Wernicke, C., 1874, Der aphasische Symptomencomplex, Breslau, Max Cohn und Weigert.

Wildhagen, F. K., 1954, "Der Wert des Audiogramms bei zentrale Hörstörungen," Arch. Ohr. Heilk. Z. Hals. Hielk., 166:59-66.

Wohlfart, G., Lindgren, A., and Jernelius, B., 1952, "Clinical picture and morbid anatomy in a case of pure word deafness," J. Nerv. Ment. Dis., 116:818-827.

Wollard, H. H., and Harpman, J. A., 1940, "The connections of the inferior colliculus and of the dorsal nucleus of the lateral lemniscus," J. Anat. (London), 74:441-458.

Wright, H. N., 1967, "An artifact in the measurement of temporal summation at the threshold of audibility," J. Speech Hearing Res., 4:354-360.

Wright, H. N., 1968, "The effect of sensori-neural hearing loss on threshold-duration functions," J. Speech Hearing Res., 11:842-852.

Zhukovich, A. V., 1966, Special Otoneurology, Leningrad, Meditsina.

Zhukovich, A. V., and Khortseva, G. A., 1964, "Differential threshold of perception of the strength of sound in patients with lesions of the central nervous system," Vestn. Otorinolaring., No. 1, pp. 7-12.

Zvorykin, V. P., 1963, "Some cytoarchitectonic and quantitative principles governing the system of subcortical formations of the central auditory system in a comparative series of mammals," Candidate's Dissertation, Moscow, Academy of Medical Sciences of the USSR.

Zwislocki, J., 1960, "Theory of temporal auditory summation," J. Acoust. Soc. Amer., 32:1046-1060.

Wilhelm Flügge

Viscoelasticity

Second Revised Edition

Springer-Verlag
Berlin · Heidelberg · New York 1975

Dr.-Ing. Wilhelm Flügge
Professor of Applied Mechanics, emeritus
Stanford University

With 85 Figures

ISBN 3-540-07344-2 Springer-Verlag Berlin Heidelberg New York
ISBN 0-387-07344-2 Springer-Verlag New York Heidelberg Berlin

Printed in Germany
Library of Congress Cataloging in Publication Data.

Flügge, Wilhelm, 1904 –
Viscoelasticity.

Includes bibliographies and index.
1. Viscoelasticity. I. Title.
TA418.2.F53 1975 620.1'1232 75–23129

Offsetprinting: fotokop wilhelm weihert kg, Darmstadt · Bookbinding: Konrad Triltsch, Würzburg

Preface

No mathematical theory can completely describe the complex world around us. Every theory is aimed at a certain class of phenomena, formulates their essential features, and disregards what is of minor importance. The theory meets its limits of applicability where a disregarded influence becomes important. Thus, rigid-body dynamics describes in many cases the motion of actual bodies with high accuracy, but it fails to produce more than a few general statements in the case of impact, because elastic or anelastic deformation, no matter how local or how small, attains a dominating influence.

For a long time mechanics of deformable bodies has been based upon Hooke's law - that is, upon the assumption of linear elasticity. It was well known that most engineering materials like metals, concrete, wood, soil, are not linearly elastic or, are so within limits too narrow to cover the range of practical interest. Nevertheless, almost all routine stress analysis is still based on Hooke's law because of its simplicity.

In the course of time engineers have become increasingly conscious of the importance of the anelastic behavior of many materials, and mathematical formulations have been attempted and applied to practical problems. Outstanding among them are the theories of ideally plastic and of viscoelastic materials. While plastic behavior is essentially nonlinear (piecewise linear at best), viscoelasticity, like elasticity, permits a linear theory. This theory of linear viscoelasticity is the subject of the present book.

The book is intended for an introductory course and for self-study. The reader should be familiar with the basic concepts of mechanics, including stress and strain in two dimensions, and the technique of deriving differential equations from the consideration of the mechanics of an infinitesimal element. On the mathematical side, the prerequisite is calculus and a brief exposure to complex numbers and to linear ordinary differential equations. In many places the text uses more advanced mathematical methods (Laplace transformation, integral equations, partial differential equations, complex contour integration), but they are explained as far as needed and the reader may postpone their study in depth until later. In Chapter 8 a previous exposure to the theory of elasticity will be helpful.

The book presents the theory of viscoelasticity as an instrument of logical analysis. Basic assumptions are plausibly explained, and mathematical reasoning is used to derive results from them, which are deemed of interest for engineering tasks. There is, however, no reference to specific applications or materials, which, in our fast-changing world, are here today and gone tomorrow, to make room for others.

The problems, that have been inserted in may places, serve various purposes. Some suggest numerical work leading to results illustrating the physical content of the formulas. Others let the reader come to grips with mathematical techniques of problem solving, introduce additional subject matter, or establish cross connections with related fields in which the reader may have experience. It is suggested that he solve as many of these problems as he can handle, but leave aside those related to an outside field with which he is not sufficiently familiar.

The first edition of this book, which appeared in 1967 with the Blaisdell Publishing Company, represented the content of a graduate course, which the author has been giving for many years at Stanford University. In the present, second, edition, new material has been added at various places. In particular, there is a new chapter on beams resting on a continuous support, and a substantial expansion of the chapter on wave propagation.

Los Altos, California W. Flügge

Contents

Introduction

The mechanics of continuous media deals with three kinds of quantities: stresses, strains, and displacements. Stresses describe forces acting inside a body. Usually they are defined as forces (or force components) per unit of area of an infinitesimal section. However, the bending and twisting moments in a plate, the membrane forces in a shell, the bending moment and the shear force in a beam, and the torque in a shaft are also quantities of the same kind. They all describe forces or moments transmitted from one side of a section to the other; and they all come in pairs, equal in magnitude but opposite in sense, as they are acting on both parts of the body separated by the section.

Strains describe local deformations - for example, the increase in length of a line element divided by its original length (tensile strain), or the decrease of the right angle between two line elements (shear strain). There are more sophisticated definitions of strain quantities, like the tensorial strain derived from the change of the square of the line element, or the logarithmic strain. On the other hand, the curvature of a bent beam or plate and the twist of a shaft are also strain quantities, since they describe local change of form without reference to an external coordinate system.

Displacements describe the movement of a point or a line element during the process of deformation, with reference to a fixed coordinate system outside the deformable body. The displacements u, v, and w of the theory of elasticity and the deflection of a beam or a plate are linear displacements; the rotation of a beam element (the "slope" of the textbooks) is an angular displacement.

The stresses, strains, and displacements are connected by three kinds of equations expressing laws of nature:

The equilibrium conditions are relations between the stress quantities, usually containing their space derivatives. They are written for an infinitesimal element of the body or, occasionally, for a finite part. On the right-hand side they may contain a load quantity. In linear problems these equations do not contain strains or displacements; in nonlinear problems they often do. In problems of dynamics, the equilibrium equations are replaced by the equations of motion, which contain second-order time derivatives of the displacements.

Since the deformation of a body is completely known when the displacement of every point is known, it must be possible to calculate the strains from the displacements. Those equations which express the strains in terms of the displacements are known as the kinematic relations and are the second set of equations. There is one for each strain quantity.

Depending on the problem, there may be more kinematic relations than displacement components. In this case, it is possible to eliminate the displacements between these equations and thus to arrive at a smaller number of equations, which contain only strains. These are called compatibility equations. They are derived from a more fundamental set, and therefore they are not part of the basic equations.

Neither the conditions of equilibrium nor the kinematic relations depend on the particular material of which the body is made. The influence of this material is expressed by a third set of equations, the constitutive equations. They describe the relation between stress and strain. In the simplest case they are six algebraic equations giving the strain components in terms of the stresses, or vice versa. If they are linear, they are known as Hooke's law.

Actual materials show a great variety of behavior. Several idealized materials have been invented which typify various aspects of material behavior. For an elastic material there exists a one-to-one coordination between stress and strain. Many materials show the phenomenon of plastic flow, which may be defined by the following statements:

(i) The material is elastic until it reaches the yield limit, that is, until a certain function of the stress components reaches a certain value. (ii) Then additional strain is possible without increase of stress. (iii) This additional strain is permanent, that is, it remains when the stresses are removed. (iv) The time derivative of the strain (the rate of strain) does not appear in the equations.

Some materials show a pronounced influence of the rate of loading, the strain being larger if the stress has grown more slowly to its final value. The same materials display creep, that is, an increasing deformation under sustained load, the rate of strain depending on the stress. Such materials are called viscoelastic. Among them are metals at elevated temperatures, concrete, and plastics.

The constitutive equations of these materials may be either linear or nonlinear. This book develops the linear theory of viscoelasticity.

Chapter 1

Viscoelastic Models

The behavior of viscoelastic materials in uni-axial stress closely resembles that of models built from discrete elastic and viscous elements. We shall see how such models can be used to describe viscoelastic materials and to establish their differential equations.

1.1 The Basic Elements: Spring and Dashpot

Consider a helical spring (Fig.1.1a). When a force P is applied, the length of the spring increases by a certain amount u, and when the force is removed the spring returns to its original length. The same phenomenon is observed in a tension test performed on an elastic bar (Fig.1.1b). We prefer in this case to speak of the stress σ and the strain ϵ, because this removes the particular values of the length and the cross section of the bar from our considerations and thus gives them more generality.

If the material is linear-elastic, we have the relation

$$\sigma = E\epsilon , \qquad (1.1)$$

that is, Hooke's law, in which E is Young's modulus.

Now consider the "dashpot" of Fig.1.1c. A piston is moving in a cylinder with a perforated bottom so that no air is trapped inside. Between the cylinder and the piston wall there is a rather viscous lubricant so that a force P is needed to displace the piston. The stronger this force, the faster the piston will move. If the relation is linear, we have $P = k(du/dt)$. A similar deformation may be found in a tension bar of certain materials: When a load is applied, the bar is stretched. However, it is not its elongation ϵl that is proportional to the force, but its time rate of change $d(\epsilon l)/dt$. Writing in terms of stress and strain, we have

$$\sigma = F\, d\epsilon/dt = F\, \dot{\epsilon}. \tag{1.2}$$

Here and elsewhere we shall employ the dot to designate ordinary or partial derivatives with respect to time t. The quantity $\dot{\epsilon}$ is called the strain rate. A material whose stress is proportional to the strain rate is called a viscous material.

When (1.2) is translated into shear stress and shear strain,

$$\tau = \mu \dot{\gamma},$$

we have precisely the constitutive equation of a viscous liquid as it is used in lubrication theory, and μ is the viscosity coefficient.

The behavior of viscoelastic materials is a mixture of the two simple cases described by (1.1) and (1.2) and by the models illustrated by Fig. 1.1a and c. We shall now proceed to build up more complicated

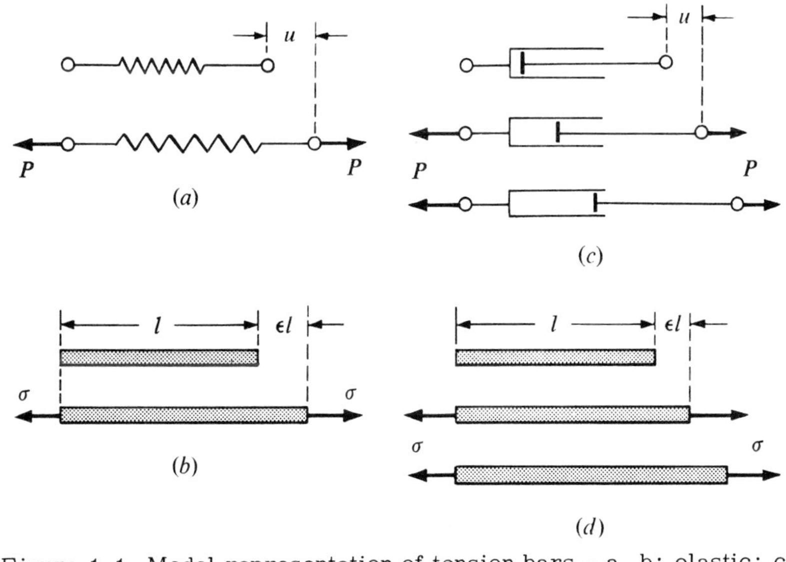

Figure 1.1. Model representation of tension bars - a, b: elastic; c, d: viscous.

models by combining springs and dashpots, and to read from them possible patterns of viscoelastic behavior. Whether a given material performs according to one or another of these patterns is a question to be resolved by testing. If it does, we can apply our theory.

Since our models will be used to derive relations between stress and strain, all forces in springs and dashpots will be written as σ, and all extensions as ϵ.

1.2 Maxwell Fluid and Kelvin Solid

The first composite model to be studied is shown in Fig. 1.2. The extension ϵ' of the spring follows from (1.1):

$$\sigma = E\epsilon', \tag{a}$$

while ϵ'' in the dashpot obeys the law (1.2):

$$\sigma = F\dot{\epsilon}''. \tag{b}$$

Since both elements are connected in series, the total elongation is

$$\epsilon = \epsilon' + \epsilon''. \tag{c}$$

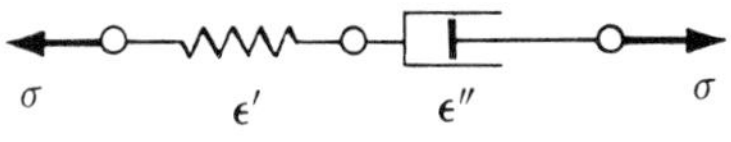

Figure 1.2. Spring and dashpot in series: Maxwell material.

We differentiate (a) and (c) and introduce $\dot{\epsilon}'$ and $\dot{\epsilon}''$ into (c) to find a relation between σ and ϵ, the force and the elongation of the spring-dashpot model:

$$\frac{\dot{\sigma}}{E} + \frac{\sigma}{F} = \dot{\epsilon}' + \dot{\epsilon}'' = \dot{\epsilon}.$$

This equation suggests that a similar relation might hold true as the the constitutive relation of some viscoelastic material. We write it in the standard form

$$\sigma + p_1\dot{\sigma} = q_1\dot{\epsilon}. \tag{1.3}$$

To understand what this equation implies in terms of the behavior of a tension bar under load, we subject such a bar to a two-stage standard test.

In the first stage, we apply at $t = 0$ a constant stress $\sigma = \sigma_0$ and ask for $\epsilon(t)$. In this case, (1.3) is a differential equation for ϵ and has the solution

$$\epsilon = \frac{\sigma_0}{q_1} t + C_1, \qquad t > 0. \tag{1.4}$$

To find C_1, an initial condition is needed. The sudden application of the stress σ_0 at $t = 0$ means that $\dot{\sigma}(t)$ has a singularity at this point. To deal with it, we integrate (1.3) across this point:

$$\int_{-\tau}^{+\tau} \sigma \, dt + p_1[\sigma(+\tau) - \sigma(-\tau)] = q_1[\epsilon(+\tau) - \epsilon(-\tau)].$$

When $\tau \to 0$, the first term goes to zero and we are left with

$$p_1\sigma_0 = q_1\epsilon_0, \quad \text{that is,} \quad \epsilon_0 = \frac{p_1\sigma_0}{q_1} = \frac{\sigma_0}{E_0}, \tag{1.5}$$

where $\epsilon_0 = \epsilon(0^+)$ is the value of the ϵ immediately to the right of $t = 0$. When we now write (1.4) for $t = 0^+$ and introduce this value for ϵ, we find that

$$C_1 = \epsilon_0 = p_1\sigma_0/q_1,$$

and hence

$$\epsilon = \frac{\sigma_0}{q_1}(p_1 + t). \tag{1.6}$$

This result is represented in Fig. 1.3 by the curves for $0 < t < t_1$.

In the second stage, which begins at $t = t_1$, the strain ϵ is fixed at whatever value ϵ_1 it has, that is, the ends of the test bar are fixed and we ask, what happens to the stress?

With $\epsilon = \epsilon_1$, $\dot{\epsilon} = 0$, (1.3) is a homogeneous differential equation for the stress σ and has the solution

$$\sigma = C_2 \exp(-t/p_1), \quad t > t_1. \tag{1.7}$$

To find C_2, we need $\sigma(t_1)$ or, more precisely, $\sigma(t_1^+)$, that is, the value which σ assumes just beyond a possible discontinuity. Any jump in the value of σ would mean an infinite value of $\dot{\sigma}$ and, from (1.3), an infinite $\dot{\epsilon}$. Since we see from Fig.1.3 that the strain rate is finite everywhere, we conclude that $\sigma(t^-) = \sigma(t^+)$ and hence $= \sigma_0$. Introducing this into (1.7), we find C_2 and then

$$\sigma = \sigma_0 \exp[-(t - t_1)/p_1]. \tag{1.8}$$

In the first stage, ϵ increases under constant stress. This phenomenon is called creep, and we shall speak of the creep phase of the test. In the second stage, the strees decreases under constant strain, that is, the material relaxes. This phase is called the relaxation phase.

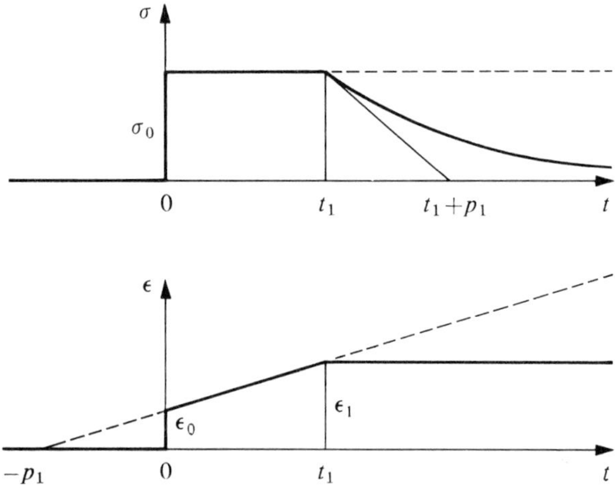

Figure 1.3. Standard test of the Maxwell fluid.

In Fig.1.3, dotted lines indicate what would happen if the creep phase were to be extended beyond $t = t_1$. The strain would increase beyond all bounds. Physically speaking, this would, of course, soon lead us out of the domain of linear relations, and we would have to look for a more realistic representation of the actual behavior. Within the realm of the linear constitutive equation (1.3), however, the material shows a typical property of a fluid: its capability of unlimited deformation under finite stress. The material described by (1.3) and Fig. 2.3 is therefore known as the Maxwell fluid. However, (1.5) shows that the response immediately after load application is elastic with a modulus E_0, the initial or impact modulus.

Another simple example is shown in Fig. 1.4. While Fig. 1.4a represents the usual way of displaying the model, it should be understood that the force σ is not to be distributed on the spring and the dashpot following the law of levers, but that really an arrangement is meant which is shown in more detail in Fig. 1.4b. At all times the elongation ϵ of the two elements is the same, and the total force σ will be split into σ' (spring) and σ'' (dashpot) in whichever way it is necessary to make ϵ the same.

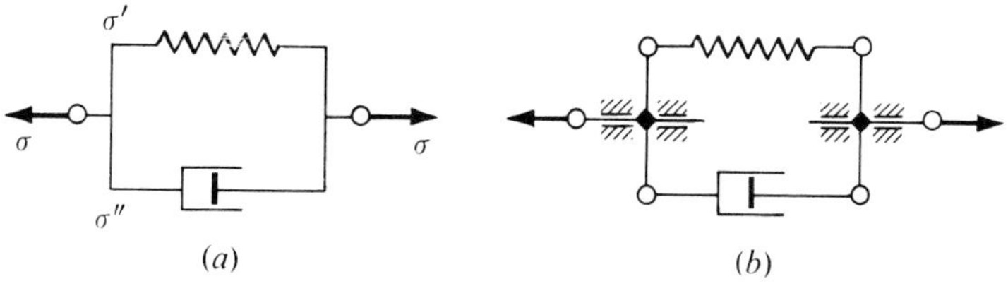

Figure 1.4. Spring and dashpot parallel: Kelvin material.

When applied to this model, (1.1) and (1.2) are

$$\sigma' = E\,\epsilon, \qquad \sigma'' = F\,\dot{\epsilon},$$

and from them we find

$$\sigma = \sigma' + \sigma'' = E\,\epsilon + F\,\dot{\epsilon},$$

which we write in the standard form

$$\sigma = q_0\epsilon + q_1\dot{\epsilon}. \tag{1.9}$$

Again, the constitutive equation is interpreted by performing the standard test.

When we let $\sigma = \sigma_0$, (1.9) has the solution

$$\epsilon = \frac{\sigma_0}{q_0} + C_1 e^{-\lambda t}, \qquad \lambda = \frac{q_0}{q_1}. \tag{1.10a,b}$$

When, at t = 0, σ jumps from 0 to σ_0, it remains finite and then (1.9) requires that $\dot{\epsilon}$ does the same. Therefore, ϵ cannot jump and the initial condition for (1.10a) is $\epsilon(0^+) = 0$. This leads to $C_1 = -\sigma_0/q_0$ and hence to

$$\epsilon = \frac{\sigma_0}{q_0}\left(1 - e^{-\lambda t}\right), \tag{1.11}$$

as illustrated by Fig. 1.5. If, following the dotted lines, the creep phase is extended to $t \to \infty$, the strain does not grow indefinitely, but approaches the limit

$$\epsilon_\infty = \frac{\sigma_0}{q_0} = \frac{\sigma_0}{E_\infty}, \tag{1.12}$$

which is proportional to the stress. This is almost the behavior of an elastic solid, the difference being that here the strain does not at once assume the final value, but approaches it gradually (delayed elasticity).

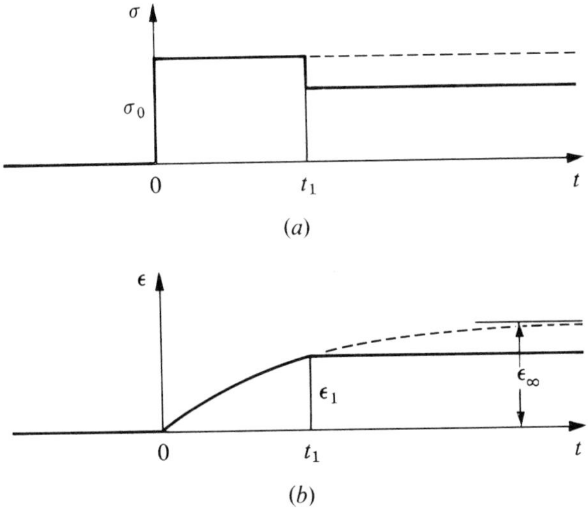

Figure 1.5. Standard test of the Kelvin solid.

The material represented by (1.9) and Fig. 1.5 is therefore a solid and is known as the Kelvin solid or the Voigt solid. The quantity E_∞ is called the asymptotic modulus.

In the relaxation phase $t > t_1$ we keep $\epsilon = \epsilon_1$ and we find from (1.9) and (1.11)

$$\sigma = q_0 \epsilon_1 = \sigma_0 [1 - \exp(-\lambda t_1)], \tag{1.13}$$

which is less than σ_0. When the strain is fixed, the stress is immediately relaxed by a certain amount and then remains forever at this value; that is, the relaxation is incomplete.

1.3 Unit Step Function, Dirac Function, Laplace Transformation

So far we have described the sudden application of a stress σ by simply stating that $\sigma = 0$ for $t < 0$ and $\sigma = \sigma_0$ for $t > 0$, splitting the t axis in two parts, to which different stress formulas apply. There is a way of writing this in a more compact form and thus facilitating mathematical manipulation.

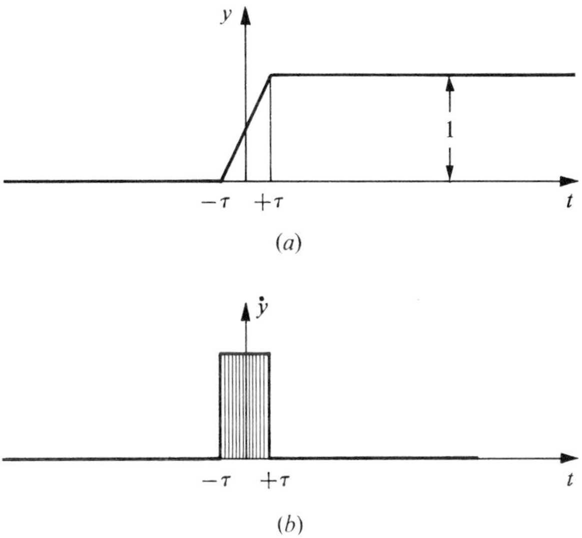

Figure 1.6. Derivation of $\Delta(t)$ and $\delta(t)$.

The unit step function $\Delta(t)$ is defined by the two equations

$$\Delta(t) = 0 \quad \text{for} \quad t < 0,$$
$$\Delta(t) = 1 \quad \text{for} \quad t > 0. \tag{1.14a,b}$$

For $t = 0$, the function is undefined unless we distinguish between $t = 0^-$ and $t = 0^+$ as the last point of negative time and the first point of positive time.

With the help of this function, the creep phase is defined by putting $\sigma = \sigma_0 \Delta(t)$. In order to introduce this into differential equations, we need the time derivative of $\Delta(t)$. Figure 1.6 shows how $\Delta(t)$ may be conceived as the limiting case of a continuous function $y(t)$. It also shows the derivative $\dot{y}$, which equals zero except in a small interval around $t = 0$. The integral over any part of the t axis including this interval, that is, the area of the shaded rectangle, equals unity. If we let $\tau \to 0$, this rectangle will degenerate into a spike, infinitely thin and infinitely high, but still of unit area. It represents a highly singular function, $\delta(t)$, which is the derivative of $\Delta(t)$ and which may be defined by the following equations:

$$\delta(t) = 0 \qquad \text{for} \quad t \neq 0, \tag{1.15a}$$

$$\delta(t) = +\infty \qquad \text{for} \quad t = 0, \tag{1.15b}$$

$$\int_{-\infty}^{+\infty} \delta(t)\,dt = \int_{0^-}^{0^+} \delta(t)\,dt = 1. \tag{1.15c}$$

This is known as the Dirac delta function. The process that led from $\Delta(t)$ to $\delta(t)$ may be repeated and leads to a sequence of rather exotic singular functions. The next one of them, $\dot{\delta}(t)$, has a positive spike at $-\tau$ and a negative one at $+\tau$. It is left to the reader to work out the details, in particular the integrability statement which corresponds to (1.15c). All these functions may be differentiated and integrated if they are defined as limiting cases of sufficiently smooth functions.

After these preparations, let us return to Fig. 1.5. We maintain the value of ε_1, but propose to reach the same strain in a shorter time, ultimately letting $t_1 \to 0$. We rewrite (1.11), using the series expansion of the exponential function:

$$\epsilon_1 = \frac{\sigma_0}{q_0}[1 - \exp(-\lambda t_1)] = \frac{\sigma_0}{q_0}\left[1 - 1 + \lambda t_1 - \frac{1}{2}(\lambda t_1)^2 + - \dots\right] = \frac{\sigma_0}{q_1} t_1 + \dots .$$

We see that in the limit $\sigma_0 t_1 = \epsilon_1 q_1$, and that σ_0 must tend to infinity as t_1 tends to zero while the first part of Fig. 1.5a degenerates into a Dirac spike $\sigma = \epsilon_1 q_1 \delta(t)$. Beyond the spike, (1.13) still holds true, and when we combine everything, we have

$$\sigma = \epsilon_1 q_1 \delta(t) + \epsilon_1 q_0 \Delta(t) \quad \text{for} \quad \epsilon = \epsilon_1 \Delta(t). \qquad (1.16)$$

This equation represents the stress response of the Kelvin solid to an enforced sudden stretching. The Dirac part points to a high stress peak at the beginning. Such a peak occurs in all those materials that do not have an initial elastic response to a suddenly applied stress, that is, for which $E_0 = \infty$.

For our further operations a knowledge of the elements of the Laplace transformation will be necessary. For details beyond the brief introduction offered here the reader is referred to textbooks on the subject [5-11].

Take any function $f(t)$, such as stress or strain, and define its Laplace transform

$$\overline{f}(s) = \int_0^\infty f(t) e^{-st} dt. \qquad (1.17)$$

Since we have integrated over t between fixed limits, $\overline{f}$ depends only on the rather meaningless variable s. The following facts are important:

(i). The values of $f(t)$ for $t < 0$ do not influence $\overline{f}(s)$.

(ii). The transforms of the derivatives of $f(t)$ have a simple relation to $\overline{f}(s)$.

To find this relation, we apply the transformation (1.17) to $\dot{f}(t)$ and integrate by parts:

$$\int_0^\infty \dot{f}(t)e^{-st}dt = \left[f(t)e^{-st}\right]_0^\infty - \int_0^\infty f(t)(-s)e^{-st}dt = -f(0) + s\bar{f}(s). \tag{1.18a}$$

Continuing this process, one easily verifies that

$$\int_0^\infty \ddot{f}(t)e^{-st}dt = -\dot{f}(0) - sf(0) + s^2\bar{f}(s),$$

$$\int_0^\infty \dddot{f}(t)e^{-st}dt = -\ddot{f}(0) - s\dot{f}(0) - s^2f(0) + s^3\bar{f}(s). \tag{1.18b,c}$$

When $f(t)$ or its derivatives have a singularity at $t = 0$, it is necessary to choose between taking either 0^+ or 0^- as the lower limit of the integral in (1.17). In most cases we shall deal with functions which vanish for all $t < 0$, and when we then choose 0^- as a base, all the f terms

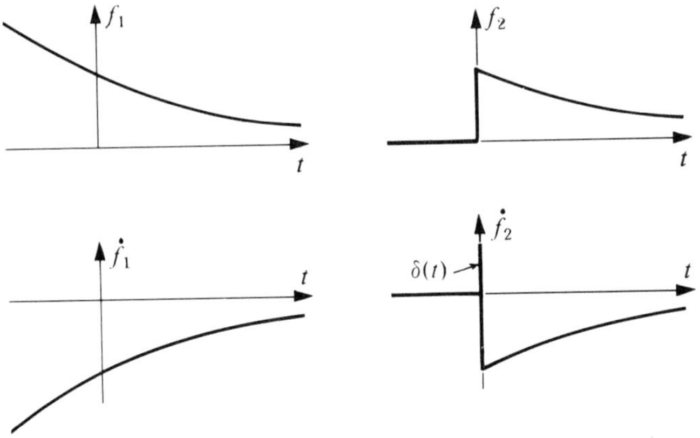

Figure 1.7. Two interpretations of a function $f(t)$.

in (1.18) vanish and the nth derivative of $f(t)$ has as its Laplace transform $s^n\bar{f}(s)$. The importance of the Laplace transformation as a tool for solving problems rests on the fact that a differentiation in the physical plane t, f is turned into an algebraic operation in the Laplace plane s, $\bar{f}$ and hence a differential equation is turned into an algebraic one, which is easier to solve. There is, however, the difficulty of transforming the solution $\bar{f}(s)$ back into the physical plane, that is, of finding the corresponding $f(t)$. The many methods to cope with this problem are one of the main subjects of books on the Laplace transformation.

As an example, consider the function $f(t) = e^{-\alpha t}$. From (1.17) we find

$$\bar{f}(s) = \int_0^\infty e^{-\alpha t} e^{-st}\, dt = -\frac{1}{\alpha + s}\left[e^{-(\alpha+s)t} \right]_0^\infty = \frac{1}{\alpha + s} .$$

Since the values of f for $t < 0$ do not enter the Laplace integral, we may identify $f(t)$ with either f_1 or f_2 shown in Fig.1.7. There is, however, a great difference in the derivatives of these functions. For f_1, (1.18a) yields the transform

$$\bar{\dot{f}}_1(s) = -1 + s\frac{1}{\alpha + s} = -\frac{\alpha}{\alpha + s} ,$$

but for f_2 it makes a difference whether 0^- or 0^+ is chosen as the lower limit in (1.17), since this means that the Dirac spike which corresponds to the jump in f_2 is either included or excluded. Based on 0^-, (1.18a) yields

$$\bar{\dot{f}}_2(s) = -f_2(0^-) + s\frac{1}{\alpha + s} = \frac{s}{\alpha + s} ,$$

but based on 0^+ it yields

$$\bar{\dot{f}}_2(s) = -f_2(0^+) + s\frac{1}{\alpha + s} = -1 + \frac{s}{\alpha + s} = -\frac{\alpha}{\alpha + s} .$$

As another example we study the unit step function $f(t) = \Delta(t)$. In this case, (1.17) yields

$$\bar{\Delta}(s) = \int_0^\infty \Delta(t) e^{-st} dt = -\frac{1}{s}\left[e^{-st} \right]_0^\infty = \frac{1}{s} .$$

Based on 0^-, (1.18a) then yields the derivative

$$\bar{\delta}(s) = -\delta(0^-) + \frac{s}{s} = 1 .$$

The same result follows from direct integration:

$$\bar{\delta}(s) = \int_{0^-}^{\infty} \delta(t)e^{-st}dt = \int_{0^-}^{0^+} \delta(t)dt \cdot e^0 + \int_{0^+}^{\infty} 0 \cdot e^{-st}dt = 1.$$

These results and a few others have been compiled in Table 1.1. All entries in this table are based on 0^- and on the assumption that functions like $e^{-\alpha t}$ are interpreted like f_1 in Fig. 1.7. More detailed tables may be found in [5] - [15] in the References.

Table 1.1

Laplace Transform Pairs

	$f(t)$	$\bar{f}(s)$
(1)	$\Delta(t)$	$1/s$
(2)	$\delta(t)$	1
(3)	$e^{-\alpha t}$	$1/(\alpha + s)$
(4)	$\frac{1}{\alpha}(1 - e^{-\alpha t})$	$1/s(\alpha + s)$
(5)	$\frac{t}{\alpha} - \frac{1}{\alpha^2}(1 - e^{-\alpha t})$	$1/s^2(\alpha + s)$
(6)	t^n	$n!s^{-n-1}, \quad n = 0, 1, \ldots$
(7)[1]	$J_0(a\sqrt{t^2 - b^2}) \cdot \Delta(t - b)$	$\frac{1}{\sqrt{s^2 + a^2}} \exp(-b\sqrt{s^2 + a^2})$
(8)[1]	$2\sqrt{\frac{t}{\pi}} \exp\left(-\frac{n^2}{4t}\right) - n\left(1 - \operatorname{erf}\frac{n}{2\sqrt{t}}\right)$	$\frac{1}{s\sqrt{s}} \exp(-n\sqrt{s})$

[1] J_0 is the Bessel function, commonly denoted in this way, and erf is the error function.

1.4 Kelvin Chains and Maxwell Models

We now return to our subject of spring-dashpot models of visco-elastic materials. Figure 1.8 shows a spring and a Kelvin element in series. For the strains of both parts we have

$$\sigma = E\epsilon', \qquad \sigma = q_0''\epsilon'' + q_1''\dot{\epsilon}'' .$$

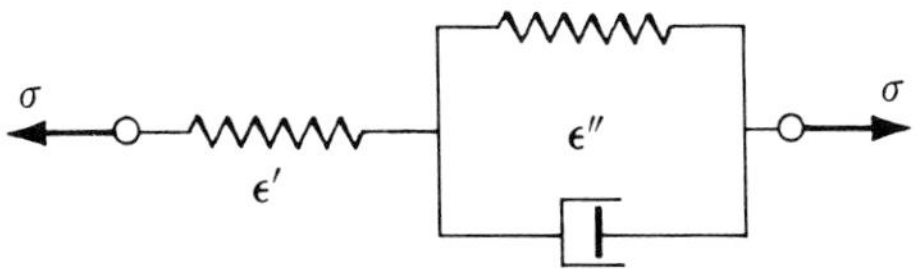

Figure 1.8. Three-parameter solid.

To both equations, the Laplace transformation is applied on both sides. Since E, q_0'', and q_1'' are constants, this yields

$$\bar{\sigma} = E\overline{\epsilon'}, \qquad \bar{\sigma} = (q_0'' + sq_1'')\overline{\epsilon''} .$$

Multiplying each of these equations with a suitable constant and adding, we find

$$\bar{\sigma}(q_0'' + sq_1'') + E\bar{\sigma} = E(q_0'' + sq_1'')(\overline{\epsilon'} + \overline{\epsilon''}) = E(q_0'' + sq_1'')\bar{\epsilon} ,$$

where $\bar{\epsilon}$ is the transform of the total strain. Transforming back into the physical plane means removing bars and replacing every factor s by a differentiation:

$$(q_0'' + E)\sigma + q_1''\dot{\sigma} = Eq_0''\epsilon + Eq_1''\dot{\epsilon}.$$

This is written in the normalized form

$$\sigma + p_1\dot{\sigma} = q_0\epsilon + q_1\dot{\epsilon}. \qquad (1.19)$$

Comparing the coefficients of both equations, one sees that

$$p_1 = q_1''/(E + q_0''), \quad q_0 = Eq_0''/(E + q_0''), \quad q_1 = Eq_1''/(E + q_0''),$$

and from these relations it follows that

$$\frac{q_1}{p_1} - q_0 = \frac{E^2}{E + q_0''}$$

is always positive, that is, that

$$q_1 > p_1 q_0. \tag{1.20}$$

If this inequality is not satisfied, it is not possible to derive (1.19) from the model, Fig. 1.8, with real, positive values of the constants of its component parts. At present, it might appear that some other model could enable us to circumvent the inequality (1.20). We shall soon see, however, that this inequality is a physical necessity.

We explore the properties of the material by again subjecting it to the standard test. In the creep phase we have

$$\sigma = \sigma_0 \Delta(t), \qquad \bar{\sigma} = \sigma_0/s.$$

From the Laplace transform of (1.19) we have

$$\sigma_0\left(\frac{1}{s} + p_1\right) = (q_0 + q_1 s)\bar{\varepsilon},$$

whence

$$\bar{\varepsilon} = \sigma_0 \frac{1 + p_1 s}{s(q_0 + q_1 s)} = \frac{\sigma_0}{q_1}\left[\frac{1}{s(s+\lambda)} + \frac{p_1}{s+\lambda}\right]$$

with $\lambda = q_0/q_1$. In the last member of this equation, the function of s has been split into two parts which can readily be recognized in Table 1.1. Using this table backwards, we find the strain

$$\varepsilon = \frac{\sigma_0}{q_1}\left[\frac{1}{\lambda}(1 - e^{-\lambda t}) + p_1 e^{-\lambda t}\right],$$

which may be written as

$$\varepsilon = \frac{\sigma_0}{q_0}\left[1 - \left(1 - \frac{p_1 q_0}{q_1}\right)\right]\exp(-q_0 t/q_1). \tag{1.21}$$

Because of (1.20), the coefficient in parentheses is positive and $\varepsilon(t)$ looks as shown in Fig. 1.9. The material has instant elasticity with

$$\varepsilon(0^+) = \varepsilon_0 = \sigma_0 p_1/q_1 = \sigma_0/E_0$$

and also asymptotic elastic behavior,

$$\varepsilon(\infty) = \varepsilon_\infty = \sigma_0/q_0 = \sigma_0/E_\infty .$$

Therefore, it qualifies as a solid, the three-parameter solid. It is also known as the standard linear material. If (1.20) is violated, $\varepsilon_\infty < \varepsilon_0$, that is, a tension bar would, under sustained load, become gradually shorter!

For the relaxation phase, we shift our time scale and introduce a new time $\tau = t - t_1$. For $\tau \geqslant 0$ we may then write $\varepsilon = \varepsilon_1 \Delta(\tau)$, $\bar{\varepsilon} = \varepsilon_1/s$, and the Laplace transform of (1.19) then reads

$$\bar{\sigma} + p_1(s\bar{\sigma} - \sigma_0) = q_0\bar{\varepsilon} + q_1(s\bar{\varepsilon} - \varepsilon_1) = q_0\varepsilon_1/s.$$

Solving for $\bar{\sigma}$, we find

$$\bar{\sigma} = \frac{q_0\varepsilon_1}{s(1 + p_1 s)} + \frac{p_1\sigma_0}{1 + p_1 s} .$$

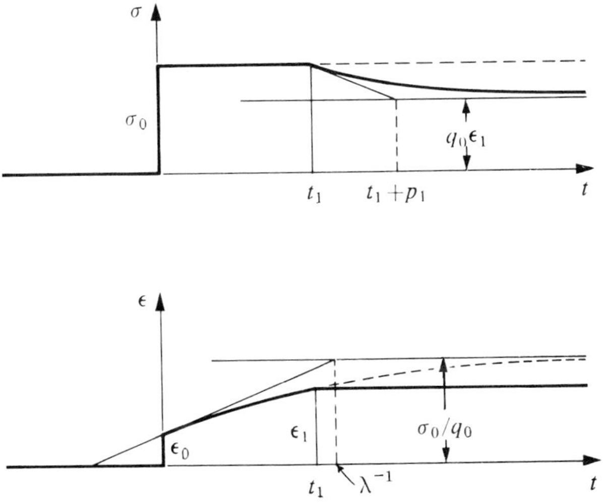

Figure 1.9. Standard test of the three-parameter solid.

Using the transformation pairs (3) and (4) of Table 1.1, we find from this the stress

$$\sigma = q_0 \epsilon_1 [1 - \exp(-\tau/p_1)] + \sigma_0 \exp(-\tau/p_1). \qquad (1.22)$$

This is the right half of the σ curve in Fig. 1.9. The material relaxes gradually to $\sigma_\infty = q_0 \epsilon_1 = E_\infty \epsilon_1$. Note the meaning of $\lambda^{-1} = q_1/q_0$ and p_1 as abscissas of the intersections of initial tangents and asymptotes. Because of (1.20), $\lambda^{-1} > p_1$.

There are two ways of systematically building up more complicated models: the Kelvin chain and the Maxwell model. In the former (Fig. 1.10a) an arbitrary number of different Kelvin units are connected in series, possibly including the degenerated units s and d. Presence of s leads to impact response ($E_0 \neq \infty$) and presence of d to fluid behavior ($E_\infty = 0$). In the Maxwell model, Maxwell units are connected in parallel (Fig. 1.10b). In this case the absence of a degenerated unit d assures impact response and the absence of s leads to fluid behavior.

In Table 1.2 some models are shown with their differential equations and other information to be explained later.

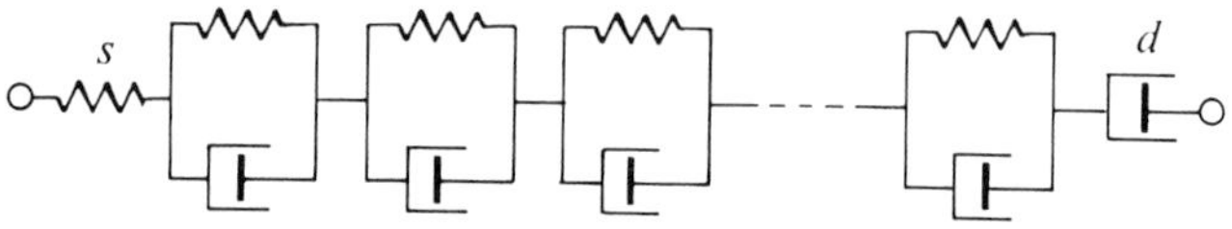

(a)

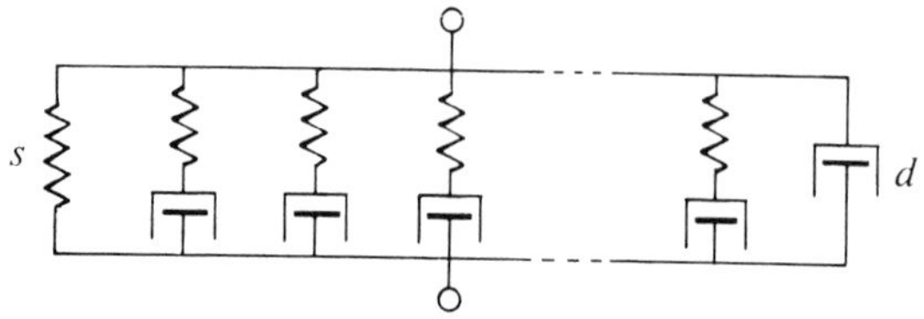

(b)

Figure 1.10. Spring-dashpot models - a: Kelvin chain; b: Maxwell model.

Obviously, the differential equation of any model of the Kelvin or Maxwell type has the form

$$\sigma + p_1\dot{\sigma} + p_2\ddot{\sigma} + \dots = q_0\epsilon + q_1\dot{\epsilon} + q_2\ddot{\epsilon} + \dots \tag{1.23a}$$

or

$$\sum_0^m p_k \frac{d^k\sigma}{dt^k} = \sum_0^n q_k \frac{d^k\epsilon}{dt^k}\,. \tag{1.23b}$$

Since we may divide the equation by a constant without changing its meaning, we shall always set $p_0 = 1$.

Equation (1.23b) may also be written as

$$\mathbf{P}\sigma = \mathbf{Q}\epsilon\,, \tag{1.23c}$$

where $\mathbf{P}$ and $\mathbf{Q}$ are differential operators:

$$\mathbf{P} = \sum_0^m p_k \frac{d^k}{dt^k}\,, \qquad \mathbf{Q} = \sum_0^n q_k \frac{d^k}{dt^k}\,. \tag{1.24a,b}$$

Equation (1.23) in any of its forms is the mathematical description of the mechanical behavior of a viscoelastic material. It is called its *constitutive equation*. Just as a book on the Theory of Elasticity does not discuss which materials obey Hooke's law, but describes what happens in those which do, so this book is not concerned with the question which materials can be represented by the viscoelastic law (1.23), but shows what happens in those which can, In both cases singularities in the solutions are typical pointers at situations in which even small (and often enough unknown) deviations from the postulated constitutive equation may exert an important influence.

When (1.23b) is subjected to the Laplace transformation, there results the following algebraic relation between the Laplace transforms $\bar{\sigma}(s)$ and $\bar{\epsilon}(s)$ of stress and strain:

$$\sum_0^m p_k s^k \bar{\sigma} = \sum_0^n q_k s^k \bar{\epsilon}\,. \tag{1.25a}$$

TABLE

Viscoelastic

Model	Name	Differential equation / Inequalities	Creep compliance $J(t)$
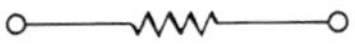	elastic solid	$\sigma = q_0 \epsilon$	$1/q_0$
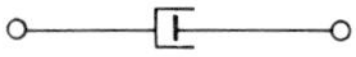	viscous fluid	$\sigma = q_1 \dot{\epsilon}$	t/q_1
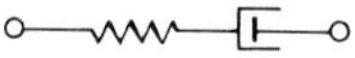	Maxwell fluid	$\sigma + p_1 \dot{\sigma} = q_1 \dot{\epsilon}$	$(p_1 + t)/q_1$
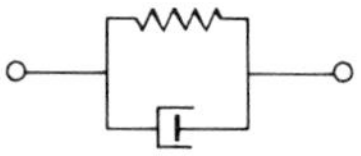	Kelvin solid	$\sigma = q_0 \epsilon + q_1 \dot{\epsilon}$	$\frac{1}{q_0}(1 - e^{-\lambda t}), \ \lambda = \frac{q_0}{q_1}$
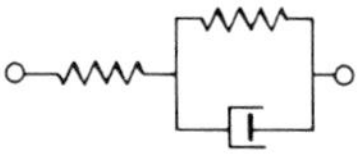	3-parameter solid	$\sigma + p_1 \dot{\sigma} = q_0 \epsilon + q_1 \dot{\epsilon}$ $q_1 > p_1 q_0$	$\frac{p_1}{q_1} e^{-\lambda t} + \frac{1}{q_0}(1 - e^{-\lambda t}),$ $\lambda = q_0/q_1$
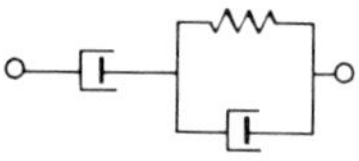	3-parameter fluid	$\sigma + p_1 \dot{\sigma} = q_1 \dot{\epsilon} + q_2 \ddot{\epsilon}$ $p_1 q_1 > q_2$	$\frac{t}{q_1} + \frac{p_1 q_1 - q_2}{q_1^2}(1 - e^{-\lambda t}),$ $\lambda = q_1/q_2$
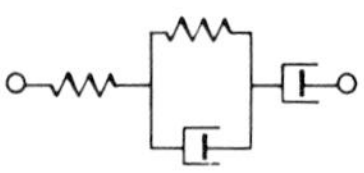	4-parameter fluid	$\sigma + p_1 \dot{\sigma} + p_2 \ddot{\sigma} = q_1 \dot{\epsilon} + q_2 \ddot{\epsilon}$ $p_1^2 > 4 p_2$ $p_1 q_1 q_2 > p_2 q_1^2 + q_2^2$	$\frac{t}{q_1} + \frac{p_1 q_1 - q_2}{q_1^2}(1 - e^{-\lambda t}) +$ $+ \frac{p_2}{q_2} e^{-\lambda t}, \ \lambda = q_1/q_2$
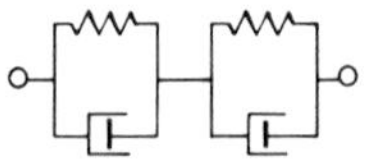	4-parameter solid	$\sigma + p_1 \dot{\sigma} = q_0 \epsilon + q_1 \dot{\epsilon} + q_2 \ddot{\epsilon}$ $q_1^2 > 4 q_0 q_2$ $q_1 p_1 > q_0 p_1^2 + q_2$	$\frac{1 - p_1 \lambda_1}{q_2 \lambda_1 (\lambda_2 - \lambda_1)}(1 - e^{-\lambda_1 t}) +$ $+ \frac{1 - p_1 \lambda_2}{q_2 \lambda_2 (\lambda_1 - \lambda_2)}(1 - e^{-\lambda_2 t})$ where λ_1, λ_2 are roots of $q_2 \lambda^2 - q_1 \lambda + q_0 = 0$

1.2
Materials

Relaxation modulus $Y(t)$	Complex compliance	
	Real part $G_1(\omega)$	Imaginary part $G_2(\omega)$
q_0	$1/q_0$	0
$q_1\delta(t)$	0	$-\dfrac{1}{q_1\omega}$
$\dfrac{q_1}{p_1}e^{-t/p_1}$	$\dfrac{p_1}{q_1}$	$-\dfrac{1}{q_1\omega}$
$q_0 + q_1\delta(t)$	$\dfrac{q_0}{q_0^2 + q_1^2\omega^2}$	$-\dfrac{q_1\omega}{q_0^2 + q_1^2\omega^2}$
$\dfrac{q_1}{p_1}e^{-t/p_1} + q_0(1 - e^{-t/p_1})$	$\dfrac{q_0 + p_1q_1\omega^2}{q_0^2 + q_1^2\omega^2}$	$-\dfrac{(q_1 - q_0p_1)\omega}{q_0^2 + q_1^2\omega^2}$
$\dfrac{q_2}{p_1}\delta(t) + \dfrac{1}{p_1}\left(q_1 - \dfrac{q_2}{p_1}\right)e^{-t/p_1}$	$\dfrac{p_1q_1 - q_2}{q_1^2 + q_2^2\omega^2}$	$-\dfrac{q_1 + p_1q_2\omega^2}{(q_1^2 + q_2^2\omega^2)\omega}$
$\dfrac{1}{\sqrt{p_1^2 - 4p_2}}\Big\vert(q_1 - \alpha q_2)e^{-\alpha t} - (q_1 - \beta q_2)e^{-\beta t}\Big\vert,$ $\left.\begin{matrix}\alpha\\ \beta\end{matrix}\right\} = \dfrac{1}{2p_2}\left(p_1 \pm \sqrt{p_1^2 - 4p_2}\right)$	$\dfrac{(p_1q_1 - q_2) + p_2q_2\omega^2}{q_1^2 + q_2^2\omega^2}$	$-\dfrac{q_1 + (q_2p_1 - p_2q_1)\omega^2}{(q_1^2 + q_2^2\omega^2)\omega}$
$\dfrac{q_2}{p_1}\delta(t) + \dfrac{q_1p_1 - q_2}{p_1^2} - \dfrac{1}{p_1^2}(q_1p_1 - q_0p_1^2 - q_2)(1 - e^{-t/p_1})$	$\dfrac{q_0 + (p_1q_1 - q_2)\omega^2}{q_0^2 + (q_1^2 - 2q_0q_2)\omega^2 + q_2^2\omega^4}$	$-\dfrac{(q_1 - p_1q_0)\omega + q_2p_1\omega^3}{q_0^2 + (q_1^2 - 2q_0q_2)\omega^2 + q_2^2\omega^4}$

It may be written in the form

$$\mathcal{P}(s) \cdot \bar{\sigma} = \mathcal{Q}(s) \cdot \bar{\epsilon}, \tag{1.25b}$$

in which $\mathcal{P}$ and $\mathcal{Q}$ are polynomials in s,

$$\mathcal{P}(s) = \sum_0^m p_k s^k, \qquad \mathcal{Q}(s) = \sum_0^n q_k s^k, \tag{1.26}$$

which have the same coefficients as the differential operators **P** and **Q**.

When studying a few simple models of viscoelastic materials, we have seen that some of them display an instantaneous response and some do not, and that there are solids, which, under constant stress σ, ultimately settle down at a finite strain ϵ, and fluids, which ultimately creep at a constant strain rate $\dot{\epsilon}$. Table 1.3 shows how these types of behavior are connected with the pattern of nonzero coefficients. If $q_0 = 0$, there are only derivatives on the right-hand side of (1.23), and at least the lowest of them must be nonzero if there is a stress σ. Such materials are fluids. If $q_0 \neq 0$, stress and strain approach finite values for $t \to \infty$ and then all derivatives on both sides of (1.23) vanish. In the limit we have $\sigma = q_0 \epsilon$, and the asymptotic modulus is

$$E_\infty = q_0 . \tag{1.27}$$

An initial eleastic response with modulus E_0 occurs if $n = m$, and it is absent if $n = m + 1$. In (1.23b) we may replace the summation limit m by n and still include both cases if we reserve the right to let $p_n = 0$.

The first two columns of Table 1.3 show how the different viscoelastic materials may be represented by Kelvin or Maxwell models, consisting of at most one spring (s) and one dashpot (d) and an arbitrary number of Kelvin elements in series or a spring, a dashpot, and an arbitrary number of Maxwell elements (m) in parallel.

When we integrate $d^k\sigma/dt^k$ from 0^- to some variable upper limit t, we obtain $d^{k-1}\sigma/dt^{k-1}$ at t. When we integrate again and repeat the procedure to a total of k integrations, we obtain $\sigma(t)$, which may have a step discontinuity, and the next and any following integration will yield

Table 1.3
Kelvin and Maxwell Models

Kelvin model	Maxwell model	Nonzero coefficients of **P**	Nonzero coefficients of **Q**	Number of parameters	E_0	Solid or fluid
s	s	p_0	q_0	1	E_0	solid
d	d	p_0	q_1	1	-	fluid
k	s/d	p_0	q_0q_1	2	-	solid
s-d	m	p_0p_1	q_1	2	E_0	fluid
s-k	s/m	p_0p_1	q_0q_1	3	E_0	solid
d-k	d/m	p_0p_1	q_1q_2	3	-	fluid
k-k	s/d/m	p_0p_1	$q_0q_1q_2$	4	-	solid
s-d-k	m/m	$p_0p_1p_2$	q_1q_2	4	E_0	fluid
s-k-k	s/m/m	$p_0p_1p_2$	$q_0q_1q_2$	5	E_0	solid
d-k-k	d/m/m	$p_0p_1p_2$	$q_1q_2q_3$	5	-	fluid
k-k-k	s/d/m/m	$p_0p_1p_2$	$q_0q_1q_2q_3$	6	-	solid
s-d-k-k	m/m/m	$p_0p_1p_2p_3$	$q_1q_2q_3$	6	E_0	fluid
s-k-k-k	s/m/m/m	$p_0p_1p_2p_3$	$q_0q_1q_2q_3$	7	E_0	solid

an entirely continuous function. Its value for $t = 0^-$ and 0^+ is the same, and if $t = 0^+$ is chosen as the upper limit of the last integration, all these integrals are zero. The same happens if we apply the procedure on the right-hand side of (1.23b) to the derivatives of ϵ. Therefore, when this equation is integrated n times and, in the last integral the upper limit is made to be $t = 0^+$, on each side only the term $k = n$ survives, and this leads to the relation

$$p_n \sigma(0^+) = q_n \epsilon(0^+) .$$

Clearly, if $p_n = 0$, the step discontinuity in σ does not lead to one in ϵ and the material does not display an instantaneous elastic response. On the other hand, if $p_n \neq 0$, the values of stress and strain at $t = 0^+$ are related by the equation

$$\epsilon(0^+) = \frac{p_n}{q_n} \sigma(0^+) \tag{1.28a}$$

which may be written in the form of Hooke's law

$$\sigma(0^+) = E_0 \varepsilon(0^+)$$

where

$$E_0 = q_n/p_n \tag{1.29}$$

is the impact modulus.

If we integrate the differential equation only (n-1) times, we obtain on each side two nonvanishing contributions:

$$p_{n-1}\sigma(0^+) + p_n\dot{\sigma}(0^+) = q_{n-1}\varepsilon(0^+) + q_n\dot{\varepsilon}(0^+),$$

and we may use this relation to calculate $\dot{\varepsilon}(0^+)$ if $\sigma(t)$ is completely known or vice versa. In the first case we have

$$\dot{\varepsilon}(0^+) = \frac{p_{n-1}q_n - p_n q_{n-1}}{q_n^2}\sigma(0^+) + \frac{p_n}{q_n}\dot{\sigma}(0^+). \tag{1.28b}$$

Stepping back once more and integrating only (n-2) times, we find the relation

$$p_{n-2}\sigma(0^+) + p_{n-1}\dot{\sigma}(0^+) + p_n\ddot{\sigma}(0^+) = q_{n-2}\varepsilon(0^+) + q_{n-1}\dot{\varepsilon}(0^+) + q_n\ddot{\varepsilon}(0^+),$$

which, in combination with the results just obtained, yields

$$\ddot{\varepsilon}(0^+) = \begin{vmatrix} p_n & q_n & 0 \\ p_{n-1} & q_{n-1} & q_n \\ p_{n-2} & q_{n-2} & q_{n-1} \end{vmatrix} \frac{\sigma(0^+)}{q_n^3} - \begin{vmatrix} p_n & q_n \\ p_{n-1} & q_{n-1} \end{vmatrix} \frac{\dot{\sigma}(0^+)}{q_n^2} + \frac{p_n}{q_n}\ddot{\sigma}(0^+). \tag{1.28c}$$

In this way one may calculate the initial values of ε and its derivatives and write the initial conditions which the solution of the differential equation (1.23) for the strain ε must satisfy. A similar procedure is possible when $\varepsilon(t)$ is known and (1.23) has to be solved for the stress $\sigma(t)$ in the domain $t > 0$.

Following the procedure shown on pp. 17-20, one may verify any of the differential equations in the third column of Table 1.2. The inequalities to which the coefficients p_k and q_k are subjected, follow from the requirement that the coefficients E_r, F_r of the elements of the Kelvin chain must be positive. One may extend the procedure to Kelvin chains of any length as shown in Fig. 1.10a. The longer the chain is, the more coefficients p_k, q_k there are in (1.23a).

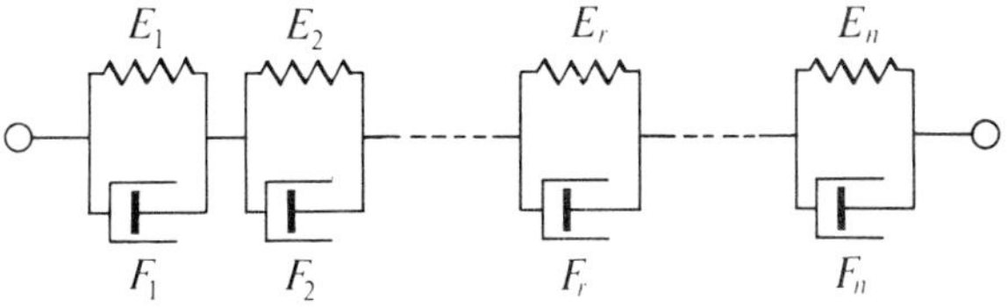

Figure 1.11. Kelvin chain.

Conversely, we may wish to construct a Kelvin chain which models an equation (1.23a) with prescribed coefficients. To solve this problem, consider the chain shown in Fig. 1.11. If in any of its Kelvin elements $F_r = 0$, it represents an isolated spring, and if $E_r = 0$, the element is reduced to an isolated dashpot. Hence, the Kelvin chain of Fig. 1.11 is as general as the one of Fig. 1.10a and may represent any of the models listed in Table 1.3.

The analysis is best done on the Laplace transforms. Using the equation preceding (1.9), we write for the r-th element

$$\bar{\sigma} = (E_r + sF_r)\bar{\varepsilon}_r$$

and for the entire chain

$$\bar{\varepsilon} = \bar{\varepsilon}_1 + \bar{\varepsilon}_2 + \dots + \bar{\varepsilon}_n = \bar{\sigma}\left[\frac{1}{E_1 + sF_1} + \frac{1}{E_2 + sF_2} + \dots + \frac{1}{E_n + sF_n}\right]. \quad (1.30)$$

This compares with (1.25a):

$$\bar{\varepsilon} = \bar{\sigma}\,\frac{\sum_{k=0}^{m} p_k s^k}{\sum_{k=0}^{n} q_k s^k} = \bar{\sigma}\,\frac{\mathcal{P}(s)}{\mathcal{Q}(s)}. \quad (1.31)$$

Evidently, the bracketed term in (1.30) is the partial fraction expansion of the quotient $\mathcal{P}(s)/\mathcal{Q}(s)$, which may be obtained by routine procedures commonly tought in textbooks on calculus. The result is unique with the exception that it does not specify the order in which the terms appear in (1.30) and, consequently, the order in which the elements of the Kelvin model follow each other.

From well known facts about partial fractions we may draw the following conclusions:

(i) The sum of partial fractions looks exactly as written in (1.30) if $m < n$ in (1.31). The polynomial $\mathcal{Q}(s)$ is of the n-th degree and has (n+1) coefficients, while $\mathcal{P}(s)$ is at most of degree (n-1) and has, with $p_0 = 1$, at most (n-1) nontrivial coefficients. The total of 2n coefficients in (1.31) corresponds to an equal number of constants E_r, F_r in (1.30). Either set may be chosen and the other set calculated from it.

(ii) The partial fractions in (1.30) make sense physically only if all the E_r and F_r are real and positive. This will be the case if the equation $\mathcal{Q}(s) = 0$ has only real, nonnegative roots. One vanishing value E_r may be admitted. It occurs when $q_0 = 0$ and indicates the presence of an isolated dashpot in the Kelvin chain and fluid behavior of the material it represents. The limits imposed upon the constants in (1.30) are equivalent to inequalities which the p_k and q_k must satisfy.

(iii) If $m = n$, long-hand division splits the quotient $\mathcal{P}/\mathcal{Q}$ into a constant p_n/q_n and a fraction with a numerator of degree (n-1). The constant is an additional term to be added to the partial fractions in (1.30) and represents an isolated spring of modulus $E_0 = q_n/p_n$.

(iv) If $m > n$, further terms $Bs + Cs^2 + \dots$ appear in addition to the partial fractions. They cannot be interpreted as Laplace transforms of differential operators and cannot be represented by Kelvin elements. Therefore, constitutive equations (1.23) with $m > n$ do not represent viscoelastic materials.

Equation (1.31) has the form

$$\bar{\sigma} = \bar{\epsilon}\, \mathcal{E}(s) \quad \text{with} \quad \mathcal{E}(s) = \mathcal{Q}(s)/\mathcal{P}(s), \tag{1.32}$$

in which it resembles Hooke's law. This indicates that there exists a strong formal tie between the behavior of elastic and viscoelastic materials. This is the basis of the Correspondence Principle, which we shall later explore and put to good use.

At present let us state a few properties of the function $\mathcal{E}(s)$. From its definition we see that it is a rational function and has real values for real arguments s. Comparison of (1.30) and (1.32) shows that

$$\frac{1}{\mathcal{E}(s)} = \sum_{k=1}^{n} \frac{1}{E_k + sF_k} \tag{1.33}$$

with positive, real E_k and F_k. When we take all the fractions to a common denominator, this denominator equals some constant multiple of $\mathfrak{Q}(s)$, and we see that $\mathfrak{Q}(s)$ and hence $\mathcal{E}(s)$ have n zeros which are all nonpositive. In fluid materials there is $E_1 = 0$ and hence $\mathcal{E}(0) = 0$; otherwise all zeros of $\mathcal{E}(s)$ are negative and real, and $\mathcal{E}(0) = q_0 = E_\infty$.

The zeros of $\mathfrak{P}(s)$ are singularities of $\mathcal{E}(s)$. To locate them, we use (1.33) to calculate $d\mathcal{E}/ds$:

$$\frac{d\mathcal{E}(s)}{ds} = \mathcal{E}^2(s) \sum_{k=1}^{n} \frac{F_k}{(E_k + sF_k)^2} \, . \tag{1.34}$$

For real s, this is obviously positive with the possible exception of the points where $\mathcal{E}(s) = 0$. These are the points where $s = -E_k/F_k$ with $k = 1, 2, \ldots n$. In the vicinity of these points one term in (1.33) dominates and

$$\mathcal{E}(s) \to E_k + sF_k \quad \text{and} \quad \frac{d\mathcal{E}(s)}{ds} = F_k ,$$

which again is positive. At the singular points of $\mathcal{E}(s)$, also its derivative is infinite. With this information, we may begin a qualitative sketch of $\mathcal{E}(s)$. Starting at any one of its zeros, it increases monotonically until it comes to the next zero. This is possible only if in between $\mathcal{E}(s)$ grows to $+\infty$ and returns from $-\infty$ as shown in Fig. 1.12. Hence, zeros and poles alternate on the negative s-axis. There are n zeros and (n-1) poles between them.

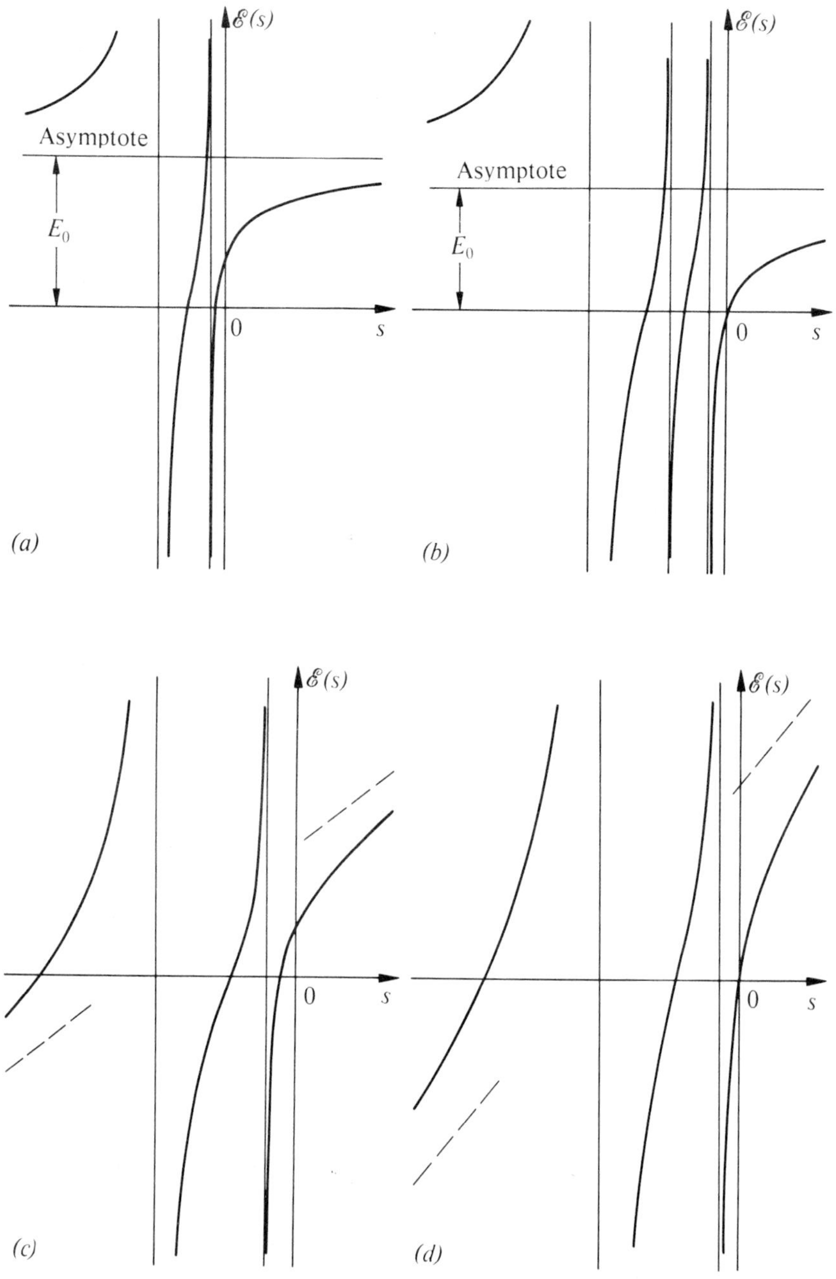

Figure 1.12. Function $\mathscr{E}(s)$ for different materials - a: $E_0 \neq 0$, solid; b: $E_0 \neq 0$, fluid; c: $E_0 = 0$, solid; d: $E_0 = 0$, fluid.

To complete the sketch, we need the limit of $\mathcal{E}(s)$ for $s \to \pm\infty$. It is different, depending upon whether or not the material has an impact modulus E_0. If $E_0 \neq 0$, then $m = n$ and

$$\lim_{s \to \pm\infty} \mathcal{E}(s) = \frac{q_n}{p_n} = E_0 > 0 .$$

For such materials, $\mathcal{E}(s)$ has another pole to the left of its last zero (Fig. 1.12a,b). On the other hand, if $E_0 = 0$, then $m = n-1$ and

$$\lim_{s \to \pm\infty} \mathcal{E}(s) = \lim \frac{q_n s}{p_{n-1}} = \pm\infty .$$

The corresponding diagrams for a solid and a fluid are shown in Fig. 1.12c,d.

Problems

1.1. Verify the differential equations for the three last models in Table 1.2. If you are not familiar with the use of the Laplace transformation, you may write differential equations for the component parts and eliminate from them all those stresses or strains which cannot be measured at the terminals of the model. Verify also the inequalities.

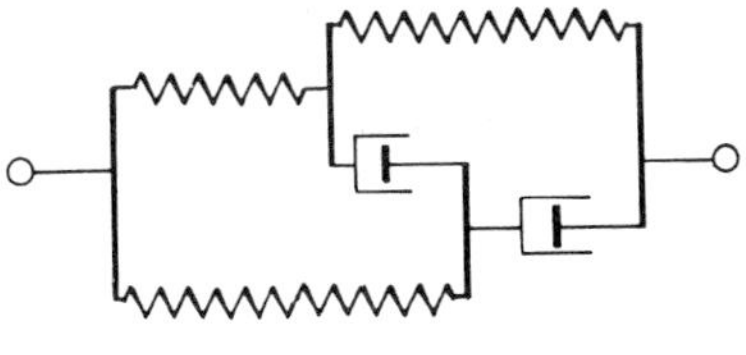

Figure 1.13.

1.2. Subject any of the three last models of Table 1.2 to the standard test.

1.3. Take any one of the four last models in Table 1.2 and consult Table 1.3 for the corresponding Maxwell model. Derive its differential equation and compare it with the entry in Table 1.2.

1.4. Show that the four-parameter solid degenerates into the Kelvin material when its component parts are made equal or when $E_1/F_1 = E_2/F_2$.

1.5. Figure 1.13 shows a model which fits neither into the Kelvin nor into the Maxwell scheme. Derive its differential equation and the associated inequalities and show that the model represents the four-parameter solid.

1.6. For the three-parameter solid, express the constants p_1, q_0, q_1 in terms of the moduli of the two springs and the dashpot. Assume that the moduli of the springs are in the ratio of 10:1, the spring inside the Kelvin element having the lower modulus. Show that, for step loading, such a material behaves for some time almost like a Maxwell fluid, but ultimately turns out to be a solid.

References

The following works are surveys of the field and may serve for collateral reading

1. E.H. Lee: Viscoelastic Stress Analysis, in J.N. Goodier and N.J. Hoff (eds.) Structural Mechanics, Proceedings of the 1st Symposium on Naval Structural Mechanics, Stanford, 1958 (London, Pergamon, 1960), pp. 456-482.

2. D.R. Bland: The Theory of Linear Viscoelasticity (London, Pergamon, 1960). (Monograph on the subject contains many cases of stress analysis problems.)

3. R.M. Christensen: Theory of Viscoelasticity, an Introduction (New York, Academic Press, 1971). (Another monograph, mathematically more demanding than the present book.)

Spring-dashpot models are studied in the following report:

4. J.M. Burgers: Mechanical Considerations, Model Systems, Phenomenological Theories, in Akademie van Wetenschappen, First Report on Viscosity and Plasticity (Amsterdam: 1935), pp. 21-33.

The Laplace transformation is described in the following books, which should be consulted for depth and further detail:

5. R.V. Churchill: Operational Mathematics (3rd ed.)(New York, McGraw-Hill, 1972).

6. W.T. Thomson: Laplace Transformation (2nd ed.)(Englewood Cliffs, N.J., Prentice-Hall, 1960).

7. H.S. Carslaw and J.C. Jaeger: Operational Methods in Applied Mathematics (2nd ed.)(Oxford, Oxford University Press, 1947; also New York, Dover Publications, 1963).

8. E.J. Scott: Transform Calculus with an Introduction to Complex Variables (New York, Harper & Row, 1955).

9. C.R. Wylie: Advanced Engineering Mathematics (2nd ed.)(New York, McGraw-Hill, 1960), Chap. 8.

10. E.J. Scott: Laplace Transformation, in W. Flügge (ed.), Handbook of Engineering Mechanics (New York, McGraw-Hill, 1962), Chap. 19.

11. G. Doetsch: Guide to the Application of the Laplace and Z-Transforms (2nd ed.)(New York, Van Nostrand, 1971).

Tables of various size of Laplace transform pairs are contained in References [5] through [11], the largest among them with 261 entries in [11]. For farther going needs, the following tables may be used:

12. A. Erdélyi, W. Magnus, F. Oberhettinger and F. Tricomi: Tables of Integral Transforms (New York, McGraw-Hill, 1954), Vol. 1, Chaps. 4 and 5.

13. G.A. Campbell and R.M. Foster: Fourier Integrals for Practical Applications (Princeton, N.J., D. Van Nostrand, 1948). (With proper precautions, this table may be used for Laplace transforms. It is easy to use and contains much material.)

14. W. Magnus and F. Oberhettinger: Formeln und Sätze für die speziellen Funktionen der mathematischen Physik (Berlin, Springer-Verlag, 1943) pp. 122-136. (Part of a book containing much additional information about some of the exotic functions occurring as inverses of simple Laplace transforms.)

15. G. Doetsch: Tabellen zur Laplace-Transformation (Berlin, Springer-Verlag, 1947).

The discussion of the function $\mathcal{S}(s)$ on pp. 28-31 has been taken from the following dissertation, where further details may be found:

16. H. Ramsey: Problems of Related Elastic and Viscoelastic Buckling in one and two Dimensions. Ph. D. Diss., Stanford, 1962.

Chapter 2

Hereditary Integrals

Thus far, we have described viscoelastic materials by their differential equations. We shall now learn to describe them by another means, the hereditary integrals. Each of them can express all the facts contained in the differential equation (1.23) and even has the advantage of greater flexibility when it comes to rendering the measured properties of an actual material.

2.1 Creep Compliance, Relaxation Modulus

To study the behavior of viscoelastic models, we have used a standard test consisting of a creep phase and a relaxation phase. In the creep phase we applied a stress $\sigma = \sigma_0 \Delta(t)$ and calculated the time-dependent strain ϵ. Since we are considering only linear materials, the strain is always proportional to σ_0 and may be written as

$$\epsilon(t) = \sigma_0 J(t) . \tag{2.1}$$

The function $J(t)$ is the strain per unit of applied stress, and is different for each material. It describes, in a certain way, its stress-strain behavior, and we shall see soon that it describes it completely. For $t < 0$, $J(t) \equiv 0$, and since, under sustained load, a tension bar will never get shorter, $J(t)$ is for $t > 0$ a monotonically increasing function. It is called the *creep compliance*. In Table 1.2 it is listed for those materials which can be represented by simple models.

To obtain $J(t)$ from the differential equation of a material, we let $\sigma = \Delta(t)$ and $\epsilon = J(t)$, and solve for the latter with the initial condition that ϵ and all its derivatives (as far as needed) vanish for $t = 0^-$. This is most conveniently done with the help of the Laplace transformation, that is, by introducing $\bar{\sigma}(s) = s^{-1}$ in (1.25b) and solving it for $\bar{\epsilon} = \bar{J}(s)$. This yields

$$\bar{J}(s) = \frac{\mathcal{P}(s)}{s\mathcal{Q}(s)} \,. \tag{2.2}$$

The result is transformed back into the physical plane to yield $J(t)$. Since the quotient of two polynomials can always be split into partial fractions, the transformation pairs of Table 1.1 are sufficiently extensive in scope and $J(t)$ always appears as a sum of exponentials plus, possibly, a linear term.

As an example, take a Kelvin model consisting of three Kelvin units in series, as shown in Fig. 1.10a, but without the spring s and the dashpot d. It represents a solid and does not show impact response. Its differential equation must contain six parameters, among them q_0, and therefore must be

$$\sigma + p_1\dot{\sigma} + p_2\ddot{\sigma} = q_0\epsilon + q_1\dot{\epsilon} + q_2\ddot{\epsilon} + q_3\dddot{\epsilon} \,,$$

which is in agreement with the entry in Table 1.3. From (2.2) we find

$$\bar{J}(s) = \frac{1 + p_1 s + p_2 s^2}{s(q_0 + q_1 s + q_2 s^2 + q_3 s^3)} \,.$$

This may be split into partial fractions if the roots of the denominator are known. Let

$$q_0 + q_1 s + q_2 s^2 + q_3 s^3 = q_3(s - \lambda_1)(s - \lambda_2)(s - \lambda_3) \,,$$

then

$$\bar{J}(s) = \frac{1}{q_3}\,\frac{1}{s}\left(\frac{a_1}{s - \lambda_1} + \frac{a_2}{s - \lambda_2} + \frac{a_3}{s - \lambda_3}\right) ,$$

where

$$a_1 = \frac{1 + p_1\lambda_1 + p_2\lambda_1^2}{(\lambda_1 - \lambda_2)(\lambda_1 - \lambda_3)} \,, \quad \text{etc.}$$

Using the transform pair (4) of Table 1.1, one finds

$$J(t) = \frac{1}{q_3} \sum_{n=1}^{3} \frac{a_n}{-\lambda_n} \left(1 - e^{\lambda_n t}\right).$$

Obviously, the exponentials must be decreasing functions of time, and this requires that $\lambda_1, \lambda_2, \lambda_3 < 0$. One of the inequalities that can be found by a detailed analysis of the model guarantees that this is the case.

We may invert the procedure which led to $J(t)$, prescribing $\epsilon = \epsilon_0 \Delta(t)$ and asking for the corresponding stress. This amounts to applying at $t = 0$ whatever stress is needed (possibly even a Dirac spike) to produce the desired extension, then fixing the terminals of the model or the ends of the tension bar and watching what stress will develop. Since the equations are linear, σ will be proportional to ϵ_0:

$$\sigma(t) = \epsilon_0 Y(t). \tag{2.3}$$

The function $Y(t)$ is called the relaxation modulus and is always a monotonically decreasing or, at least, a nonincreasing function of time. Letting $\bar{\epsilon} = s^{-1}$ and $\bar{\sigma} = \bar{Y}(s)$ in (1.25b) leads to

$$\bar{Y}(s) = \frac{\mathcal{Q}(s)}{s\mathcal{P}(s)}, \tag{2.4}$$

from which $Y(t)$ may be found.

The relaxation modulus and the creep compliance are connected by a simple relation between their Laplace transforms, which results from a comparison of (2.2) and (2.4):

$$\bar{J}(s)\bar{Y}(s) = s^{-2}. \tag{2.5}$$

Formulas for the relaxation moduli of simple materials have been listed in Table 1.2. As may be seen there, $Y(t)$ contains a Dirac function if the material is lacking impact response. This is quite understandable, because if a finite stress is not sufficient to produce at once a finite strain, an infinite one will be needed.

It should be noted that by their very definition both $J(t)$ and $Y(t)$ are zero for all $t < 0$, and that the formulas given in Table 1.2 are therefore applicable only for $t > 0$.

2.2 Hereditary Integrals

Since all our materials are linear, we may use the rule of linear superposition to calculate the strain produced by the common action of several loads. For the tension bars considered thus far, "several loads" cannot mean anything but tensile stresses of different magnitudes applied successively. As an example, consider the case shown in Fig. 2.1. At $t = 0$ a stress σ_0 is applied suddenly, which produces

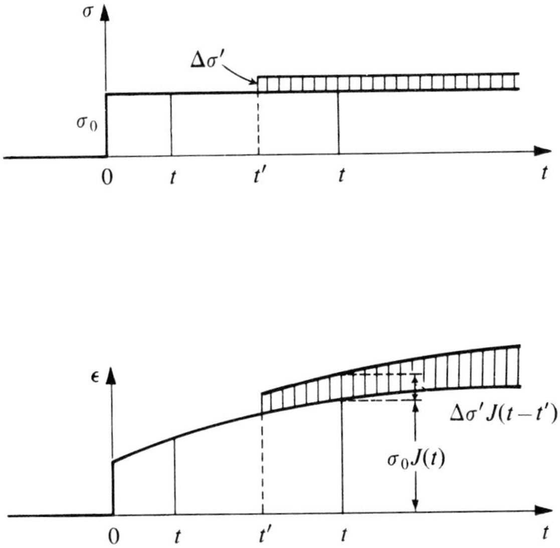

Figure 2.1. Linear superposition of step inputs.

a strain $\epsilon = \sigma_0 J(t)$. If the stress σ_0 is maintained unchanged, this equation will describe the strain for the entire future; but if, at $t = t'$, some more stress is added, then for $t > t'$ additional strain will be produced which is proportional to $\Delta\sigma'$ and which depends on the same creep compliance. However, for this additional strain, time is measured by a clock that starts running at $t = t'$. The total strain for $t > t'$ is, therefore,

$$\epsilon(t) = \sigma_0 J(t) + \Delta\sigma' J(t - t').$$

From this equation it is but one step to a very general case. Assume that, as before, a stress σ_0 is suddenly applied at $t = 0$, but that σ

then varies as an arbitrary function $\sigma(t)$. As shown in Fig.2.2, this stress diagram can be broken up into the basic part $\sigma_0 \Delta(t)$ and a sequence of infinitesimal step functions $d\sigma' \cdot \Delta(t - t')$ where $d\sigma' = (d\sigma/dt)_{t=t'}\, dt'$, which we shall write as $(d\sigma'/dt')dt'$. The corresponding strain at time t is then the sum of the strain caused by all the steps that have taken place at times $t' < t$, that is,

$$\varepsilon(t) = \sigma_0 J(t) + \int_0^t J(t - t') \frac{d\sigma'}{dt'}\, dt'. \tag{2.6a}$$

This formula shows how the strain at any given time depends on all that has happened before - on the entire stress history $\sigma'(t'), t' < t$. This is quite different from what happens in an elastic material, whose strain depends at any time solely on the stress acting at that time.

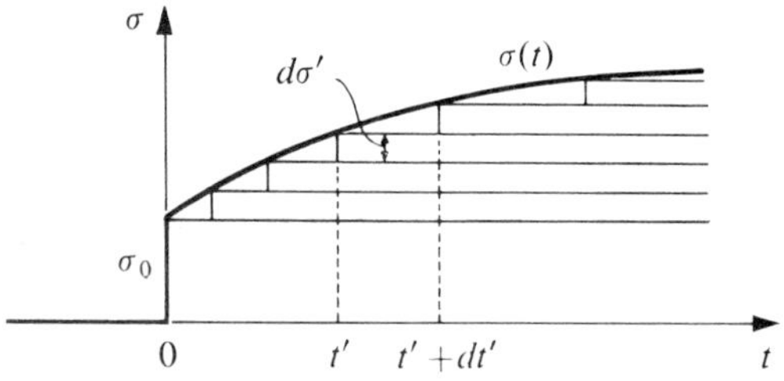

Figure 2.2. Derivation of the hereditary integral.

The integral in (2.6a) is called a hereditary integral. Through integration by parts it may be brought into another, often useful form:

$$\varepsilon(t) = \sigma_0 J(t) + \Big[J(t - t') \cdot \sigma(t')\Big]_0^t - \int_0^t \sigma(t') \frac{dJ(t - t')}{dt'}\, dt'.$$

It should be noted that all the zeros in these equations mean 0^+. Therefore when the bracketed boundary term is evaluated, it combines with the first term. On the other hand, we may write $dJ(t - t')/dt' =$ $= -dJ(t - t')/d(t - t')$ and thus arrive at the following, second version of the hereditary integral:

$$\varepsilon(t) = \sigma(t)J(0) + \int_0^t \sigma(t') \frac{dJ(t-t')}{d(t-t')}\, dt'. \tag{2.6b}$$

While (2.6a) separates the strains caused by the initial load σ_0 and by later load increases, (2.6b) shows the strain that would occur if the total stress σ were applied right now at t, and the additional strain stemming from the fact that much or all of the stress has been applied earlier and has had time to produce some creep.

The hereditary integral (2.6a) may be subjected to some formal changes which, at times, make it easier to use. First, since $J(t) = 0$ for all $t < 0$, it does not make any difference if the upper limit of the integral is raised above $t' = t$, even to $t' = \infty$, since in the added integration interval $J(t - t')$ has a negative argument. If this change is made in the upper limit, it must, of course, not be forgotten that any analytic expressions for $J(t)$ - for example, those listed in Table 1.2 - are not valid for negative arguments.

Another formal change may be made as follows: Instead of $(d\sigma'/dt')dt'$ we may simply write $d\sigma'$ or $d\sigma(t')$ and integrate over all increments of stress, using with each one the proper time t' in the argument of $J(t - t')$. It then makes no difference when many increments $d\sigma'$ occur in rapid succession or even all at the same time, adding up to a finite step $\Delta\sigma_1$ at some time $t = t_1$. We may then also absorb the initial step σ_0 into the integral, and even move its lower limit to $t' = -\infty$, since for $t' < 0$ there is no $\sigma(t')$ and hence no contribution to the integral. In this way we arrive at the following form of the hereditary integral:

$$\epsilon(t) = \int_{t'=-\infty}^{t'=+\infty} J(t - t')\, d\sigma(t') \,. \tag{2.6c}$$

Integrals of this form are known as S t i e l t j e s i n t e g r a l s .

As an example, we may consider the stress history of Fig. 2.3. With $\sigma_0 = 0$ and $\sigma = \sigma_1 t/t_1$ we find from (2.6b) for a Maxwell material in the range $t < t_1$:

$$\epsilon(t) = \frac{\sigma_1 t}{t_1} \cdot \frac{p_1}{q_1} + \frac{\sigma_1}{t_1} \int_0^t t' \cdot \frac{1}{q_1} dt' = \frac{\sigma_1}{q_1 t_1} \left(p_1 t + \frac{t^2}{2} \right) .$$

For $t > t_1$, the integral must be broken into two parts:

$$\epsilon(t) = \sigma_1 \cdot \frac{p_1}{q_1} + \frac{\sigma_1}{t_1}\int_0^{t_1} t' \cdot \frac{1}{q_1}\, dt' + \sigma_1 \int_{t_1}^{t} \frac{1}{q_1}\, dt' = \frac{\sigma_1}{q_1}\left(p_1 - \frac{t_1}{2} + t\right).$$

If the total stress σ_1 had been applied suddenly at $t = t_1$, the strain would be

$$\epsilon(t) = \sigma_1 J(t - t_1) = \frac{\sigma_1}{q_1}(p_1 + t - t_1),$$

which is less, and if the load had been applied all at once at $t = 0$, we would have

$$\epsilon(t) = \sigma_1 J(t) = \frac{\sigma_1}{q_1}(p_1 + t),$$

which is more. The differences between these three load histories will be felt undiminished no matter how much time elapses.

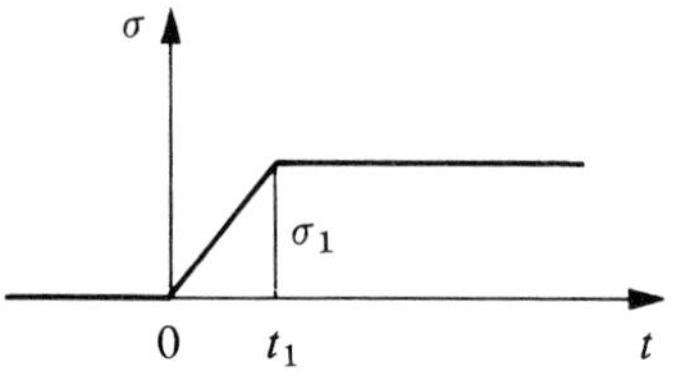

Figure 2.3. Stress history.

A quite different result is found for the Kelvin material. With $\sigma(t)$ from Fig. 2.3, we then have for $t > t_1$:

$$\epsilon(t) = \frac{\sigma_1}{t_1 q_1}\int_0^{t_1} t' e^{-q_0(t-t')/q_1}\, dt' + \frac{\sigma_1}{q_1}\int_{t_1}^{t} e^{-q_0(t-t')/q_1}\, dt'$$

$$= \frac{\sigma_1}{q_0}\left[1 + \frac{q_1}{q_0 t_1}\left(1 - e^{q_0 t_1/q_1}\right) e^{-q_0 t/q_1}\right].$$

For $t \to \infty$, this goes to $\epsilon = \sigma_1/q_0$, and the same limit would be approached if σ_1 were to be applied suddenly at $t = t_1$ or at $t = 0$, that is, the differences of stress history are wiped out if enough time has elapsed. The two examples show the typical difference between fluid and solid behavior.

The hereditary integrals (2.6a-c) have been derived from the definition of the creep compliance contained in (2.1). A similar argument may start from the concept of the relaxation modulus Y(t) in (2.3). If

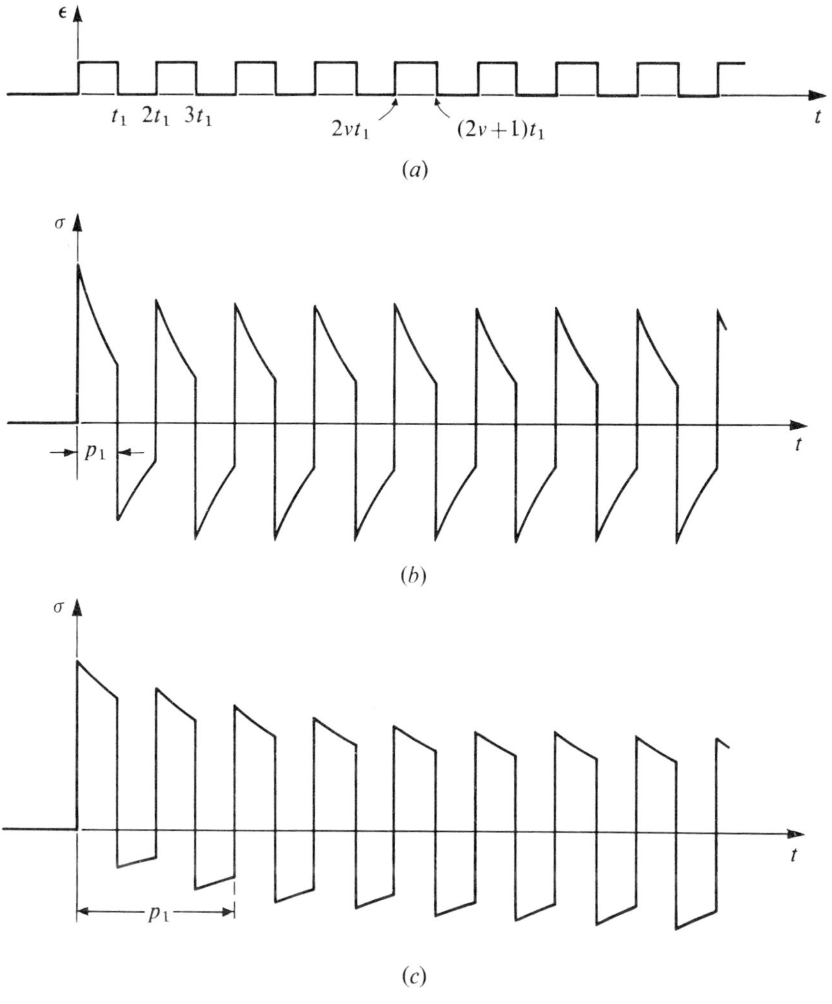

Figure 2.4. Maxwell material - a: prescribed strain history; b,c: stress histories for t_1/p_1 = 1.0 and 0.25, respectively.

the strain of a tension bar is known as a function of time (strain history) the stress follows from

$$\sigma(t) = \epsilon_0 Y(t) + \int_0^t Y(t-t')\frac{d\epsilon'}{dt'}\,dt' \tag{2.7a}$$

$$= \epsilon(t)Y(0) + \int_0^t \epsilon(t')\frac{dY(t-t')}{d(t-t')}\,dt' \tag{2.7b}$$

$$= \int_{t'=-\infty}^{t'=+\infty} Y(t-t')\,d\epsilon(t')\,. \tag{2.7c}$$

The following example illustrates the use of (2.7a-c). The ends of a tension bar made of a Maxwell material are moved so as to produce the strain history shown in Fig.2.4a. To calculate the ensuing stress, we apply (2.7b). The term before the integral is either $= \epsilon_0 q_1/p_1$ or $= 0$, depending on whether the bar is stretched or not. At $t = (2nt_1)^-$, that is, immediately before a new cycle of stretching and unstretching begins, the integral yields

$$\sigma = \sum_{\nu=0}^{n-1} \int_{2\nu t_1}^{(2\nu+1)t_1} \frac{-q_1\epsilon_0}{p_1^2} \exp\left(-(2nt_1 - t')/p_1\right)dt'\,.$$

which may be evaluated by first performing the integration and then summing a geometric series. The result is

$$\sigma = -\frac{\epsilon_0 q_1}{p_1}\,\frac{1 - e^{-2nt_1/p_1}}{1 + e^{t_1/p_1}}\,.$$

Similarly, (2.7b) may be evaluated for other points t within each cycle The result is shown in Fig.2.4b and c for two choices of t_1 in terms of the relaxation time p_1 of the material. One sees how the bar adjusts itself to a system of alternating positive and negative stresses of the same magnitude. If $t_1 = p_1$, the steady state has almost been reached after four cycles, while for $t_1 = 0.25p_1$ more cycles are needed.

2.3 Integral Equations

The differential equation (1.23) describes a viscoelastic material completely. If the stress history $\sigma(t)$ is known, we may solve (1.23) for $\varepsilon(t)$, and if the strain history is known, we may use the same equation to find the stress.

We shall now see that each of the hereditary integrals (2.6) and (2.7), taken alone, can do the same service. Let us assume that $\sigma(t)$ is known. Then (2.6b) obviously leads to $\varepsilon(t)$, and we used it in this way when we calculated the strain produced by the stress history of Fig.2.3. Now let $\varepsilon(t)$ be known and $\sigma(t)$ be unknown. Then (2.6b) has the form

$$\sigma(t) + \int_0^t \sigma(t')\,K(t,t')\,dt' = f(t), \tag{2.8}$$

where $f(t) = \varepsilon(t)/J(0)$ and the kernel

$$K(t,t') = \frac{1}{J(0)}\,\frac{dJ(t-t')}{d(t-t')}$$

are known fuctions of their arguments. Equation (2.8) is called an integral equation, more precisely an integral equation of the second kind of the Volterra type[1]. It has a unique solution and thus determines the stress when the strain is known. We shall later repeatedly encounter Volterra's integral equation, and then learn more about it. At present it suffices to know that knowledge of one function, $J(t)$, through the double use of (2.6), permits finding ε from σ and σ from ε, that is, that this function describes the material as completely as does the differential equation (1.23). The same statement applies to the relaxation modulus $Y(t)$, since the hereditary integral (2.7) can be used "forward" to find $\sigma(t)$ from $\varepsilon(t)$ and "backward", that is, as an integral equation, to find ε from σ.

---

[1] In an integral equation of the first kind the term $\sigma(t)$ outside the integral is missing. In the Volterra type the upper limit of the integral is the independent variable t.

Problems

2.1. The right end A of a Scotch yoke mechanism (Fig. 2.5) has the horizontal displacement $r \sin \omega t$. At $t = 0$ it makes contact for the first time with the left end B of the viscoelastic bar BC. Find the stress in the bar as a function of time. At what time do the points A and B cease to be in contact? What happens next? Continue the investigation to cover many periods of the motion of the yoke. The problem may be solved in general terms or for a Maxwell or Kelvin material.

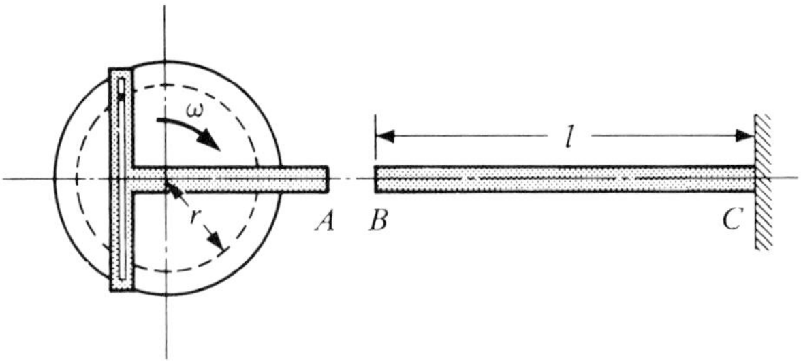

Figure 2.5.

2.2. A viscoelastic material is represented by a chain of three Kelvin elements. Let q be a reference constant of the dimension of a stress and T a reference time, and assume the following viscoelastic coefficients for the Kelvin elements: first element $q_0 = 2q$, $q_1 = 2qT$; second element: $q_0 = q$, $q_1 = 4qT$; third element: $q_0 = 1.5q$, $q_1 = 16.5qT$. Find $\bar{J}(s)$ and from it $J(t)$. Then calculate and plot $\epsilon(t)$ for the following two stress histories:

$$\text{(i)} \quad \sigma = \sigma_0[\Delta(t) - \Delta(t - 0.8T)].$$

$$\text{(ii)} \quad \sigma = \sigma_0[\Delta(t) - \Delta(t - 3T)].$$

Study on the graphs to which extent the different Kelvin elements get into action.

2.3. For the same material as in the preceding problem, find $\bar{Y}(s)$ and then $Y(t)$. Is the material solid or fluid? Does it have impact response?

References

Hereditary integrals are discussed to some extent in most of the references given in Chapter 1; see [1], p. 462. See also the following handbook article:

17. E.H. Lee: Viscoelasticity, in W. Flügge (ed.), Handbook of Engineering Mechanics (New York, McGraw-Hill, 1962), Chap. 53, pp. 8-9.

The following sources may be consulted for integral equations. They will be useful to readers who wish to go beyond the few simple facts needed for the understanding of this book:

18. W.V. Lovitt: Linear Integral Equations (New York, Dover Publications, 1950).

19. F.B. Hildebrand: Methods of Applied Mathematics (Englewood Cliffs, N.J., Prentice-Hall, 1952), Chap. 4.

20. M.A. Heaslet: Integral equations, in W. Flügge (ed.), Handbook of Engineering Mechanics, (New York, McGraw-Hill, 1962), Chap. 17.

Chapter 3

Viscoelastic Beams

We are now prepared to solve some simple stress problems involving a viscoelastic material. The subject of our study will be a structure, that is, a deformable body of known shape to which external forces, the loads, are applied. We shall use the term "structure" to cover anything, as simple as a tension bar or as complicated as an entire bridge or an entire airplane. The structures to be considered in this chapter are straight beams of constant cross section, but the results obtained apply to any structure in uni-axial stress.

3.1 The Correspondence Principle

For any structure the general problem of stress analysis is this: Given the dimensions and the material of the structure and a set of loads applied to it, what are the stresses in it and how will it be deformed? Very often only part of the complete problem is solved. In many cases only the stresses are of interest and the deformation is either not asked for at all or is investigated only to the extent that it influences the stress distribution, as for example in statically indeterminate structures.

The general problem is the same for elastic and for viscoelastic structures. In both cases the three basic sets of equations must be satisfied; the equilibrium conditions, the kinematic relations, and the constitutive equations, as explained on p. 2, the only difference being that for viscoelastic structures Hooke's law is to be replaced by another equation.

Since we have, so far, formulated the viscoelastic law only for the case of uni-axial tension or compression, we must restrict here our attention to structures in which only uni-axial stress occurs. Besides simple tension and compression members, these are trusses and beams. For these the constitutive equation is a single relation between the stress σ and the strain ϵ, and we may choose either the differential equation (1.23) or one of the hereditary integrals (2.6) or (2.7).

Obviously, we could easily extend the scope of our operations to the torsion of prismatic bars and of circular shafts of variable diameter [21], since in these cases the stress system consists at each point of one pair of shear stresses τ_{ij} and for these and the corresponding shear strain γ_{ij} we might write a constitutive equation of the same kind. Of course, the numerical values of the coefficients p_k, q_k and the fuctions $J(t)$ and $Y(t)$ would be different. This chapter, however, will be restricted to the study of beams.

Consider first an elastic beam carrying certain loads P_i, $i = 1, 2, \ldots$ There are bending stresses $\sigma(x,y,z)$ that satisfy the equilibrium conditions for every element of the beam. Then there are strains $\epsilon(x,y,z)$, which (i) are connected with the stresses by Hooke's law

$$\epsilon(x,y,z) = \sigma(x,y,z)/E$$

and which (ii) are so distributed that plane cross sections remain plane and that the beam curvature calculated from them yields, after two integrations, a deflection $w(x)$ that satisfies all support conditions.

Now consider a beam of the same shape, but made of a viscoelastic material. Assume that the same loads are applied to it at $t = 0$ and then held constant, that is, that the beam carries the loads

$$P_i(t) = P_i\,\Delta(t).$$

Consider as a tentative solution of its stress problem the time-dependent stresses

$$\sigma(x,y,z;t) = \sigma(x,y,z)\Delta(t),$$

where σ on the right-hand side is the stress in the elastic beam. In the viscoelastic material there would then be strains

$$\epsilon(x,y,z;t) = \sigma(x,y,z)J(t).$$

At any time t they would be distributed like the strains in an elastic beam of modulus $E = 1/J(t)$, and hence they would satisfy all the kinematic conditions of the problem. From this we conclude that our tentative solution is the correct solution for the viscoelastic beam, and we have the following first version of the correspondence principle: If a viscoelastic beam is subjected to loads which are all applied simultaneously at $t = 0$ and then held constant, its stresses are the same as those in an elastic beam under the same load, and its strains and displacements depend on time and are derived from those of the elastic problem by replacing E by $1/J(t)$.

Now let us turn to a beam problem in which not the loads but the displacements of selected points are prescribed. As an example, we might think of a cantilever beam whose free end is suddenly deflected by a certain amount w_0 and then held in this position. For a tentative solution, we start from the deflections $w(x)$ of the elastic beam. Through certain kinematic relations they are connected with strains $\epsilon(x,y,z)$ and through Hooke's law with stresses $\sigma(x,y,z)$, which satisfy all equilibrium conditions. If we adopt for the viscoelastic beam deflections $w(x,t) = w(x) \cdot \Delta(t)$ and strains

$$\epsilon(x,y,z;t) = \epsilon(x,y,z)\Delta(t),$$

they will satisfy the kinematic conditions and also our boundary condition prescribing the displacement $w_0 \cdot \Delta(t)$ at the end. In the viscoelastic beam these strains would be accompanied by stresses

$$\sigma(x,y,z;t) = \epsilon(x,y,z)Y(t)$$

which, being proportional to the elastic stresses, would satisfy the same zero-load equilibrium conditions and hence would be acceptable for the viscoelastic beam. This leads us to the second version of the correspondence principle: If a viscoelastic beam is subjected to forced displacements of certain points, which are all imposed at $t = 0$ and then held constant, the displacements of all points and all the strains are the same as in the corresponding elastic beam, and the stresses are derived from those of the elastic problem by multiplying them by $Y(t)/E$.

Both forms of the correspondence principle apply in the same form to trusses and to beam structures like portal frames and arches. They may be extended to the torsion problem mentioned before if E is replaced by the shear modulus G, and J(t) and Y(t) are replaced by the shear creep compliance and the shear relaxation modulus.

As an example consider the beam shown in Fig.3.1. It is originally straight, and at t = 0 a deflection w_0 is forced upon its midspan point.

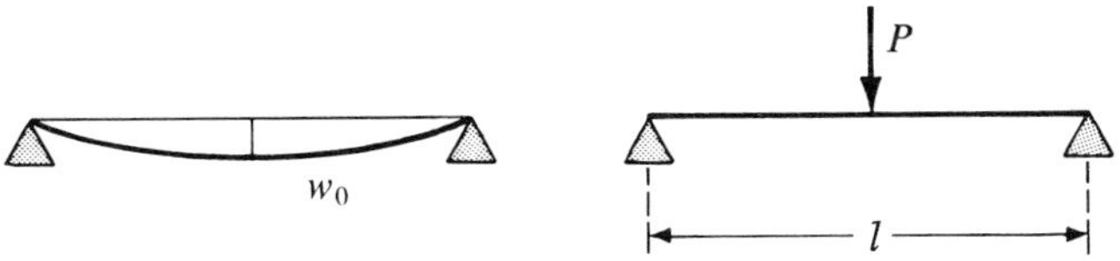

Figure 3.1. Viscoelastic beam with prescribed deflection w_0.

To do this, a still unknown force P is needed. For an elastic beam we may find in any handbook the relation

$$w_0 = \frac{Pl^3}{48\,EI} .$$

We solve for P and replace E by the relaxation modulus to find

$$P = \frac{48\,Iw_0}{l^3}\,Y(t) .$$

Using formulas from Table 1.2, the results plotted in Fig.3.2 may be obtained.

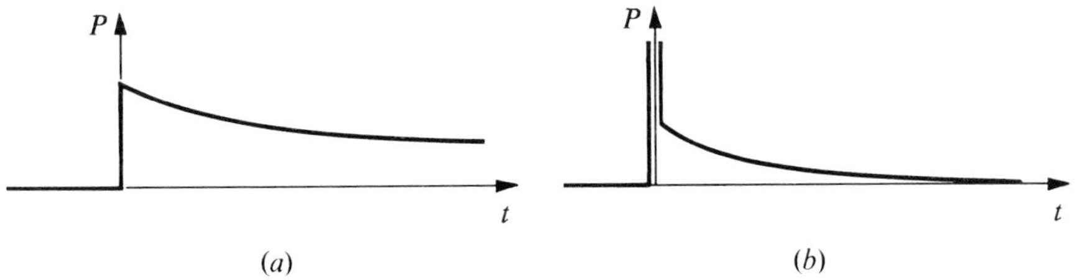

Figure 3.2. Force P needed for the beam in Figure 3.1 - a: three-parameter solid; b: three-parameter fluid.

If the beam material is a three-parameter solid, the force needed to hold the beam is less than the one needed for first pushing it down, both being connected by a gradual transition.

The three-parameter fluid does not at once deform under a finite load, and a Dirac spike

$$P = \frac{48\, Iw_0}{l^3} \frac{q_2}{p_1} \delta(t)$$

is needed to make the beam deflect; but after a length of time the force needed to hold it down relaxes and tends to zero. The beam "gets used" to being bent and will not spring back when released if it has been held down long enough.

3.2 Hereditary Integrals

Let $\mathfrak{w}(x)$ be the deflection of a beam under a load $p(x)$, assuming an elastic material of modulus $E = 1$. Then, because of the correspondence principle,

$$w(x,t) = \mathfrak{w}(x) J(t)$$

is the deflection for the same beam, but made of a viscoelastic material and subjected to the step fuction load $p(x,t) = p(x) \cdot \Delta(t)$. We may easily generalize this statement to an arbitrary load history

$$p(x,t) = p(x) f(t)$$

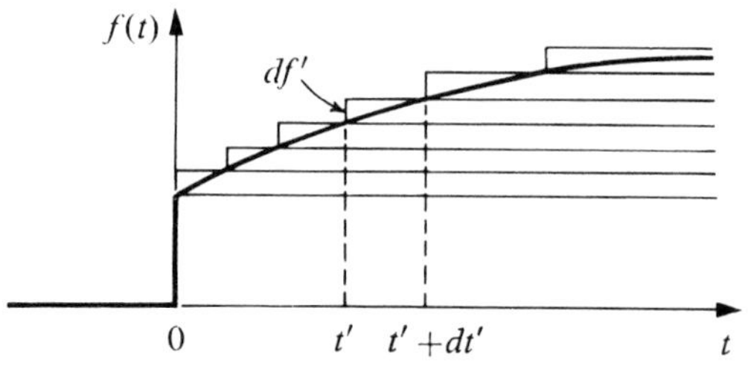

Figure 3.3. Hereditary integral for beams.

by breaking it down into a sequence of infinitesimal steps as shown in Fig.3.3. We have then

$$w(x,t) = \mathfrak{w}(x) \left[f(0^+) \cdot J(t) + \int_{0^+}^{t} J(t-t') \frac{df(t')}{dt'} dt' \right], \qquad (3.1a)$$

which is the same hereditary integral as (2.6a). Integration by parts will bring it again into the form

$$w(x,t) = \mathfrak{w}(x)\left[f(t)J(0^+) + \int_{0^+}^{t} f(t')\,\frac{dJ(t-t')}{d(t-t')}\,dt' \right], \qquad (3.1b)$$

and a form corresponding to (2.6c) is also possible.

As an example, consider a beam carrying a uniform load p, but with one of the histories shown in Fig. 3.4b,c. The elastic deflection with E = 1 is

$$\mathfrak{w}(x) = \frac{16\,\mathfrak{w}_0}{5l^4}\,(x^4 - 2lx^3 + l^3x)\,,$$

where

$$\mathfrak{w}_0 = \frac{5\bar{p}l^4}{384\,I}$$

is the midspan deflection. For the load history of Fig. 3.4b we find from (3.1a) for $0 < t < t_1$:

$$w(\tfrac{1}{2}l, t) = \frac{5\bar{p}l^4}{384\,It_1}\int_{0^+}^{t} J(t-t')\,dt'$$

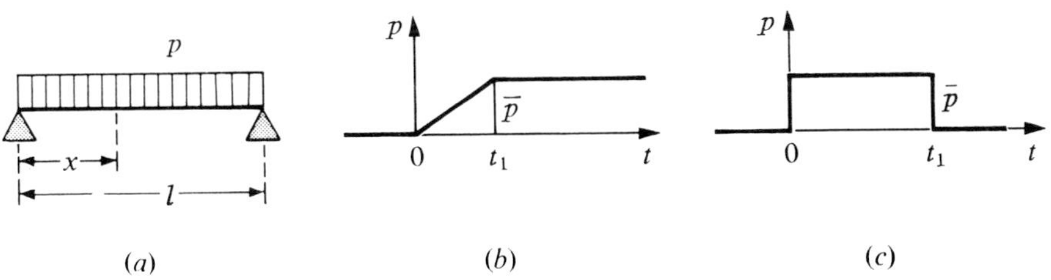

Figure 3.4. Beam with two load histories.

and for $t > t_1$:

$$w(\tfrac{1}{2}l, t) = \frac{5\bar{p}l^4}{384\,It_1}\int_{0^+}^{t_1} J(t-t')\,dt'\,.$$

For a Kelvin material, evaluation of the integrals yields the following formulas, which lead to the curves shown in Fig.3.5a:
for $0 < t < t_1$:

$$w(\tfrac{1}{2}l,t) = \frac{5\bar{p}l^4}{384\, Iq_0 t_1}\left[t - \frac{q_1}{q_0}(1 - e^{-\lambda t})\right]$$

and for $t > t_1$:

$$w(\tfrac{1}{2}l,t) = \frac{5\bar{p}l^4}{384\, Iq_0 t_1}\left[t_1 - \frac{q_1}{q_0}\left(e^{\lambda t_1} - 1\right)e^{-\lambda t}\right].$$

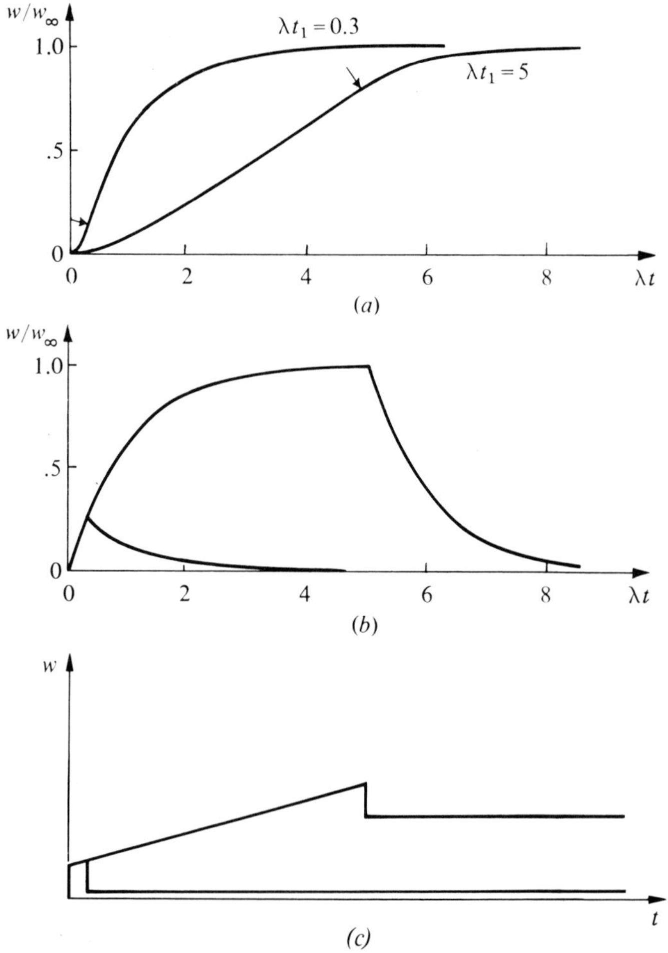

Figure 3.5. Deflection of the beam shown in Fig.3.4a - a: load history of Fig.3.4b, Kelvin material; b, c: load history of Fig.3.4c, Kelvin and Maxwell materials.

The two curves represent extreme cases. The time $\lambda^{-1} = q_1/q_0$ is characteristic for the creep of the material. It is the time at which the initial tangent to the creep curve in Fig.1.5b reaches the asymptote $\epsilon = \epsilon_\infty$. If $\lambda t_1 = 0.3$, the time t_1 needed for applying the full load $\bar{p}$ is only a fraction of λ^{-1}, and therefore not much deformation takes place during this time. Of the ultimate deflection, 86% comes from creep under full load. The behavior of the beam approaches the case of sudden loading. The second curve in Fig.3.5a belongs to a load that is very gently applied. After a short transient the deflection increases almost linearly with the load, reaching 80% of its ultimate value when the loading is accomplished.

Now to the load history of Fig.3.4c. In this case we use (3.1b) and find for $0 < t < t_1$:

$$w(\tfrac{1}{2}l, t) = \frac{5\bar{p}l^4}{384I}\left[J(0) + \int_0^t \frac{dJ(t-t')}{d(t-t')}\,dt'\right] = \frac{5\bar{p}l^4}{384I}J(t),$$

a result which we might have obtained more easily by applying the correspondence principle for step loading, and for $t > t_1$:

$$w(\tfrac{1}{2}l, t) = \frac{5\bar{p}l^4}{384I}\int_0^{t_1} \frac{dJ(t-t')}{d(t-t')}\,dt' = \frac{5\bar{p}l^4}{384I}(J(t) - J(t-t_1)).$$

A plot of the deflection for a Kelvin beam is shown in Fig.3.5b. If, compared with λ^{-1}, the load is only for a short time on the beam, not much happens; but if t_1 is substantially larger than λ^{-1}, the loading and unloading are clearly separated phenomena.

Figure 3.5c shows the corresponding behavior of a Maxwell beam. As long as the load is present the deflection increases at an even rate; and when the load is removed it at once drops by a certain amount and then remains constant.

Since in all these examples the load was prescribed, the bending moments and the stresses are exactly the same as in an elastic beam, while the deformation is controlled by a hereditary integral. The opposite is true when we prescribe the deflection at one or several points of the structure. Consider the case shown in Fig.3.6a. A beam is supported at three points and carries some load, in which we are not interested since we can evaluate its effect separately and superpose it to the solution that we are about to study here. Under the influence of this load and the ensuing reaction at B, this support sinks slowly and steadily until it has reached a certain displacement w_0, that is, we have

$$\text{for} \quad 0 < t < w_0/c: \qquad w_B = ct ,$$
$$\text{for} \quad t > w_0/c: \qquad w_B = w_0 . \tag{3.2a,b}$$

This function may be represented by a diagram, Fig.3.6b, and may be resolved into a sequence of step functions

$$dw'_B = c\,\Delta(t - t')dt' \quad 0 < t' < w_0/c ,$$

as we have done before. We may then expect that the beam deflects exactly as an elastic beam would do under the same circumstances, and that all stresses, bending moments, shear forces, and reactions are controlled by hereditary integrals of the type (2.7). In particular, the deflection dw'_B would, in an elastic beam, produce at B the reaction

$$dR'_B = \frac{6EI}{l^3}\, dw'_B$$

and in a viscoelastic beam

$$dR'_B = \frac{6I}{l^3}\, Y(t - t')\, \frac{dw'_B}{dt'}\, dt' .$$

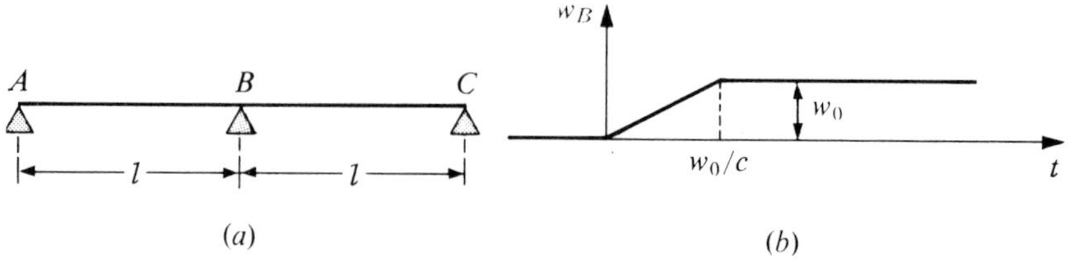

Figure 3.6. Continuous beam - a: the beam; b: prescribed displacement of support B.

Introduction of dw_B' from (3.2) and integration yields

$$R_B = \frac{6\,Ic}{l^3} \int_0^{w_0/c} Y(t - t')\,dt' . \qquad (3.3)$$

For $t < w_0/c$, one might argue that the upper limit of the integral should rather be t; however, for values of $t' > t$, the relaxation modulus has negative argument and hence equals zero.

To illustrate this formula, we evaluate it for the two simplest materials, using the formulas for $Y(t)$ given in Table 1.2.

For the Maxwell material we find for $t < w_0/c$:

$$R_B = \frac{6\,Ic}{l^3}\frac{q_1}{p_1}\int_0^t e^{-(t-t')/p_1}\,dt' = \frac{6\,Icq_1}{l^3}\left(1 - e^{-t/p_1}\right),$$

and for $t > w_0/c$:

$$R_B = \frac{6\,Icq_1}{l^3}\left(e^{w_0/cp_1} - 1\right)e^{-t/p_1} .$$

This is represented in Fig. 3.7 for two values of the speed c with which the deflection is produced. The maximum of R_B, and hence of all bending moments and of all stresses, occurs when the maximum deflection has just been reached; thereafter the beam relaxes and will ultimately be without stress. Each of the last pair of formulas is applicable at $t = w_0/c$ and yields

$$R_{B\max} = \frac{6\,Icq_1}{l^3}\left(1 - e^{-w_0/cp_1}\right) .$$

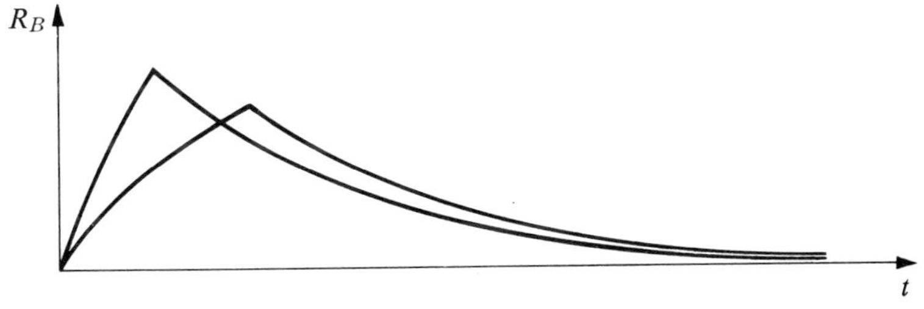

Figure 3.7. Reaction at B for the beam in Fig. 3.6.

This maximum depends on c and increases as c is increased. When the total deflection w_B is produced instantaneously, that is, for $c \to \infty$, the right-hand side is an indefinite expression. Expanding the exponential, we find

$$R_{B\max} = \frac{6\,Iq_1}{l^3}\,c\left[1 - 1 + \frac{w_0}{cp_1} - \frac{1}{2}\left(\frac{w_0}{cp_1}\right)^2 + - \cdots\right]$$

and in the limit

$$R_{B\max} = \frac{6\,Iq_1}{l^3 p_1}\,w_0\,.$$

The example shows how, in a Maxwell beam, the same deflection needs less force the slower it is applied.

For a Kelvin beam a similar integration yields for $t < w_0/c$:

$$R_B = \frac{6\,Ic}{l^3}\int_0^{t^+}(q_0 + q_1\delta(t - t'))dt' = \frac{6\,Ic}{l^3}(q_0 t + q_1),$$

for $t > w_0/c$:

$$R_B = \frac{6\,Ic}{l^3}\int_0^{w_0/c} q_0\,dt' = \frac{6\,Iq_0}{l^3}\,w_0\,.$$

It is left to the reader to plot and discuss this result.

3.3 Structures Made of Two Materials

In the foregoing examples we used different forms of the correspondence principle, that is, we replaced the actual structure by one of the same dimensions, but made of an elastic material, and then we replaced in all formulas the modulus E by $1/J(t)$ or $Y(t)$ or by an integral operator. This procedure is no longer possible when more than one material is involved. We shall now see what can be done in such cases.

Figure 3.8a shows a continuous beam resting on two rigid supports A and C and on a deformable support B. We assume that the beam is made of some viscoelastic material described by the differential equation (1.23) or by the creep compliance J(t) or the relaxation modulus Y(t), and that the spring is elastic and has the spring constant k.

The beam may carry any load. To keep the equations simple, the symmetric load arrangement shown in the figure is chosen and the loads are assumed to be applied suddenly at t = 0.

This beam is statically indeterminate, that is, the reactions at A, B, and C, and hence the bending moments in the beam, cannot be cal-

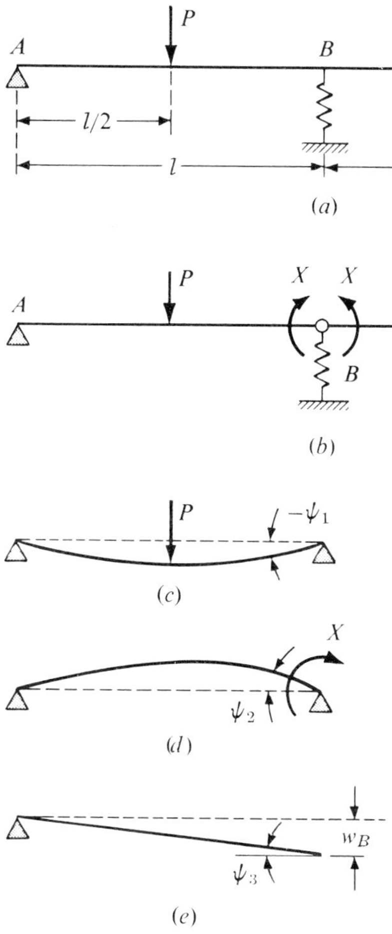

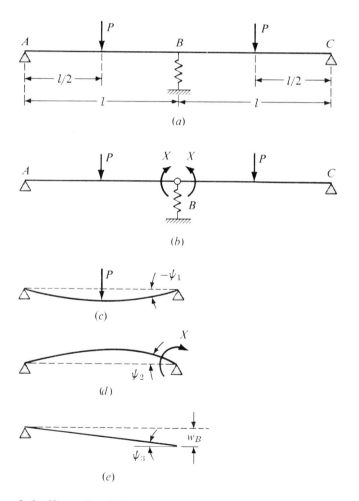

Figure 3.8. Viscoelastic beam on elastic support - a: actual system; b: primary system; c-e: deformation of the primary system.

culated from the equilibrium conditions alone, but depend on the deformation of the structure. There are several methods of dealing with statically indeterminate structures. We choose the one based on a primary system as shown in Fig. 3.8b. This system differs from the actual structure by the presence of a frictionless hinge at B. This has two important consequences: (i) While in the actual continuous beam there is a certain bending moment M_B in the cross section at B, the primary structure, because of the hinge, has at this point a zero moment - unless we apply external couples X as shown to the ends of the beams AB and BC. If we do so, we have $M_B = -X$. (ii) In the actual structure, the tangent to the deflection line has at every point a unique direction. This is not true at the point B of the primary structure, where the ends of the two adjacent spans can and usually do have different slopes. Evidently, the stresses and the deformation of the primary structure (b) and of the actual system (a) will be the same if the magnitude of X is such that there is no discontinuity in the slope of the deflection line at B.

Since the primary structure consists of two simple beams AB and BC, we can easily calculate its deformation. It consists of three parts: (i) the bending of the beams caused by the load P, (ii) the bending of the beams caused by the external couples X, and (iii) the compression of the spring support. The first two of these are deformations of the viscoelastic part of the structure, and hence they are subject to the correspondence principle.

We calculate the slope of the right end of the left beam and call it positive when it represents a clockwise rotation of the tangent from the undeformed into the deformed position. Figures 3.8c-e show the three contributions.

Let I be the moment of inertial of the beam's cross section; then, for an elastic beam of modulus E,

$$\psi_1 = -\frac{Pl^2}{16EI}, \qquad \psi_2 = \frac{Xl}{3EI},$$

formulas which may be found in many books on elementary mechanics of materials. Since P is supposed to be a step function in time, ψ_1 for the viscoelastic beam is

$$\psi_1 = -\frac{Pl^2}{16I} J(t) .$$

The moment X is an unknown function of time with, of course, $X(t) \equiv 0$ for $t < 0$. Therefore, ψ_2 must be calculated from the hereditary integral (3.1). We choose (3.1b), write $\psi_2(t)$ for $w(x,t)$, $1/3I$ for $\mathfrak{w}$, and X for f, and have

$$\psi_2 = \frac{1}{3I}\left[X(t)J(0^+) + \int_{0^+}^{t} X(t')\,\frac{dJ(t-t')}{d(t-t')}\,dt'\right] .$$

Both the loads P and the external couples X lead to a reaction at B. It is

$$R_B = P + \frac{2X(t)}{l}$$

and causes a compression of the spring, that is, a downward displacement of the point B by the amount R_B/k and hence a rigid-body rotation of the entire beam AB in the amount of

$$\psi_3 = \frac{R_B}{kl} = \frac{P}{kl} + \frac{2X(t)}{kl^2} .$$

The total, time dependent, rotation of the right end of the beam AB is $\psi = \psi_1 + \psi_2 + \psi_3$. Because of the symmetry, the left end of BC rotates by the same amount in the opposite sense so that there is a *relative* rotation 2ψ of one end with respect to the other. In the actual beam, Fig.3.8a, there is no such relative rotation because there is no hinge to allow it, and therefore we must choose $X(t)$ such that it makes at all times $\psi \equiv 0$. This is the equation from which X can be calculated. Written out in detail, it reads

$$-\frac{Pl^2}{16I} J(t) + \frac{1}{3I} X(t)J(0^+) + \frac{1}{3I}\int_{0^+}^{t} X(t')\,\frac{dJ(t-t')}{d(t-t')}\,dt' + \frac{P}{kl} + \frac{2}{kl^2} X(t) = 0 .$$

This equation is similar to (2.8), that is, it is also a Volterra integral equation of the second kind. In the standard form it reads

$$\left(J(0^+) + \frac{6I}{kl^3} \right) X(t) + \int_{0^+}^{t} X(t') \frac{dJ(t-t')}{d(t-t')} dt' = \frac{3Pl}{16} \left(J(t) - \frac{16I}{kl^3} \right). \quad (3.4)$$

3.4 Solution of the Integral Equation

There are several ways to find the solution of (3.4). A straightforward one is to subject it to the Laplace transformation. To do this, we need the *convolution theorem*, which we shall now derive.

The integral in (3.4) has the form

$$h(t) = \int_0^t f(t')g(t - t')dt'. \quad (3.5)$$

Its Laplace transform is

$$\bar{h}(s) = \int_0^\infty e^{-st} \int_0^t f(t')g(t - t')dt'dt.$$

The integration interval is the shaded area in Fig. 3.9. When we interchange the order of integrations, we have

$$\bar{h}(s) = \int_0^\infty \int_{t'}^\infty e^{-st} f(t')g(t - t')dt\,dt'$$

$$= \int_0^\infty \int_{t'}^\infty e^{-s(t-t')} e^{-st'} f(t')g(t - t')dt\,dt'.$$

Since in the inner integral t' is held constant, we can replace dt by $d(t - t')$ and, with $t - t' = \tau$, we can write

$$\bar{h}(s) = \int_0^\infty e^{-st'} f(t')dt' \int_0^\infty e^{-st} g(\tau)d\tau = \bar{f}(s)\bar{g}(s).$$

The integral (3.5) is called the convolution of f(t) and g(t), and the convolution theorem states that the Laplace transform of the convolution is the product of the two transforms $\bar{f}$ and $\bar{g}$.

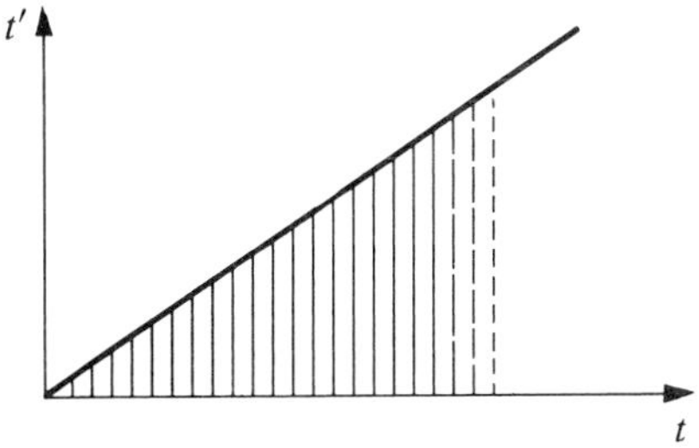

Figure 3.9. Integration domain.

With the help of this theorem the Laplace transform of (3.4) may now be written:

$$\left[J(0^+) + \frac{6I}{kl^3}\right]\bar{X}(s) + \bar{X}(s)[s\bar{J}(s) - J(0^+)] = \frac{3Pl}{16}\left[\bar{J}(s) - \frac{16I}{kl^3 s}\right]. \quad (3.6)$$

This is an algebraic equation for $\bar{X}(s)$. After solving it, the inverse Laplace transformation is applied to obtain X(t).

For a Maxwell material, we have

$$J(t) = \frac{p_1 + t}{q_1}, \qquad \bar{J}(s) = \frac{p_1 s + 1}{q_1 s^2},$$

and (3.6) assumes the following form:

$$\left[\frac{p_1}{q_1} + \frac{6I}{kl^3} + \frac{1}{q_1 s}\right]\bar{X}(s) = \frac{3Pl}{16}\left[\frac{p_1 s + 1}{q_1 s^2} - \frac{16I}{kl^3 s}\right].$$

We solve for $\bar{X}(s)$ and collect terms to obtain

$$\bar{X}(s) = \frac{3Pl}{16} \frac{\left(p_1 kl^3 - 16Iq_1\right)s + kl^3}{s\left[\left(p_1 kl^3 + 6Iq_1\right)s + kl^3\right]}.$$

To transform this back to the variable t, we use pairs (3) and (4) of Table 1.1 and, after a few lines of algebra, arrive at the following result:

$$X(t) = \frac{3Pl}{16}\left[1 - \frac{22Iq_1}{p_1kl^3 + 6Iq_1}\exp\left(-\frac{kl^3t}{p_1kl^3 + 6Iq_1}\right)\right]. \qquad (3.7)$$

To understand this formula, we compare the viscoelastic beam with an elastic one. In an elastic beam, the moment X is, of course, independent of time, and we could easily find its value by repeating the analysis, using for ψ_1 and ψ_2 the elastic formulas given on p. 58. The use of the Laplace transformation is then, of course, not necessary. However, we may use a limiting process to extract the elastic solution from (3.7).

The Maxwell model degenerates into a simple spring if the dashpot is immobilized. Correspondingly, the differential equation of the Maxwell fluid assumes the form $\dot{\sigma} = E\dot{\epsilon}$ if we let $p_1 \to \infty$ while keeping $q_1/p_1 = E$ constant. When we perform this process in (3.7), the argument of the exponential function goes to zero and we obtain

$$X = \frac{3Pl}{16}\left[1 - \frac{22EI}{kl^3 + 6EI}\right] = \frac{3Pl}{16}\,\frac{kl^3 - 16EI}{kl^3 + 6EI}. \qquad (3.8)$$

Returning to the Maxwell beam, we see that X(0) equals the value from (3.8) if we use for E the impact modulus $E_0 = q_1/p_1$ of the Maxwell material. As time goes by, the moment X increases and tends to the limit

$$X(\infty) = 3Pl/16.$$

As may readily be seen from (3.8), this is the moment to occur in an elastic beam for $k \to \infty$, that ist, for a *rigid* support at B.

The physical background of these results is easy to understand. We saw on p. 9 that at the instant of loading the Maxwell fluid behaves like an elastic solid of modulus E_0, and that if the load persists, the deformation is unbounded. Therefore the beam behaves initially like an elastic beam, but ultimately the deformation of the elastic spring (which necessarily is bounded) becomes negligible compared to the ever increasing deflection of the beam.

It should be kept in mind that all our formulas are based on the assumption of small deflections and hence ultimately become invalid when the deflection of the beam keeps growing.

The reader who is not familiar enough with the Laplace transformation may solve the integral equation (3.4) in the following way: Since we have seen that many viscoelastic processes are exponential in time, it is plausible that X might have the form

$$X(t) = C_1 + C_2 e^{-\lambda t} .$$

When one introduces this together with $J(t)$ for the Maxwell fluid in (3.4), the integral may be evaluated and one finds an equation containing terms linear in t, terms with $e^{-\lambda t}$, and constants. Each of these must separately add up to zero, and this yields three equations, from which one calculates C_1, C_2, and λ. The result is in agreement with (3.7).

3.5 Differential Equation of the Beam

We solved the last problem by applying the correspondence principle to the viscoelastic part of the structure. If the solution for the corresponding elastic problem is readily available, this is the proper thing to do. Otherwise, however, it seems to be a detour to find first the solution to a problem in which we are not interested and then to derive from it the one for the problem at hand. To avoid this detour, we need the differential equation of the viscoelastic beam.

In any beam, we have the well-known equilibrium relations:

$$V' = -p, \quad M' = V, \quad M'' = -p, \qquad (3.9a\text{-}c)$$

where, as usual, M and V are bending moment and shear force as shown in Fig.3.10a, p is the load per unit length of the beam, and the primes stand for derivatives with respect to x. Since in a viscoelastic beam all quantities depend also on time, the primes should be understood as indicating partial differentiation.

Besides (3.9a-c) we have for the elastic beam the elastic relation

$$w'' = -M/EI. \tag{3.10}$$

We now derive its equivalent under the assumption that the beam material obeys the viscoelastic law (1.23).

Figure 3.10b shows in heavy lines a beam element before deformation, and in thin lines its deformed shape. The cross sections at its ends were originally both vertical, but on the deformed element they make an angle $d\psi = \varkappa\, dx$, where $\varkappa$ is the curvature of the beam axis. If the deflection w of the beam is small enough to make $(w')^2 \ll 1$, then

$$\varkappa = -w'',$$

as is known from elastic beams.

We choose in the cross section, Fig.3.10c, an arbitrary area element $dA = dy \cdot dz$ and consider the corresponding "fiber" of length dx in the beam element. In the deformed state it is stretched by the amount $z\, d\psi$, whence its strain

$$\epsilon = \frac{z\, d\psi}{dx} = z\varkappa.$$

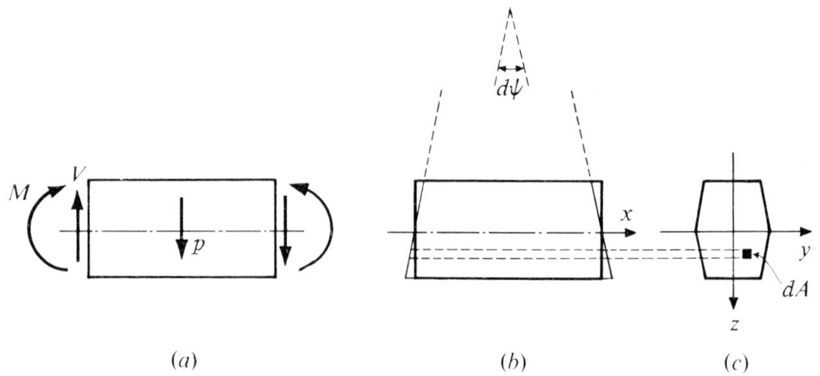

Figure 3.10. Beam element.

Across the area element dA a stress σ is acting, which is related to ε by (1.23). The force σ dA makes a contribution to the bending moment M transmitted in the cross section,

$$M = \int_A \sigma z \, dA .$$

To this equation we apply the operator $\mathbf{P}$ of (1.23c) and then replace $\mathbf{P}(\sigma)$ by $\mathbf{Q}(\varepsilon)$ to obtain

$$\mathbf{P}(M) = \int_A \mathbf{P}(\sigma) z \, dA = \int_A \mathbf{Q}(\varepsilon) z \, dA = \int_A \mathbf{Q}(\varkappa z) z \, dA .$$

$\mathbf{Q}$ is a linear operator containing only time derivatives. Therefore, we may pull z out from under it and then $\mathbf{Q}(\varkappa)$ out of the integral, which yields

$$\mathbf{P}(M) = \int_A \mathbf{Q}(\varkappa) z^2 \, dA = \mathbf{Q}(\varkappa) \int_A z^2 \, dA = \mathbf{Q}(\varkappa) \cdot I ,$$

where I is the moment of inertia of the cross section with respect to the y axis, which must pass through the centroid for the same reason as in an elastic beam. When we still express the curvature in terms of the deflection, we arrive finally at the differential equation

$$I\mathbf{Q}(w'') = -\mathbf{P}(M). \tag{3.11}$$

It may be combined with (3.9c) to yield

$$I\mathbf{Q}(w^{iv}) = \mathbf{P}(p), \tag{3.12}$$

which corresponds to the well-known equation

$$EI\, w^{iv} = p$$

of the elastic beam. In x it is of the fourth order, but its order in time derivatives depends on the special choice of the operators $\mathbf{P}$ and $\mathbf{Q}$.

Once the deflection $w(x,t)$ of a beam is known, M and V may be found from (3.11) and (3.9b), respectively. Solving the problem for a viscoelastic beam of length l (no matter how supported) means finding the solution of (3.12) for a semi-infinite strip in the x, t-plane which is bounded by the x axis and the lines $x = 0$ and $x = l$, Fig.3.11. Just as in the elastic case, we need to know two boundary conditions at each end of the beam, prescribing there w or V and w' or M. In addition, we need initial conditions for $t = 0$ and $0 \leqslant x \leqslant l$, their number depending on the operator **Q** (which is never lower than the order of **P**, see Tables 1.1 and 1.3, pp. 16 and 25).

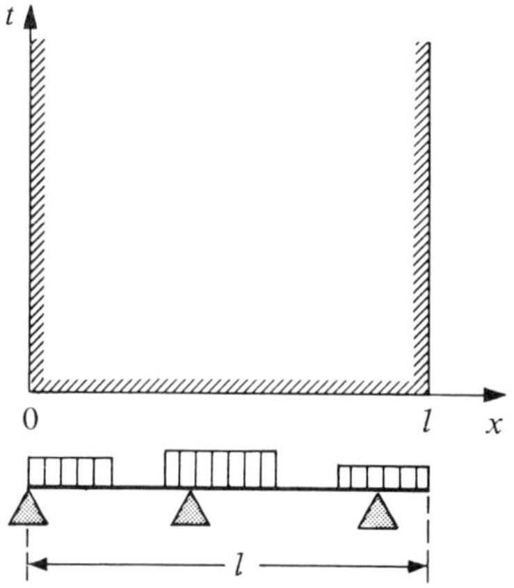

Figure 3.11. Semi-infinite strip in the x,t plane.

3.6 General Correspondence Principle

We use an example to explain the general form of the correspondence principle, considering again the beam of Fig.3.8, but replacing the concentrated forces by a distributed load $p(x,t)$, of which we require only that it by symmetric with respect to the point B in Fig.3.12. This symmetry allows us to restrict our attention to the left span AB.

The deflection $w(x,t)$ in this span is governed by the partial differential equation (3.12). There are four boundary conditions. At the left end the deflection and the bending moment are zero for all times t:

$$x = 0: \quad w = 0, \quad M = 0.$$

At the right end, symmetry requires a zero slope, and the shear force must be equal to half the reaction $R_B = kw$. With due consideration of the sign convention of the shear force, this yields

$$x = l: \quad w' = 0, \quad V = M' = -\frac{1}{2}kw.$$

As initial conditions we assume that w and as many of its time derivatives as needed are zero at $t = 0$ and for $0 \leqslant x \leqslant l$.

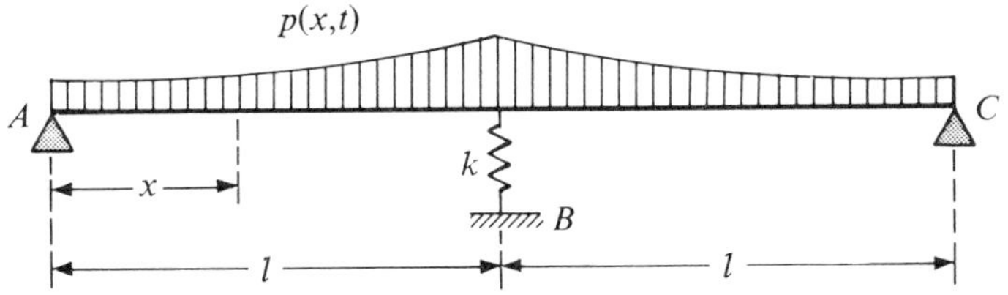

Figure 3.12. Viscoelastic beam on elastic support.

We now subject the differential equation and the boundary conditions to the Laplace transformation. On the right-hand side of (3.12) we have

$$\mathbf{P}(p) = \left(p_0 + p_1\frac{\partial}{\partial t} + p_2\frac{\partial^2}{\partial t^2} + \cdots\right)p.$$

When we apply the Laplace transformation to each of these terms, we obtain

$$(p_0 + p_1 s + p_2 s^2 + p_3 s^3 + \ldots)\bar{p} = \mathcal{P}(s)\cdot\bar{p},$$

and similarly the left hand side yields $\mathcal{Q}(s)\cdot\bar{w}^{iv}$, where $\mathcal{P}(s)$ and $\mathcal{Q}(s)$ are the polynomials defined by (1.26).

With this notation the Laplace transforms of our equations may be written as follows:

$$I\mathcal{Q}(s)\bar{w}^{iv}(x,s) = \mathcal{P}(s)\bar{p}(x,s), \tag{3.13a}$$

$$x = 0: \quad \bar{w} = 0, \tag{3.13b}$$

$$\mathcal{P}(s)\overline{M} = -I\mathcal{Q}(s)\bar{w}'' = 0, \quad \therefore \bar{w}'' = 0 \tag{3.13c}$$

$$x = l: \quad \bar{w}' = 0, \tag{3.13d}$$

$$-\frac{1}{2}k\mathcal{P}(s)\bar{w} = \mathcal{P}(s)\bar{M}' = -I\mathcal{Q}(s)\bar{w}''',$$

$$\therefore \bar{w}''' - \frac{k}{2I}\frac{\mathcal{P}(s)}{\mathcal{Q}(s)}\bar{w} = 0. \tag{3.13e}$$

For comparison we now list the equations which would apply to an elastic beam of modulus E and a time-dependent load $p(x,t)$:

$$EIw^{iv}(x,t) = p(x,t), \tag{3.14a}$$

$$x = 0: \quad w = 0, \qquad w'' = 0, \tag{3.14b,c}$$

$$x = l: \quad w' = 0, \tag{3.14d}$$

$$-\frac{1}{2}kw = V = M' = -EIw''',$$

$$\therefore w''' - \frac{k}{2EI}w = 0. \tag{3.14e}$$

These two sets of equations are identical if we let

$$E = \mathcal{Q}(s)/\mathcal{P}(s) \tag{3.15}$$

and equate $p(x,t)$, $w(x,t)$ of the elastic beam with $\bar{p}(x,s)$, $\bar{w}(x,s)$ of the viscoelastic one. Obviously, this result is not restricted to the particular case for which we have just found it. For any beam, frame, or arch we would have boundary conditions in terms of w and its first three derivatives with respect to x, and since the Laplace transform of (1.23c) and Hooke's law are related by (3.15), the Laplace transform of any boundary condition would show the same arrangement of the polynomials $\mathcal{P}(s)$ and $\mathcal{Q}(s)$ which would relate it via (3.15) to its elastic counterpart.

Thus we have arrived at the most general form of the *correspondence principle*, which we can formulate for beam structures:

To find the stresses in and the deformation of a viscoelastic structure, solve the corresponding elastic problem, replace E by $\mathcal{Q}(s)/\mathcal{P}(s)$, and the ensuing functions are the Laplace transforms of the solution of the viscoelastic problem.

As an example, we use the beam of Fig. 3.12, assuming a uniformly distributed load applied at $t = 0$ and then held constant:

$$p(x,t) = p\Delta(t).$$

The solution of the corresponding elastic problem for the left span is

$$w(x) = \frac{p}{24EI}\left[(8l^3 - 4lx^2 + x^3)x - \frac{5kl^4}{2(6EI + kl^3)}(3l^2 - x^2)x\right]$$

and it will be assumed that the reader either knows how to obtain it or that he is willing to accept it on good faith.

Now let the beam be made of a Maxwell material with

$$\mathcal{P}(s) = 1 + p_1 s, \qquad \mathcal{Q}(s) = q_1 s$$

according to the third column of Table 1.1. The Laplace transform of the step function load is $\bar{p} = p/s$, and the correspondence principle yields for $\bar{w}(x,s)$ the formula

$$\bar{w} = \frac{p}{24Iq_1}\frac{1 + p_1 s}{s^2}\left[(8l^3 - 4lx^2 + x^3)x - \frac{5kl^4(1 + p_1 s)}{2\left[6Iq_1 s + kl^3(1 + p_1 s)\right]}(3l^2 - x^2)x\right].$$

To transform this back into $w(x,t)$, we need the pairs (3), (4), (5) of Table 1.1. The calculation involves some lengthy algebra, but it does not present any other difficulties. It yields the following result:

$$w(x,t) = \frac{5p}{8kl^2}\left[1 - \frac{6Iq_1}{6Iq_1 + kl^3 p_1}e^{-\lambda t}\right](3l^2 - x^2)x + \frac{p}{48Iq_1}(p_1 + t)(l^3 - 3lx^2 + 2x^3)x$$

with

$$\lambda = \frac{kl^3}{6Iq_1 + kl^3 p_1}$$

Its physical interpretation may follow the same lines as that given on p. 62.

Problems

3.1. A cantilever beam of span l is made of a three-parameter solid. It carries at its tip a load P, which depends on time according to one or the other of the load histories shown in Fig.3.13 (the last of these is a sine curve). Find the deflection of the tip of the beam. For an elastic beam, the deflection is

$$w(l) = \frac{Pl^3}{3EI} .$$

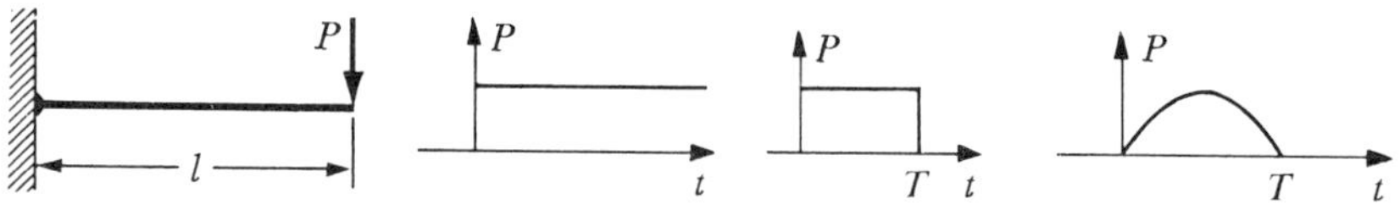

Figure 3.13.

3.2. A viscoelastic beam of span l carries a chain of three beamlets connected by hinges. Over these a load P is moving at constant speed c from left to right. For the main beam, this produces loads P_1 and P_2, which vary as shown in Fig.3.14. Find the bending moment and the deflection for the midspan point. Start from the solution of the elastic problem, which can be found in many books.

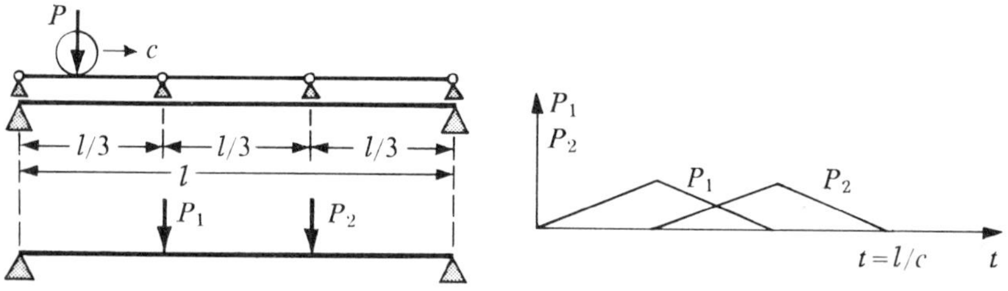

Figure 3.14.

3.3. The beam shown in Fig.3.15 has pin supports, but the rotation θ of its ends is restrained by viscoelastic springs. Let the beam be made of a Kelvin material described by (1.9), and let the reactive moment M of each spring be related to the end rotation of the beam by a Maxwell law:

$$M + m_1\dot{M} = n_1\dot{\theta} .$$

Establish an integral equation for the common value M of the moments at both ends of the beam. Solve it and plot as functions of time the bending moments at $x = 0$ and $x = l/2$ and the deflection at the midspan point.

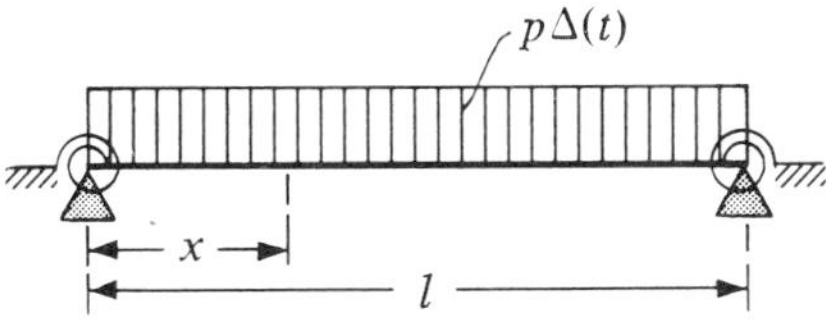

Figure 3.15.

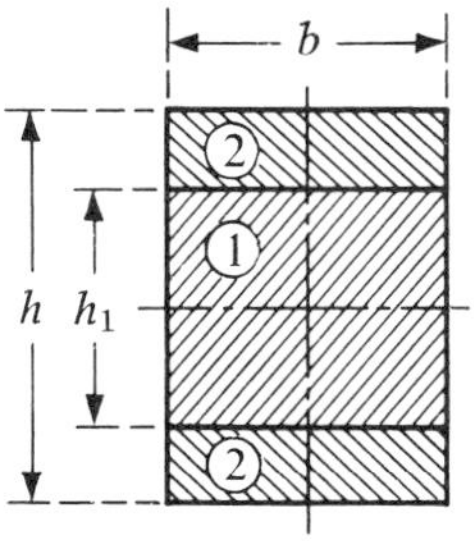

Figure 3.16.

3.4. Reconsider the beam shown in Fig.3.8, but assume that only in the left span a load P is acting. Establish the integral equation for the redundant moment X and solve it for the case that the spring obeys the Kelvin law.

3.5. A beam has a rectangular cross section built up of two different viscoelastic materials, as shown in Fig.3.16. The relaxation moduli of these materials are Y_1 and Y_2. Find the relaxation modulus of the beam, that is, a function $Y(t)$ such that the bending moment $M = Y(t)$ if the curvature is $\varkappa = \Delta(t)$.

3.6. Assume that in the beam cross section of Fig.3.16 the core material is elastic (modulus E) and that material 2 is a three-parameter solid. Derive a relation of type (3.11) between bending moment and curvature.

3.7. A cantilever beam of span l_0 is made of a Maxwell material (Fig.3.17). At $t = 0$ it receives its load p and at the same time begins to burn or to melt from its tip so that at time t its length is $l = l_0 - ct$. Find the deflection as a function of x and t.

There are two ways to solve this problem: (i) establishing the proper boundary conditions and then solving (3.12), or (ii) calculating the statically determinate bending moments, then w'' from (3.11) and by integration for constant time the deflection w.

It is suggested that the first approach be used for solving the problem, and the second for checking the solution.

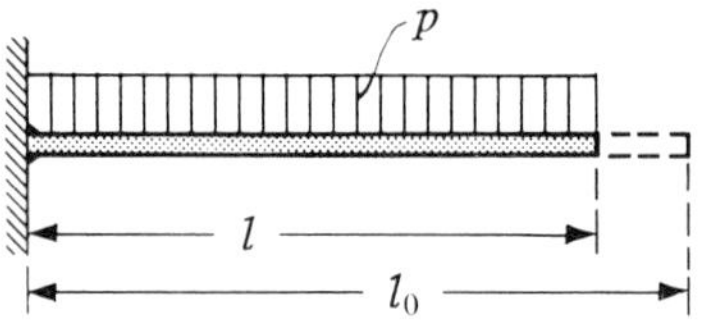

Figure 3.17.

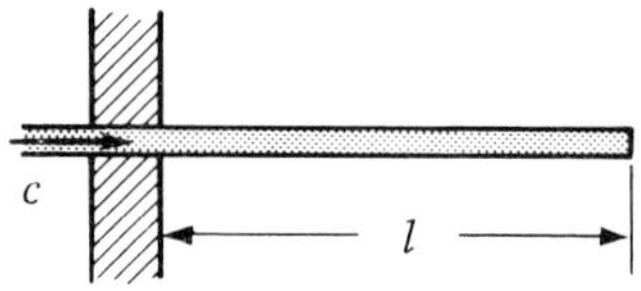

Figure 3.18.

3.8. A bar of constant cross section is extruded horizontally from an orifice (Fig.3.18). At time t its length is $l = ct$. The bar carries its own weight as a cantilever. Find the deflection.

Reference

For information on related problems in the theory of elasticity see

21. S. Timoshenko and J.N. Goodier: Theory of Elasticity (3rd ed.) (New York, McGraw-Hill, 1970), pp. 291-313 (torsion of prismatic bars), and pp. 341-349 (torsion of shafts of variable diameter).

Chapter 4

Beam on Continuous Support

In the preceding chapter we have used the hereditary integrals and the correspondence principle for the analysis of viscoelastic beams. We have seen how both approaches may be applied even to structures which consist of several materials with different kinds of viscoelastic response. We shall now have a brief look at a problem in which we may study other methods of solution.

4.1 Differential Equation

The object of our study is shown in Fig.4.1a. It is a beam supported by an elastic or viscoelastic half-space. If under some load (not shown in the figure) the beam deflects by an amount $w(x)$, the supporting medium reacts by exerting a distributed upward force on the beam. We denote by $q(x)$ this force per unit length of the beam.

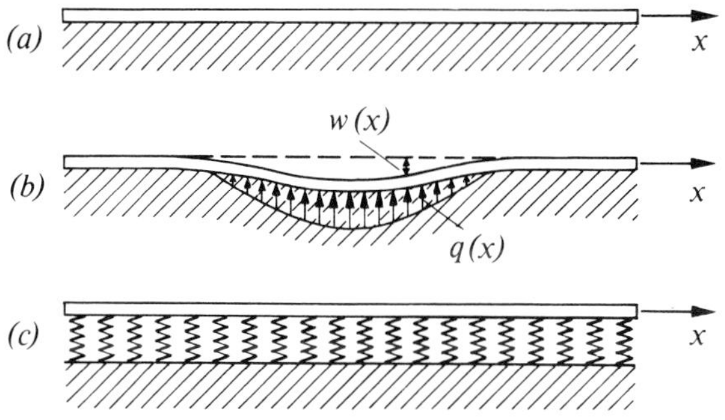

Figure 4.1. Beam on a continuous support - a,b: half-space; c: Winkler support.

The reaction $q(x_1)$ at any point x_1 depends, of course, not only upon the local value $w(x_1)$ of the deflection, but also upon that of neighbor points x_2, their influence decreasing as the distance $|x_1 - x_2|$ increases. Traditionally, this substantial complication has been swept aside by substituting for the half-space the so-called Winkler model [22], which assumes that the reaction $q(x)$ at any point depends only on the deflection $w(x)$ measured at the same place. Such a beam may be considered as resting on a kind of spring mattress (Fig.4.1c), the infinitesimal springs forming a continuum, but acting independently of each other. On p. 83 we shall discuss the limitations of this simplification. We shall use this Winkler model for our study and assume that both the beam and the supporting medium are made of viscoelastic materials. This, of course, includes elastic materials as a limiting case.[1]

To describe the material of the beam, we use (1.23), which we now write

$$\mathbf{P}_a \sigma = \mathbf{Q}_a \varepsilon \, . \tag{4.1}$$

Equation (3.11), the constitutive equation for the beam element, reads then

$$I\,\mathbf{Q}_a(w'') = -\,\mathbf{P}_a(M) \, . \tag{4.2a}$$

The beam may carry an arbitrary load $p(x,t)$, positive when directed downward. In addition, it is exposed to the reaction $q(x,t)$ from the support, which will be counted positive in the opposite direction. Therefore, the equilibrium condition (3.9c) reads now

$$M'' = -\,p + q \, . \tag{4.2b}$$

---

[1] In the English literature the name "beam on elastic foundation" has become widely used. We shall avoid it and rather speak of a continuously supported beam or a beam resting upon a continuous medium, because in one of the important applications of the theory it is the beam, which is the foundation of some building, while the supporting medium is the ground on which this foundation is resting.

Combining both these equations, we have

$$I\,\mathbf{Q}_a(w^{iv}) = \mathbf{P}_a(p - q) \tag{4.3}$$

and this replaces the differential equation (3.12) of the beam without a continuous support, but it is not yet the differential equation of our problem. To obtain this, we still have to express q in terms of w, that is, we must introduce the constitutive equation of the support. We assume it in the form

$$\mathbf{P}_b q = \mathbf{Q}_b w, \tag{4.4}$$

which is the viscoelastic counterpart to the relation written for the elastic case [23, 24].

We eliminate q between the last two equations by applying the operators $\mathbf{P}_b$ to (4.3) and $\mathbf{P}_a$ to (4.4). This leads to

$$I\,\mathbf{P}_b\mathbf{Q}_a(w^{iv}) + \mathbf{P}_a\mathbf{Q}_b(w) = \mathbf{P}_a\mathbf{P}_b(p), \tag{4.5}$$

and this is the differential equation of a viscoelastic beam resting upon a viscoelastic base of the Winkler type.

4.2 A Simple Example

Let us consider the beam shown in Fig.4.2. It is continuously supported by a Winkler medium and in addition it has rigid, hinged supports at both ends. It carries the load

$$p(x,t) = p \sin\frac{\pi x}{l}, \tag{4.6}$$

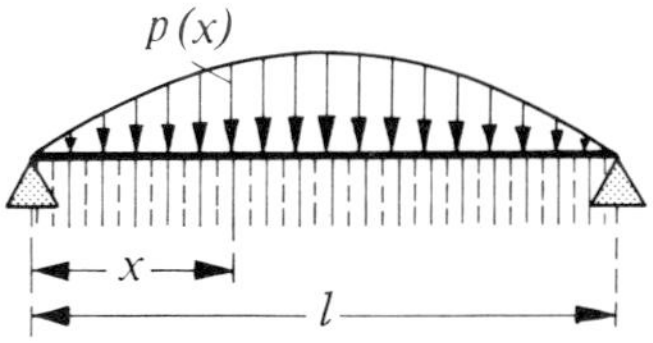

Figure 4.2. Beam with simple end support and continuous support, sinusoidal load.

applied at $t = 0$ and then maintained without change. The deflection $w(x,t)$ must satisfy the differential equation (4.5) and at the ends $x = 0$ and $x = l$ the boundary conditions

$$w(0,t) = 0, \qquad w(l,t) = 0$$

and

$$M(0,t) = 0, \qquad M(l,t) = 0,$$

whence with (4.2a)

$$w''(0,t) = 0, \qquad w''(l,t) = 0.$$

In addition, $w(x,0)$ must satisfy initial conditions, which we shall discuss later.

A solution which automatically satisfies the end conditions, may be assumed in the form

$$w(x,t) = W(t) \sin \frac{\pi x}{l} . \tag{4.7}$$

Introducing it into (4.5), we obtain an ordinary differential equation for $W(t)$:

$$\left(\frac{I \pi^4}{l^4} \mathbf{P}_b \mathbf{Q}_a + \mathbf{P}_a \mathbf{Q}_b \right) W(t) = \mathbf{P}_a \mathbf{P}_b \, p. \tag{4.8}$$

This equation has the form

$$\mathbf{Q} W = \mathbf{P} p, \tag{4.9}$$

and we may apply to it all we have learned about such equations. In our special case, p is a constant, the amplitude of the sinusoidal load defined in (4.6), and the operator on the right-hand side of (4.9) is trivial. It would not be so if we wanted to generalize (4.6), maintaining the same spanwise load distribution, but allowing its amplitude to vary in a known way with time.

The general solution of (4.9) consists of one particular solution and the sum of the solutions of the homogeneous equation $\mathbf{Q}(W) = 0$. Their number depends upon the order of the operator $\mathbf{Q}$.

If at least one of the materials involved is a solid, that is, if at leat one of the coefficients q_{a0} and q_{b0} is not zero, the simplest particular solution is a constant $W = C$, where C is found from

$$q_0 C \equiv \left(\frac{I\pi^4}{l^4} q_{a0} + q_{b0} \right) C = p. \tag{4.10a}$$

If both materials are of the fluid type, there exists a particular solution $W = Ct$, where C follows from

$$q_1 C \equiv \left(\frac{I\pi^4}{l^4} q_{a1} + q_{b1} \right) C = p. \tag{4.10b}$$

Since (4.9) has constant coefficients, the solution of the homogeneous equation may be assumed in the form

$$W(t) = \sum_r C_r e^{\lambda_r t} \tag{4.11}$$

where the λ_r are the solutions of the characteristic equation

$$\mathcal{Q}(\lambda) \equiv \frac{I\pi^4}{l^4} \mathcal{P}_b(\lambda)\mathcal{Q}_a(\lambda) + \mathcal{P}_a(\lambda)\mathcal{Q}_b(\lambda) = 0. \tag{4.12}$$

While the constant C in the particular solution follows from one of the equations (4.10), the constants C_r in (4.11) must be determined from the initial conditions at $t = 0$.

As an illustrative example, consider the case that the beam is elastic:

$$\mathbf{P}_a = 1, \qquad \mathbf{Q}_a = E, \tag{4.13a}$$

and that the support is an array of Maxwell springs with

$$\mathbf{P}_b = 1 + p_1 \frac{\partial}{\partial t}, \qquad \mathbf{Q}_b = q_1 \frac{\partial}{\partial t}. \tag{4.13b}$$

The particular solution $W_p(t) = C$ follows from (4.10a) as

$$W_p(t) = \frac{pl^4}{EI\pi^4}.$$

The characteristic equation (4.12) is linear:

$$\frac{EI\pi^4}{l^4}(1 + p_1\lambda) + q_1\lambda = 0$$

and has only one root. With the abbreviation

$$\rho = EI\pi^4/l^4$$

it leads to the complementary solution

$$W_c(t) = C_1 \exp\frac{-\rho t}{p_1\rho + q_1} .$$

The free constant C_1 is found from an initial condition prescribing $W(0^+)$. We derive it from (1.28a), replacing there ϵ and σ by W and p, respectively, and extracting the coefficients p_n and q_n to be used from the operators **P** and **Q** defined by (4.9). In terms of the present notation (in which p_1 and q_1 refer to the support operators $\mathbf{P}_b$ and $\mathbf{Q}_b$), we find the boundary condition to be

$$W(0^+) = \frac{p_1}{\rho p_1 + q_1} p .$$

It must be satisfied by the general solution

$$W(t) = W_p(t) + W_c(t),$$

and after a brief computation one easily obtains the result

$$\begin{aligned} w &= W(t) \sin\frac{\pi x}{l} \\ &= \frac{pl^4}{EI\pi^4}\left(1 - \frac{q_1}{\rho p_1 + q_1} \exp\frac{-\rho t}{\rho p_1 + q_1}\right) \sin\frac{\pi x}{l} . \end{aligned} \tag{4.14}$$

Comparison with the column J(t) of Table 1.2 shows that the system of beam plus ground behaves like a three-parameter solid. The beam undergoes an immediate deflection with the midspan value $W(0^+)$, which is exactly the one which the beam resting upon an elastic medium of stiffness q_1/p_1 would have. As time goes by, the deflection increases and tends asymptotically to the value

$$W(\infty) = \frac{pl^4}{EI\pi^4} ,$$

which indicates that in the end the beam carries the entire load without any help from the "supporting" medium.

The analysis is similar if we exchange the two materials and let a beam made of a Maxwell material with

$$\mathbf{P}_a = 1 + p_1 \frac{\partial}{\partial t} , \qquad \mathbf{Q}_a = q_1 \frac{\partial}{\partial t} \tag{4.15a}$$

rest upon an elastic support described by

$$\mathbf{P}_b = 1, \qquad \mathbf{Q}_b = k. \tag{4.15b}$$

In this case, (4.10a) yields a particular solution

$$W_p(t) = p/k$$

and the complementary solution is

$$W_c(t) = C_1 e^{-t/(p_1+\mu q_1)}$$

with

$$\mu = I\pi^4/kl^4 .$$

Again the initial condition is extracted from (1.28a) by writing it in terms of the parameters of deformation and load of the present problem:

$$W(0^+) = \frac{p}{k} \frac{p_1}{p_1 + \mu q_1}$$

and the final solution is

$$w = \frac{p}{k}\left(1 - \frac{\mu q_1}{p_1 + \mu q_1} e^{-t/(p_1+\mu q_1)}\right) \sin\frac{\pi x}{l} . \tag{4.16}$$

Also here the connection between the load p and the deflection w it produces is the same as that between stress and strain in a three-parameter solid, and $W(0^+)$ follows from elastic theory with the impact modulus $E_0 = q_1/p_1$ of the beam material, but for $t \to \infty$ the beam now relaxes completely and the load is fully carried by the underlying elastic medium.

4.3 Concentrated Load

The difference in asymptotic behavior of the two beam-support systems just studied has great consequences when we use (4.14) and (4.16) to construct solutions for a beam carrying a concentrated force P at the mid-span point.

If in (4.7) we replace l by l/n, this formula describes a load as illustrated in Fig.4.3 for $n = 3$. The corresponding deflection is obtained by replacing l by l/n in (4.14) and (4.16) and, consequently, replacing ρ by ρn^4 and μ by μn^4.

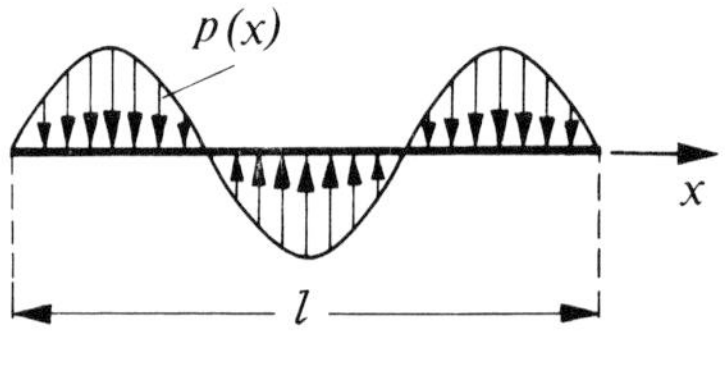

Figure 4.3. Load according to the term $n = 3$ of (4.17).

Now, a concentrated load P applied at $x = l/2$, that is, a Dirac spike $p(x) = P\delta(x)$, can, in the domain $0 \leqslant x \leqslant l$, be represented by the Fourier series[2]

$$p(x) = \frac{2P}{l} \sum_{n=1,3,\ldots}^{\infty} (-1)^{\frac{n-1}{2}} \sin\frac{n\pi x}{l}, \qquad (4.17)$$

[2] See, for example, Handbook of Engineering Mechanics, W. Flügge ed., New York 1962, p. 20-10.

in which the summation is extended over all odd integers n. This series does not converge but is summable, that is, the average of all partial sums up to a certain n converges to a limit as n increases. Such a series may be used for our purpose. If extended beyond our limited range of interest on the x axis, (4.17) represents a sequence of alternating upward and downward forces P at the points $x = \pm l/2, \pm 3l/2, \ldots$.

After these preparations we may write the solution for the beam problem shown in Fig.4.4 under either of the assumptions (4.13) and (4.15) about the materials. In the first case, we apply (4.14) to the load (4.17) and find

$$w = \frac{2Pl^3}{EI\pi^4} \sum_{n=\text{odd}}^{\infty} \frac{(-1)^{\frac{n-1}{2}}}{n^4} \left(1 - \frac{1}{1 + n^4 \rho p_1/q_1} \exp \frac{-t}{p_1 + q_1/n^4 \rho} \right) \sin \frac{n\pi x}{l} . \tag{4.18}$$

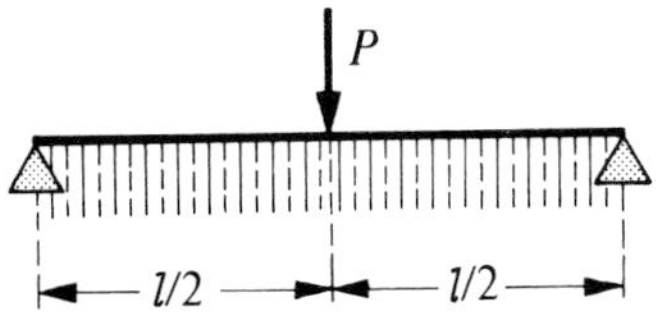

Figure 4.4. Beam with simple end support and continuous support, concentrated load.

This series is convergent and may easily be evaluated numerically. A result of such work is shown in Fig.4.5. The dimensionless para-

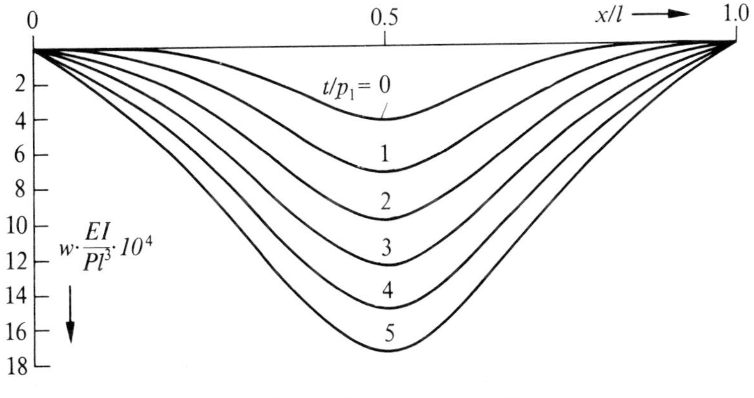

Figure 4.5. Beam of Fig.4.4, elastic beam, Maxwell supporting medium, $q_1/\rho p_1 = 81$.

meter $\rho\, p_1/q_1$ has been chosen such that for $t = 0$ the deflection does not much differ from that of an infinite beam. One can recognize how, in the course of time, the end supports make themselves felt and how the deflected beam approaches the shape of a free beam carrying the load P between the end supports. For $t \to \infty$, (4.18) yields

$$w = \frac{2P\, l^3}{EI\, \pi^4} \sum_{n=\text{odd}}^{\infty} \frac{(-1)^{\frac{n-1}{2}}}{n^4} \sin\frac{n\pi x}{l},$$

and this is the Fourier expansion of the deflection of a simple beam with a load P at mid-span.

If we now turn to the choice of materials described by (4.15), we find the deflection

$$w = \frac{2P}{kl} \sum_{n=\text{odd}}^{\infty} (-1)^{\frac{n-1}{2}} \left(1 - \frac{1}{1 + p_1/\mu q_1 n^4} \exp\frac{-t}{p_1 + n^4 \mu q_1}\right) \sin\frac{n\pi x}{l}. \tag{4.19}$$

With the exception of the limit $t \to \infty$, this Fourier series is convergent, although much less rapidly than the one in (4.18). The result of a numerical evaluation is shown in Fig.4.6. For $t = 0$, the deflection is about the same as in Fig.4.5, that is the one of an elastic beam

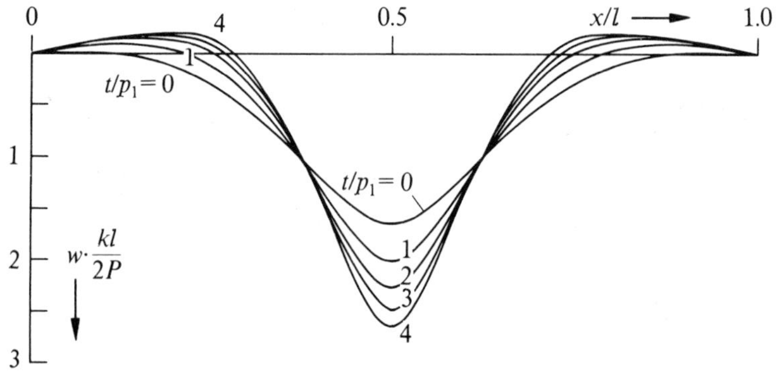

Figure 4.6. Beam of Fig.4.4, Maxwell beam, supporting medium elastic, $p_1 k l^4 / q_1 I \pi^4 = 81$.

resting upon an elastic medium[3]. But as time increases, the deflection develops in a quite different way. In stead of spreading over the entire length of the beam, it increases in the central part and decreases elsewhere, even becomes negative. This phenomenon may easily be understood if one remembers what we have found out when discussing the same system under a sinusoidal load. We saw that in the long run the Maxwell beam relaxes completely and that ultimately the load applied to the beam is, without change in magnitude or distribution, passed on to the supporting elastic medium. The same happens here again. In the limit, the series in (4.19) becomes identical with that in (4.17) and we simply have

$$\lim_{t \to \infty} w(x,t) = \frac{p}{k} .$$

Our highly singular load distribution then produces a highly singular deformation and we are clearly beyond the range of usefulness of the Winkler model for the supporting medium. We might have anticipated this from Fig.4.3. If we let n increase, the load distribution consists of a sequence of many positive and negative parts, and so does the distribution of the ground reaction $q(x)$. Under such forces a half-space must be expected to be much less deformed than a Winkler mattress. In (4.18) no harm came from this because the stiffness of the elastic beam makes the ratio q/p decrease rapidly as n increases. Therefore the Fourier series in (4.18) converges well and its higher terms, though increasingly unrealistic, do not have much influence upon the result. Thus we are on safe ground when using the Winkler model. On the other hand, the refusal of the Maxwell beam to make *in the long run* a useful contribution to the load carrying process, makes here the Winkler model unsuitable for large times t. However, we see from Fig.4.6 that for a limited time deflection lines are obtained which suggest a rather smooth distribution of $q(x)$ and for which the Winkler model may still be trusted.

---

[3] Note that the numbers on the ordinate axes in these two diagrams are not comparable since they had to be dedimensionalized by different factors.

4.4 Moving Load on an Infinite Beam

We shall now turn to a quite different problem connected with the same beam on a continuous support. This time the beam is assumed to be infinitely long and acted upon by a concentrated load P, which moves at a constant speed c from the left to the right. At the time t, it is acting at the point x = ct, as shown in Fig.4.7. For $x \neq ct$, there are no other loads and the deflection must satisfy the homogeneous form of the differential equation (4.5):

$$I \mathbf{P}_b \mathbf{Q}_a w^{iv} + \mathbf{P}_a \mathbf{Q}_b w = 0. \tag{4.20}$$

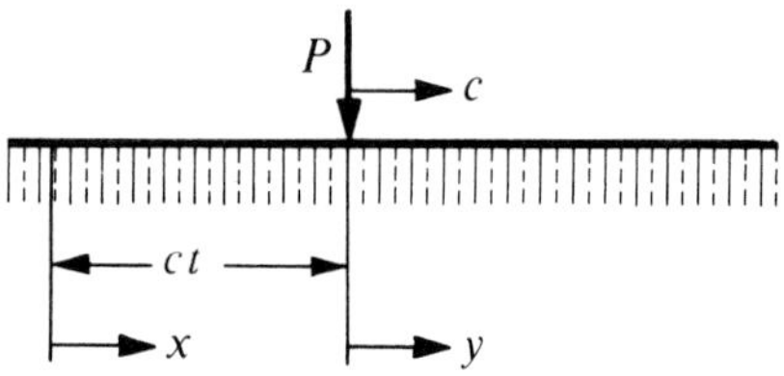

Figure 4.7. Beam on a continuous support, load moving with velocity c.

If the load came from $x = -\infty$, there will be no transients and w(x,t) depends on the single variable

$$y = x - ct,$$

that is, a certain pattern of deformation and stress moves with the load along the beam. We may write any of the operators **P** and **Q** in terms of derivatives with respect to y, for example

$$\mathbf{P} \equiv \mathcal{P}\left(\frac{\partial}{\partial t}\right) = \mathcal{P}\left(-c\frac{d}{dy}\right),$$

and (4.20) becomes an ordinary differential equation for w(y):

$$I \mathcal{P}_b\left(-c\frac{d}{dy}\right) \mathcal{Q}_a\left(-c\frac{d}{dy}\right) \frac{d^4 w}{dy^4} + \mathcal{P}_a\left(-c\frac{d}{dy}\right) \mathcal{Q}_b\left(-c\frac{d}{dy}\right) w = 0. \tag{4.21}$$

It has constant coefficients and its solution may be written as the sum of exponential functions as usual:

$$w = \sum C e^{\lambda y}, \tag{4.22}$$

the number of terms depending upon the order of the differential equation. Introduction of the generic term of the sum into (4.21) yields the characteristic equation

$$I \lambda^4 \mathcal{P}_b(-c\lambda)\, \mathcal{Q}_a(-c\lambda) + \mathcal{P}_a(-c\lambda)\, \mathcal{Q}_b(-c\lambda) = 0. \tag{4.23}$$

The solution (4.22) may be written separately, with different values for the constants C, for the domains $y < 0$ and $y > 0$. Linear equations for the calculation of the constants follow from the end conditions at $y = \pm\infty$ and from the matching of the two solutions at $y = 0$. This matching is a complicated process, which may be explored in general terms [25]. This gets rather cumbersome, and we shall content ourselves with studying the matching for a few simple examples.

Let us begin with the choice of materials described by (4.13), that is, with an elastic beam resting on a Maxwell support. In this case, the characteristic equation is

$$EI\, cp_1 \lambda^5 - EI \lambda^4 + cq_1 \lambda = 0.$$

It has the root $\lambda = \lambda_5 = 0$, leading to the solution $w = C_5$, and four others, which must be calculated from the equation

$$EI\, cp_1 \lambda^4 - EI \lambda^3 + cq_1 = 0.$$

Descartes's rule of signs indicates that there are either two real, positive roots and a complex pair, or two different pairs of conjugate complex roots. Fig.4.8 shows the location of the roots in a complex plane of the dimensionless quantity $\Lambda = \lambda l$ as a function of the dimensionless velocity parameter $\gamma = cp_1/l$, where the reference length l is defined by

$$l^4 = EI\, p_1/q_1.$$

For $\gamma < 0.570$, there exists only one pair of complex roots and we write the entire set of roots in the form

$$\lambda_{1,2} = -\varkappa_1 \pm i\mu_1,\ \lambda_3,\ \lambda_4,\ \lambda_5 = 0.$$

The deflection is then

$$w = e^{-\varkappa_1 y}(C_1 \cos \mu_1 y + C_2 \sin \mu_1 y) + C_3 e^{\lambda_3 y} + C_4 e^{\lambda_4 y} + C_5. \tag{4.24a}$$

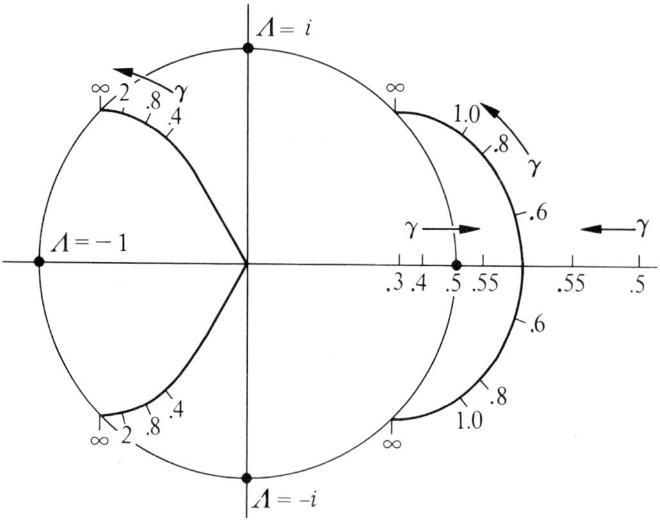

Figure 4.8. Elastic beam on a Maxwell support, location of the zeroes of the characterisitc equation in the complex Λ plane.

If $\gamma > 0.570$, there are four complex roots λ and w appears in the form

$$w = e^{-\varkappa_1 y}(C_1 \cos \mu_1 y + C_2 \sin \mu_1 y) + e^{\varkappa_2 y}(C_3 \cos \mu_2 y + C_4 \sin \mu_2 y) + C_5. \tag{4.24b}$$

One or the other of these solutions must be applied with different sets of constants C independently to the regions $y < 0$ and $y > 0$, and we need ten conditions from which to find the ten constants. On the right-hand side of the beam, we must drop the terms with C_3, C_4, C_5 because for $y \to \infty$, that is in the region where the load has not yet been and is not soon to get, the beam must be entirely undisturbed. On the other hand, when we write the solution for $y < 0$, we must discard the terms with C_1 and C_2 to keep the deflection finite for $y \to -\infty$, but we may not require that also $C_5 = 0$, because the Maxwell material under the beam may well have suffered a permanent deformation. Thus we have eliminated 5 of the 10 unknown constants from conditions at infinity. We now have

for $y > 0$:

$$w = e^{-\varkappa_1 y}(C_1 \cos \mu_1 y + C_2 \sin \mu_1 y) \tag{4.25a}$$

and for $y < 0$:

$$w = C_3 e^{\lambda_3 y} + C_4 e^{\lambda_4 y} + C_5 \tag{4.25b}$$

or

$$w = e^{\varkappa_2 y}(C_3 \cos \mu_2 y + C_4 \sin \mu_2 y) + C_5 . \tag{4.25c}$$

In either case there are five unknown constants left, which must be calculated from the matching requirements at $y = 0$.

To establish the conditions to be satisfied for the match, let us first define for the discontinuity of any function $f(y)$ at $y = 0$ the jump

$$\Delta f = f(0^+) - f(0^-) .$$

The continuity of the beam requires that[4]

$$\Delta w = 0, \qquad \Delta w' = 0 . \tag{4.26a,b}$$

Equilibrium of the beam element straddling the point $y = 0$ requires that

$$\Delta M = 0, \qquad \Delta M' = -P . \tag{4.26'}$$

[4] Here and in the following, primes may be interpreted arbitrarily as derivatives with respect to x or to y.

To translate these conditions into equations for the deflection w, we rewrite (4.2a) for the elastic beam and differentiate it once:

$$M = -EI\,w'', \qquad M' = -EI\,w'''.$$

Applying to each of these equations the jump operator Δ, we find that

$$\Delta w'' = 0, \qquad \Delta w''' = P/EI\,. \tag{4.26c,d}$$

The fifth condition is harder to find. We begin by differentiating (4.2a) once more and applying the jump operator:

$$\Delta M'' = -EI\,\Delta w^{iv}\,.$$

Then we turn to the equilibrium condition (4.2b), which with $p \equiv 0$ yields

$$\Delta M'' = \Delta q,$$

and at last we rewrite (4.4):

$$q - c p_1 q' = -c q_1 w'\,.$$

When this equation is integrated between the limits 0^- and 0^+, the first term makes no contribution and we have

$$p_1\,\Delta q = q_1\,\Delta w\,,$$

whence

$$\Delta q = 0, \qquad \Delta M'' = 0,$$

and hence

$$\Delta w^{iv} = 0. \tag{4.26e}$$

This is the last one of the matching conditions.

Applying (4.26a-e) to the solution (4.25) is a routine procedure and need not be demonstrated here. Some numerical results are shown in Fig.4.9 for two choices of γ, one involving (4.25b) and the other one (4.25c).

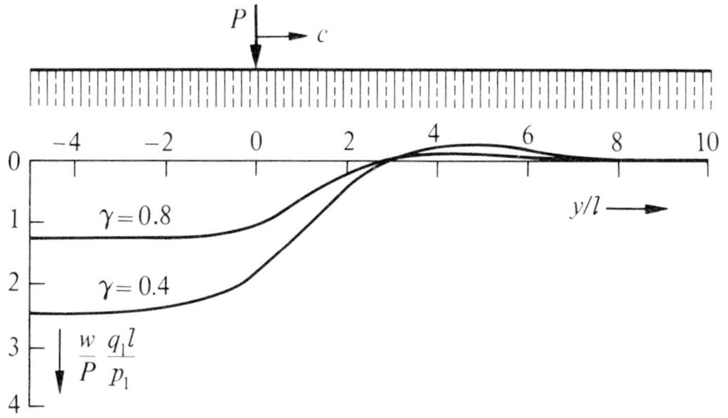

Figure 4.9. Elastic beam on a Maxwell support, deflection for two values of the velocity of the moving load.

The difference between the solutions (4.25b,c), which should show up in these curves, is completely wiped out by the high exponential damping present in both cases. The permanent sag of the beam behind the load increases as the speed of the load decreases. However, the limiting case $c = 0$ is not covered by our analysis. In this case, the independent variable y becomes equal to x and is no longer suitable to serve in the description of a time-dependent process. Correspondingly, the solution degenerates completely. Also if c gets very large, the solution, though existing, is no longer applicable, but for a quite different reason. Here as in all preceding chapters of this book, we have considered slow creep processes, but if c gets large, there appear fast changes of deformation, which are to an increasing extent influenced by the mass inertia of the beam and its supporting medium. Wave propagation phenomena similar to those described in Chapter 6, but much more complicated, come into play, and the Winkler model is no longer suitable to describe the participation of the ground. Our equations, in which inertia terms have not been included, are then losing contact with the physical reality. Between the two extremes of very large and almost vanishing load velocity there lies the domain of slow viscoelastic action covered by our equations.

For a second example, we choose a Kelvin beam resting on an elastic support. In (4.20) we have then

$$\mathbf{P}_a = 1, \qquad \mathbf{Q}_a = q_0 + q_1 \frac{\partial}{\partial t}, \tag{4.27a}$$

$$\mathbf{P}_b = 1, \qquad \mathbf{Q}_b = k . \tag{4.27b}$$

The characteristic equation (4.23) then reads

$$I\lambda^4 (q_0 - c q_1 \lambda) + k = 0 .$$

It is again of the fifth degree, but this time there is no solution $\lambda = 0$. This reflects the fact that both materials are solid and that there can be no permanent deformation for $y \to -\infty$. Descartes's rule of signs indicates that there is one real root $\lambda = \lambda_5 > 0$ and that there are two pairs of conjugate complex roots. Numerical evaluation produces the result that one of these pairs has a positive real part and the other a negative one:

$$\lambda_{1,2} = -\varkappa_1 \pm i\mu_1, \qquad \lambda_{3,4} = +\varkappa_2 \pm i\mu_2$$

with $\varkappa_1, \varkappa_2, \mu_1, \mu_2 > 0$. The general solution of the differential equation (4.20) is, therefore,

$$w = e^{-\varkappa_1 y}(C_1 \cos \mu_1 y + C_2 \sin \mu_1 y) + $$
$$+ e^{\varkappa_2 y}(C_3 \cos \mu_2 y + C_4 \sin \mu_2 y) + C_5 e^{\lambda_5 y} . \tag{4.28}$$

As in the preceding example, the first two terms of this solution apply only in the domain $y \geq 0$, since they lead to $w = 0$ for $y \to +\infty$ but would grow beyond bounds for $y \to -\infty$, while $C_3, C_4, C_5 \neq 0$ for $y \leq 0$.

At $y = 0$, the two branches of the solution must be matched. The kinematic matching conditions are the same as before:

$$\Delta w = 0, \qquad \Delta w' = 0, \tag{4.29a,b}$$

and also the static conditions (4.26') for ΔM and $\Delta M'$ still hold, but from (4.27a) we have now

$$M = -I(q_0 w'' - cq_1 w'''),$$

$$M' = -I(q_0 w''' - cq_1 w^{iv}).$$

Introducing this into (4.26') we obtain a preliminary form of the next two matching conditions:

$$q_0 \Delta w'' - cq_1 \Delta w''' = 0,$$

$$q_0 \Delta w''' - cq_1 \Delta w^{iv} = P/I.$$

However, we shall not consider these conditions as final, but use them in linear combinations with the fifth condition.

To find this one, we integrate the relation for M between the limits 0^- and 0^+. Since $\int M\,dy = 0$, this yields

$$-I(q_0 \Delta w' - cq_1 \Delta w'') = 0.$$

Because of (4.29b), we know now that

$$\Delta w'' = 0 \tag{4.29c}$$

and then the conditions called "preliminary" simplify to the statements that

$$\Delta w''' = 0, \qquad \Delta w^{iv} = -P/Icq_1. \tag{4.29d,e}$$

In (4.29a-e) we now have a set of five matching conditions, from which the free constants $C_1 \ldots C_5$ can be calculated.

What remains to be done, is again routine work. For the graphic presentation of numerical results we define a reference length l by

$$l^4 = I q_0/k$$

and a load velocity parameter

$$\gamma = cq_1/q_0 l \ .$$

Some results are shown in Fig.4.10. They represent the deflection of a beam under a load which is moving from left to right. The influence of the load velocity parameter γ is not spectacular. The beam begins to deflect well ahead of the load, and after the load has passed, the Kelvin beam relaxes again and the deflection returns gradually to zero, passing first through negative values just as an elastic beam would do. The fact that here a viscoelastic material is involved, manifests itself in the asymmetry of the picture. In particular, the deepest deflection does not occur right under the load, but a small distance behind it.

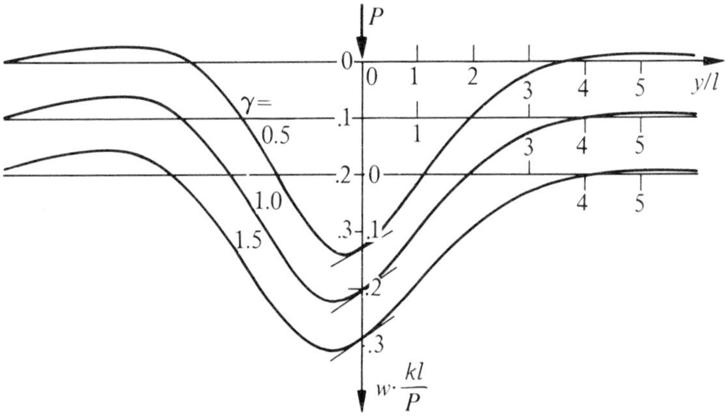

Figure 4.10. Kelvin beam on an elastic support, deflection for three values of the velocity of the moving load.

4.5 Rolling Friction

Where the load is applied, the beam has an upward slope, $dw/dy = \partial w/\partial x < 0$. This means that the load moving with the velocity c has to do work although it stays all the time at the same level. This phenomenon, well known and occurring in various situations, does not stand in the common text books and may need some explanation. Assume that the load P is applied to the axle of a wheel, which rolls from left to right over the beam. Since there is no sliding motion, the force transmitted between the wheel and the beam must be at right angles with the surface of contact and, therefore, must deviate by an angle w' from the vertical, as shown in Fig.4.11. To keep the wheel balanced, we must apply a horizontal force F = P w', which is pushing the wheel. This is the force which does work during the rolling motion and supplies the energy needed for the viscoelastic deformation.

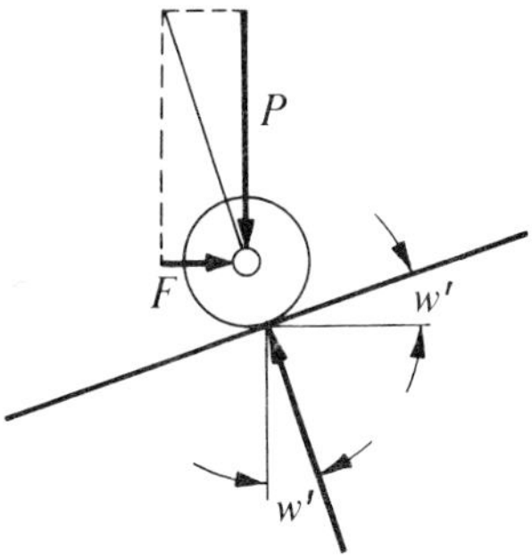

Figure 4.11. Rolling friction.

The factor w' appears to play the same role as the coefficient of dry (Coulomb) friction for a body sliding on a rough surface. There is, however, a remarkable difference. The coefficient of dry friction is, within a wide range, a constant; doubling the load P also doubles the friction force. In the present case, the deflection w(x) is proportional to the applied load P, and so is w'(0). Doubling P therefore also doubles w' and requires four times as much F. The rolling friction in this system increases (and also decreases) with the square of the load!

References

The theory of an elastic beam resting on an elastic medium goes back to

22. E. Winkler: Die Lehre von der Elastizität und Festigkeit. (Prague 1867) p. 182.

Modern presentations are the following:

23. M. Hetényi: Beams on Elastic Foundation. (Ann Arbor, University of Michigan Press, 1946).

24. M. Hetényi: "Beams on Elastic Foundation" in W. Flügge (ed.), Handbook of Engineering Mechanics (New York, McGraw-Hill, 1962), Chap. 31.

The theory of viscoelastic systems with a moving load has been developed by

25. J.M. Kelly: Moving Load Problems in the Theory of Viscoelasticity. Ph. D. Diss., Stanford 1962.

Chapter 5

Vibrations

All viscoelastic deformations vary with time, that is, there is always some motion taking place. Whenever the velocity changes, there must be an unbalance of forces producing the acceleration. However, most visoelastic motion is so slow that the product of acceleration and mass is very small compared to other forces present. It is this fact that made it possible to develop a substantial part of the theory without introducing inertia terms into the equations. It is clear that mass inertia becomes an important feature as soon as we wish to deal with vibrations, and this field we now shall enter.

5.1 Complex Compliance

Before actually introducing inertia terms and writing dynamic equations, we must examine the constitutive equation of the viscoelastic material for the special case that stress and strain are oscillating functions of time. This means essentially an interpretation of (1.23) or any of its equivalents, and this task may be approached in two different ways. Either we apply an oscillating stress $\sigma = \sigma_0 \sin \omega t$ to a tension specimen and ask for the strain it produces, or we force upon the specimen a deformation described by an oscillating strain and ask for the stress that will be produced. While the first approach may seem more natural, the second one has the advantage of not leading to minus signs at inconvenient places.

Instead of assuming ε to vary like a sine or cosine of time, it will be advantageous to write

$$\varepsilon = \varepsilon_0 e^{i\omega t} = \varepsilon_0(\cos \omega t + i \sin \omega t). \qquad (5.1)$$

In this formula the real and imaginary parts represent, each by itself, two oscillatory strains of the frequency ω. Since (1.23b) has real coefficients p_k and q_k, the real part of the stress σ will correspond to the real part of ε and similarly, the imaginary parts of σ and ε correspond to each other. In this way we get simultaneously the solutions to two closely related problems, at the same time having the additional advantage of greater simplicity of the mathematical formalism.

When we introduce ε from (5.1) into (1.23b), we see that also the stress must have a factor $e^{i\omega t}$, that is,

$$\sigma = \sigma_0 e^{i\omega t}. \tag{5.2}$$

Equation (1.23b) then reads

$$\sum_0^m p_k \sigma_0 (i\omega)^k e^{i\omega t} = \sum_0^n q_k \varepsilon_0 (i\omega)^k e^{i\omega t},$$

and after cancellation of $e^{i\omega t}$ this may be solved for the stress amplitude

$$\sigma_0 = \varepsilon_0 \frac{\sum q_k i^k \omega^k}{\sum p_k i^k \omega^k} = \varepsilon_0 \frac{\mathcal{Q}(i\omega)}{\mathcal{P}(i\omega)}, \tag{5.3}$$

where $\mathcal{P}$ and $\mathcal{Q}$ are the polynomials introduced in (1.26). Evidently, σ_0 is a complex quantity and may be written as

$$\sigma_0 = \sigma_1 + i\sigma_2, \tag{5.4}$$

whence

$$\sigma = \sigma_0 e^{i\omega t} = (\sigma_1 + i\sigma_2)(\cos \omega t + i \sin \omega t)$$

and, after separation of real and imaginary parts,

$$\sigma = (\sigma_1 \cos \omega t - \sigma_2 \sin \omega t) + i(\sigma_2 \cos \omega t + \sigma_1 \sin \omega t). \tag{5.5}$$

The real part of σ is the stress response to $\varepsilon = \varepsilon_0 \cos \omega t$, and the imaginary part is the response to a strain $\varepsilon = \varepsilon_0 \sin \omega t$. In both cases the stress is a mixture of a sine and a cosine oscillation, that is, there is a phase shift between stress and strain, and they reach their peak values at different times.

The relation between σ and ε may be visualized in a vector diagram similar to those used in other fields of vibration theory. This diagram (Fig.5.1) has two pairs of orthogonal axes, R, I and r,i. The axes R, I are a coordinate system, in which we plot points with the coordinates σ_1, σ_2 and ε_0, 0 and vectors $\boldsymbol{\sigma}$ and $\boldsymbol{\epsilon}$ which have these coordinates as their components. We call these vectors the amplitude vectors of the oscillating quantities σ and ε.

The axes r, i revolve clockwise with the angular velocity ω. When we now project at any time t the vectors $\boldsymbol{\sigma}$ and $\boldsymbol{\epsilon}$ on the axis r, we find the component vectors

$$\sigma_1 \cos \omega t - \sigma_2 \sin \omega t \quad \text{and} \quad \varepsilon_0 \cos \omega t,$$

that is, the real parts of the right-hand sides of (5.5) and (5.1). Similarly, the projections of $\boldsymbol{\sigma}$ and $\boldsymbol{\epsilon}$ on the axis i are the imaginary parts of the oscillating quantities σ and ε. The angle ψ between the two amplitude vectors describes the phase shift of the oscillations. The r axis (and also the i axis) coincides first with $\boldsymbol{\sigma}$ and by a time $t = \psi/\omega$ later with $\boldsymbol{\epsilon}$. This means that σ reaches its peak value that much earlier than ε.

So far, we have assumed that ε_0 is real, that is, that $\boldsymbol{\epsilon}$ coincides with the R axis of Fig.5.1. It would not make much of a difference if we would rotate the vectors $\boldsymbol{\epsilon}$ and $\boldsymbol{\sigma}$ by any angle, as long as we preserve the phase angle ψ between them. Stress and strain would then reach their maxima or pass through zero by a certain time earlier or later without any change in their relations to each other, that is, the whole oscillation would be shifted in phase. If we make use of this possibility of generalizing our formulas, ε_0 will become complex - let us say, $\varepsilon_0 = \varepsilon_1 + i\varepsilon_2$ - but (5.3) will not be affected.

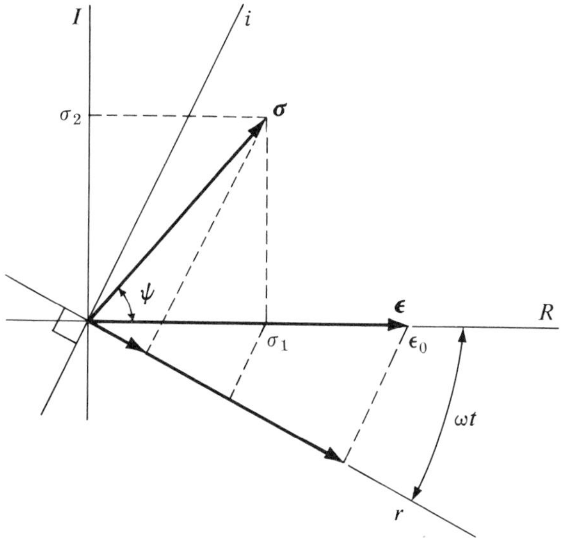

Figure 5.1. Representation of a vibration by complex vectors.

Since the differential equation (1.23) is linear, it is not surprising that (5.3) is a linear relation between σ_0 and ϵ_0. We write it in the form

$$\epsilon_0 = G(\omega) \cdot \sigma_0 \tag{5.6}$$

and call the factor

$$G(\omega) = \frac{\mathfrak{P}(i\omega)}{\mathfrak{Q}(i\omega)} = G_1(\omega) + iG_2(\omega) \tag{5.7}$$

the complex compliance. It depends on the frequency, but not on the amplitude of stress or strain or on time. Assuming the general case that both ϵ_0 and σ_0 are complex, we may write (5.6) in the form

$$(\epsilon_1 + i\epsilon_2) = (G_1 + iG_2)(\sigma_1 + i\sigma_2),$$

from which we see that

$$\epsilon_1 = G_1\sigma_1 - G_2\sigma_2, \qquad \epsilon_2 = G_2\sigma_1 + G_1\sigma_2. \tag{5.8}$$

Solving these equations for σ_1, σ_2, we find

$$\left(G_1^2 + G_2^2\right)\sigma_1 = G_1\varepsilon_1 + G_2\varepsilon_2,$$
$$\left(G_1^2 + G_2^2\right)\sigma_2 = G_1\varepsilon_2 - G_2\varepsilon_1, \qquad (5.9a,b)$$

and these two pairs of equations show us what strain is produced by a given stress and what stress by a given strain. In view of later needs we let $\sigma_1 = 1$, $\sigma_2 = 0$ and see from (5.8) that then $\varepsilon_1 = G_1$, $\varepsilon_2 = G_2$. From the real parts of (5.1) and (5.2) it then follows that a unit oscillatory stress $\sigma = \cos\omega t$ produces the strain

$$\varepsilon = G_1(\omega)\cos\omega t - G_2(\omega)\sin\omega t, \qquad (5.10a)$$

and from the imaginary parts that $\sigma = \sin\omega t$ produces

$$\varepsilon = G_2(\omega)\cos\omega t + G_1(\omega)\sin\omega t. \qquad (5.10b)$$

5.2 Dissipation

We consider an element of a tension bar of cross section A and length dx. At its ends forces σA are acting, and in the time dt the strain increases by $\dot{\varepsilon}\,dt$. This makes the forces do the work

$$\sigma A \cdot dx\,\dot{\varepsilon}\,dt = dW\,A\,dx,$$

where dW is the work done per unit volume of the bar. If the deformation continues for a finite time, the work done on a unit volume is

$$W = \int dW = \int \sigma\dot{\varepsilon}\,dt. \qquad (5.11)$$

This work comes from an outside source of energy and goes into the element. In an elastic bar it creates potential energy (strain energy), which will be recovered upon unloading. In a viscoelastic material part or even all of this energy may be lost in the sense that it is transformed into heat and therefore is not recoverable. We call such energy *dissipated*.

In (5.11), the stress may be any function of time, increasing or decreasing, or a constant. We shall now apply this formula to the special case of an oscillating stress, accompainied by an oscillating strain. However, in doing so, we cannot use the complex notation of (5.1) and (5.2). This notation represents, as we have seen, the simultaneous handling of two oscillations having a phase difference of 90°, keeping them apart by multiplying one of them by a factor i. Now, our work integral contains the product of stress and strain, and in this product the imaginary stress working on an imaginary strain would do no negative, but real, work so that the real part of W would be an unidentifiable mixture of the work done by both oscillations, while the imaginary part would be entirely meaningless. We therefore resort to writing stress and strain in real quantities, choosing

$$\sigma = \sigma_0 \cos \omega t \quad \text{and} \quad \varepsilon = \sigma_0 [G_1(\omega) \cos \omega t - G_2(\omega) \sin \omega t].$$

We then have

$$W = -\sigma_0^2 \omega \int \cos \omega t (G_1 \sin \omega t + G_2 \cos \omega t) dt. \tag{5.12}$$

It is now necessary to choose limits for the integral. Two such choices are of interest: We may integrate over one period $T = 2\pi/\omega$, or we may integrate over a unit of time.

Let us begin with the integral over one period and write

$$W = -\sigma_0^2 \omega G_1 \int_0^T \cos \omega t \sin \omega t \, dt - \sigma_0^2 \omega G_2 \int_0^T \cos^2 \omega t \, dt.$$

The first of the two integrals is zero. It represents the work done by σ on a deformation which is in phase with the stress. This is the kind of work encountered in elastic materials. Through half the period energy is pumped into the material, and in the other half it is recovered. In a viscoelastic material the strain has another component, which is by 90° out of phase with (in quadrature with) the stress and this one makes a permanent contribution:

$$W = -\sigma_0^2 \omega G_2 \frac{\pi}{\omega} = -\pi \sigma_0^2 G_2(\omega). \tag{5.13}$$

During every period of the oscillation this amount of work is done, and the corresponding energy is dissipated. Since the second law of thermodynamics requires that this dissipated energy be non-negative, we learn from (5.13) that

$$G_2(\omega) \leqslant 0, \tag{5.14}$$

and we shall see that the equal sign applies only in some limiting cases.

In applications it is of more interest to know the energy dissipated in a unit of time. We call this the dissipation D and find it by dividing W from (5.13) by $T = 2\pi/\omega$:

$$D = -\frac{1}{2}\sigma_0^2\,\omega G_2(\omega). \tag{5.15}$$

If we try to verify this formula from (5.12), we find that it checks only if there is an integer number of periods T in the time unit. Otherwise there is a small deviation, positive or negative, which depends on how the time unit is cut out of the sequence of ups and downs of the oscillation. This indicates that D is an average quantity and does not make sense when we are interested in the energy turnover within a few seconds, while the period T is of the order of minutes or hours.

5.3 Application to Specific Materials

We shall now use the concepts of complex compliance and dissipation to see how some of our standard materials behave under oscillating stress.

We begin with the three-parameter solid. From (5.7) and the differential equation (1.19) we find

$$G(\omega) = \frac{1 + p_1 i\omega}{q_0 + q_1 i\omega}, \tag{5.16}$$

which, after multiplying numerator and denominator by $(q_0 - q_1 i\omega)$, can be separated into real and imaginary parts:

$$G_1(\omega) = \frac{q_0 + p_1 q_1 \omega^2}{q_0^2 + q_1^2\omega^2}, \qquad G_2(\omega) = -\frac{(q_1 - p_1 q_0)\omega}{q_0^2 + q_1^2\omega^2}. \tag{5.17}$$

We saw that G_2 must be negative, and this leads us back to the inequality (1.20), which here acquires a new significance.

From (5.10a) we see that, in our material, a stress $\sigma = \cos \omega t$ produces a strain

$$\epsilon = \frac{q_0 + p_1 q_1 \omega^2}{q_0^2 + q_1^2 \omega^2} \cos \omega t + \frac{(q_1 - p_1 q_0)\omega}{q_0^2 + q_1^2 \omega^2} \sin \omega t. \qquad (5.18)$$

Since the sine lags in phase 90° behind the cosine, the strain is between 0° and 90° behind the stress. When we let ω approach zero or infinity, the coefficient of $\sin \omega t$ goes to zero, and the phase difference between σ and ϵ tends to disappear, that is, the material approaches elastic behavior. In particular, we have

$$\text{for} \quad \omega \approx 0: \qquad \epsilon \approx \frac{1}{q_0} \cos \omega t = \frac{1}{E_\infty} \cos \omega t,$$

$$\text{for} \quad \omega \to \infty: \qquad \epsilon \to \frac{p_1}{q_1} \cos \omega t = \frac{1}{E_0} \cos \omega t$$

with the moduli E_∞ and E_0 as defined on pp. 9 and 10.

In a coordinate system G_1, G_2, (5.17) is the parameter representation of a curve (Fig. 5.2a). It may be left to the reader to show that it is a semicircle.

The dissipation can be calculated from (5.15) and (5.17). It is

$$D = \frac{1}{2} \sigma_0^2 \frac{(q_1 - p_1 q_0)\omega^2}{q_0^2 + q_1^2 \omega^2} . \qquad (5.19)$$

For $\omega \to \infty$, it approaches a finite value, but for $\omega = 0$ it vanishes. This indicates that in the latter case the material truly approaches elastic behavior, while at high frequency there is little dissipation per cycle, but there are so many cycles per unit of time that their combined contribution does not vanish.

Our results include as limiting cases the Kelvin solid and the Maxwell fluid.

As may be seen from the third column of Table 1.2, the three-parameter solid degenerates into the Kelvin solid if we let $p_1 = 0$. This leads to quantitative changes in G_2 and D, but to a qualitative change of G_1, which is now

$$G_1(\omega) = \frac{q_0}{q_0^2 + q_1^2\omega^2}.$$

For $\omega \to \infty$ this goes to zero as ω^{-2}, while G_2 tends to zero only as ω^{-1}. This means that at high frequencies the phase shift between stress and strain approaches 90° and that the behavior of the Kelvin solid approaches that of a viscous fluid. In Fig. 5.2a, the half circle reaches at its left end the origin of the coordinate system.

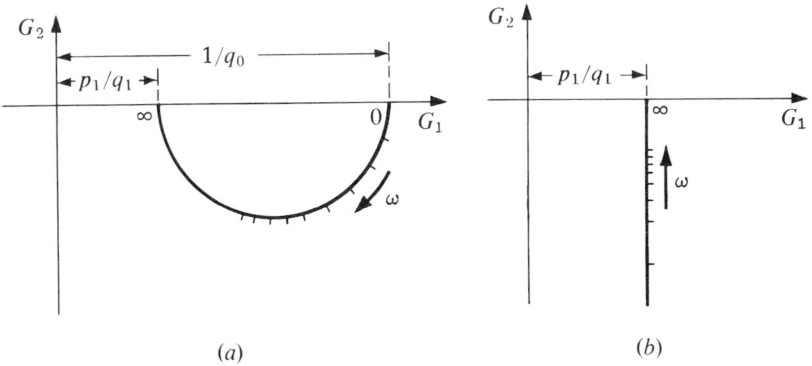

Figure 5.2. Complex compliances - a: three-parameter solid; b: Maxwell fluid.

If in (5.16) through (5.19) we keep p_1 but let $q_0 = 0$, we have the results for the Maxwell fluid. In this case the right end of the half circle in Fig. 5.2a moves to infinity and the curve becomes a vertical straight line, as is shown in Fig. 5.2b. Both parts of the complex compliance change substantially and are now

$$G_1(\omega) = \frac{p_1}{q_1}, \qquad G_2(\omega) = -\frac{1}{q_1\omega}. \tag{5.20}$$

G_2 still vanishes when $\omega \to \infty$, but for $\omega \to 0$ it becomes infinite and outweighs G_1 in importance. This means that for high frequencies the Maxwell material approaches elastic behavior, while for low ones it becomes purely viscous. The dissipation turns out to be independent of the frequency:

$$D = \sigma_0^2/2q_1 . \tag{5.21}$$

The results contained in (5.17) and (5.20) and similar expressions for other materials are listed in the last two columns of Table 1.2.

5.4 Relations Between Compliances

So far we have derived expressions for the complex compliance $G(\omega)$ from the differential equation (1.23) of the material. The existence of the hereditary integral (2.6) proves that the creep compliance $J(t)$ completely determines the strain produced by a given stress. Therefore, it must be possible to calculate $G(\omega)$ when only $J(t)$ is known. Now, as we have seen in (5.10a), the stress $\sigma = \cos\omega t$ produces the periodic strain $\epsilon = G_1 \cos\omega t - G_2 \sin\omega t$. However, if we start applying such a stress at $t = 0$, the strain my not be a simple oscillation, but may contain a transient part. We try to remove this transient by postulating that the oscillatory stress has already been acting for a very long (an infinite) time, let us say, since $t = -T$. Then, with an abvious modification, the hereditary integral (2.6a) yields the strain

$$\epsilon(t) = \sigma(-T) \cdot J(t+T) + \int_{-T}^{t} J(t-t') \frac{d\sigma(t')}{dt'}\, dt'$$

and, with $T \to \infty$, we expect this to be the strain described by (5.10a):

$$G_1(\omega) \cos\omega t - G_2(\omega) \sin\omega t$$

$$= \lim_{T\to\infty} \left\{ J(t+T) \cos\omega T - \omega \int_{-T}^{t} J(t-t') \sin\omega t'\, dt' \right\} . \tag{5.22}$$

We shall study the working of this formula by applying it to two typical materials, a solid and a fluid.

For a Kelvin solid with J(t) from Table 1.2, we have

$$G_1 \cos\omega t - G_2 \sin\omega t$$

$$= \frac{1}{q_0} \lim_{T\to\infty} \left\{ (1 - e^{-\lambda(t+T)}) \cos\omega T - \omega \int_{-T}^{t} (1 - e^{-\lambda t} e^{\lambda t'}) \sin\omega t' \, dt' \right\}$$

with $\lambda = q_0/q_1$. In the term preceding the integral, the exponential tends to zero and may be dropped immediately. After performing the integration, we then have

$$G_1 \cos\omega t - G_2 \sin\omega t = \frac{1}{q_0} \lim_{T\to\infty} \left\{ \cos\omega T + \Big[\cos\omega t' \Big]_{-T}^{t} \right.$$
$$\left. + \frac{\omega e^{-\lambda t}}{\lambda^2 + \omega^2} \Big[(\lambda \sin\omega t' - \omega \cos\omega t') e^{\lambda t'} \Big]_{-T}^{t} \right\} .$$

When the integration limits are introduced in the bracketed terms, some cancellations take place, and then the expression is reduced to

$$G_1 \cos\omega t - G_2 \sin\omega t = \frac{1}{q_0} \left\{ \cos\omega t + \frac{\lambda\omega}{\lambda^2 + \omega^2} \sin\omega t - \frac{\omega^2}{\lambda^2 + \omega^2} \cos\omega t \right\} .$$

This really is a harmonic oscillation, and by separating sine and cosine parts one obtains G_1 and G_2 as listed in Table 1.2.

For the Maxwell fluid we start out with

$$G_1 \cos\omega t - G_2 \sin\omega t$$

$$= \frac{1}{q_1} \lim_{T\to\infty} \left\{ (p_1 + t + T) \cos\omega t - \omega \int_{-T}^{t} (p_1 + t - t') \sin\omega t' \, dt' \right\} .$$

Performing the integration and collecting terms yields in this case the following expression:

$$\frac{1}{q_1} \lim_{T\to\infty} \left\{ p_1 \cos\omega t + \frac{1}{\omega} \sin\omega t - \frac{1}{\omega} \sin\omega T \right\} .$$

This has a sine and a cosine term, both of which are independent of T, and which may be equated to $G_1 \cos\omega t$ and $G_2 \sin\omega t$. This indeed yields the results found previously and listed in Table 1.2, but there is also a constant, which depends on T and which does not even approach a definite limit as $T \to \infty$. This is a "transient" that never dies out, indicating that at present, at a fixed time t, the strain still depends on the point within a period at which long, long ago the oscillating load was started. A term of this kind is to be expected whenever the spring-dashpot model has a free dashpot, that is, in all fluids. For these materials, ϵ = const is a solution of the homogeneous differential equation $\mathbf{Q}\epsilon = 0$, and this constant may appear in addition to the particular solution (5.10a).

We now reverse our problem: Can we find the creep compliance J(t) when the complex compliance $G(\omega)$ is known? To find the answer, we need a simple formula from the theory of the Fourier integral [28, 29]. It says that the unit step function can be written in the form

$$\Delta(t) = \frac{1}{2} + \frac{1}{\pi}\int_0^\infty \frac{\sin\omega t}{\omega}\,d\omega . \tag{5.23}$$

The second term on the right-hand side is a function of t and changes sign when t is replaced by -t. The equation states that, for $t > 0$, it has the constant value 1/2.

The creep compliance J(t) is the strain produced by a unit of stress applied as a step function, $\sigma = \Delta t$. Equation (5.23) shows how this stress may be resolved into an average of $\sigma = 1/2$ and the sum of infinitely many oscillations of infinitesimal amplitudes $d\omega/\pi\omega$. To these latter ones we may apply (5.10b) to find the corresponding strain, but we have still to find a way to deal with the constant average $\sigma = 1/2$. To make (5.10) applicable to it, we interpret it as a cosine oscillation of vanishing frequency,

$$\frac{1}{2} \equiv \frac{1}{2}\lim_{\omega\to 0}\cos\omega t .$$

Equation (5.10a) then yields

$$\epsilon(t) = \frac{1}{2}\lim_{\omega\to 0}\,[G_1(\omega)\cos\omega t - G_2(\omega)\sin\omega t]$$

$$+ \frac{1}{\pi}\int_0^\infty [G_1(\omega)\sin\omega t + G_2(\omega)\cos\omega t]\frac{d\omega}{\omega} , \tag{5.24}$$

and this must be equal to $J(t)$. In the first term of the first bracket the limiting process may at once be carried out, and in the second term we may at least let $\sin \omega t \approx \omega t$. We then have

$$J(t) = \frac{1}{2} G_1(0) + \frac{1}{\pi} \int_0^\infty G_2(\omega) \cos \omega t \frac{d\omega}{\omega}$$

$$- \frac{1}{2} t \lim_{\omega \to 0} [\omega G_2(\omega)] + \frac{1}{\pi} \int_0^\infty G_1(\omega) \sin \omega t \frac{d\omega}{\omega}. \qquad (5.25)$$

In this equation terms have been so arranged that the first line is an even function of t and the second an odd one. Now consider any $t < 0$. Since then $J(t) = 0$, it follows that the two lines are equal in absolute value, but opposite in sign. When we now change the sign of t to positive, all that happens is that the second line changes sign, and then both lines are equal and each of them equals $\frac{1}{2} J(t)$. Thus we obtain two formulas for the creep compliance, namely:

$$J(t) = G_1(0) + \frac{2}{\pi} \int_0^\infty G_2(\omega) \cos \omega t \frac{d\omega}{\omega} \qquad (5.26a)$$

and

$$J(t) = -t \lim_{\omega \to 0} [\omega G_2(\omega)] + \frac{2}{\pi} \int_0^\infty G_1(\omega) \sin \omega t \frac{d\omega}{\omega}. \qquad (5.26b)$$

As we have seen, a sinusoidal stress may produce a strain which, in addition to $\sin \omega t$ and $\cos \omega t$ contains an additive constant $\epsilon = c$ of undefined value. Thus the right-hand side of (5.25) may not represent $J(t)$ but rather $J(t) + c$. Since this constant is an even function of t, it would be part of the first line and hence would appear in (5.26a). We must therefore expect that (5.26b) is correct while (5.26a) may be in error by a constant.

For a viscous fluid we find from Table 1.2 that $G_1 \equiv 0$, $G_2 = -1/q_1\omega$. This we now introduce into (5.26a) and have

$$J(t) = -\frac{2}{\pi q_1} \int_0^\infty \cos \omega t \frac{d\omega}{\omega^2} = -\frac{2t}{\pi q_1} \int_0^\infty \frac{\cos \omega t \, d(\omega t)}{(\omega t)^2}.$$

This integral leads to a rare transcendental function, the sine integral, defined by the formula

$$\mathrm{Si}\, x = \int_0^x \frac{\sin y}{y}\, dy .$$

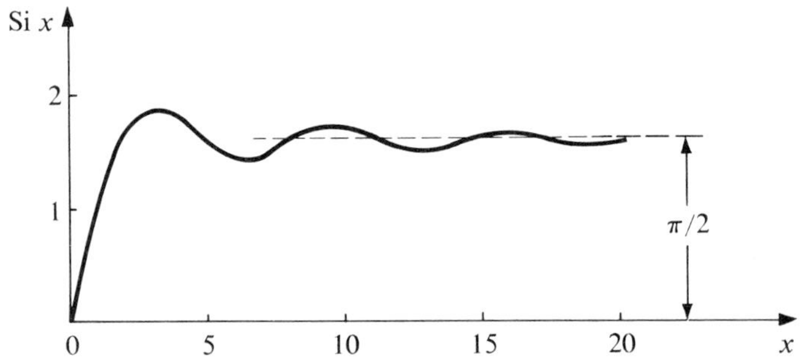

Figure 5.3. Sine integral Si x.

It has been tabulated and is shown in Fig. 5.3. An integration by parts brings our integral in a suitable form and we find easily that

$$J(t) = -\frac{2t}{\pi q_1}\left[-\frac{\cos \omega t}{\omega t} - \mathrm{Si}(\omega t)\right]_0^{\infty} = -\frac{2}{\pi q_1}\left(\infty - \frac{\pi t}{2}\right),$$

a meaningless result. We try now (5.26b) and find very easily

$$J(t) = -t \lim_{\omega \to 0}\left(-\frac{1}{q_1}\right) = \frac{t}{q_1},$$

which is correct. The Maxwell fluid may be handled in a similar way. For other materials the integrals are difficult and require complex contour integration. For readers sufficiently experienced in complex variable theory we use the Kelvin solid to demonstrate the technique.

We insert G_1 and G_2 from Table 1.2 into (5.26a).

$$J(t) = \frac{1}{q_0} - \frac{2q_1}{\pi}\int_0^{\infty} \frac{\cos \omega t}{q_0^2 + q_1^2\omega^2}\, d\omega$$

$$= \frac{1}{q_0} - \frac{2t}{\pi q_1}\int_0^{\infty} \frac{\cos \omega t}{(\lambda t)^2 + (\omega t)^2}\, d(\omega t) .$$

We must find the integral

$$H = \int_0^\infty \frac{\cos z \, dz}{a^2 + z^2} ,$$

and when we interpret $z = x + iy$ as a complex variable, our integration path is the positive part of the real axis (Fig. 5.4). Since the in-

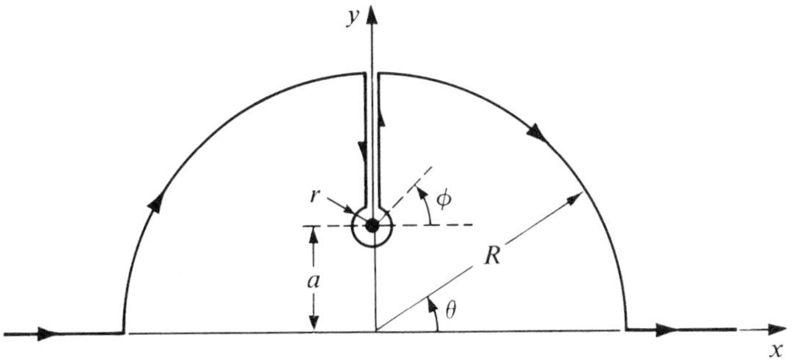

Figure 5.4. Complex contour integral.

tegrand is an even function, the integral over the entire real axis is 2H, and this does not change when we add an integral over an odd function which, by itself, equals zero:

$$2H = \int_{-\infty}^\infty \frac{\cos z \, dz}{a^2 + z^2} + i \int_{-\infty}^\infty \frac{\sin z \, dz}{a^2 + z^2} = \int_{-\infty}^\infty \frac{e^{iz} \, dz}{a^2 + z^2} .$$

In the theory of complex variables it is shown that an integral does not change its value if we change the integration path (connecting the same end points), provided that there is no singular point of the integrand between the two paths (Cauchy's integral theorem). This condition is satisfied when we switch to the path which in Fig. 5.4 is shown by a heavy line. It consists of the outer parts of the real axis and a large half-circle, but this half-circle is interrupted by a detour, which is so chosen that the singular point $z = ia$ (for which $a^2 + z^2 = 0$) still lies above the integration path. The vertical parts of this detour are supposed to coincide with the y axis. For both, the integrand is the same, but going down, dy is negative, and going up, it is positive, and the contributions to 2H cancel each other. On the big circle we write

$z = Re^{i\theta}$ and on the small one $z = ia + re^{i\phi}$. When we let $R \to \infty$, the horizontal parts of the path vanish entirely, and we have ultimately

$$2H = \lim_{R\to\infty} \int_{\pi}^{0} \frac{\exp(iRe^{i\theta})}{a^2 + R^2 e^{2i\theta}} Rie^{i\theta} d\theta + \lim_{r\to 0} \int_{\pi/2}^{5\pi/2} \frac{\exp i(ia + re^{i\phi})}{a^2 + (ia + re^{i\phi})^2} rie^{i\phi} d\phi .$$

Now let us have a close look at the first integral. In the numerator we write

$$\exp(iRe^{i\theta}) = e^{iR(\cos\theta + i\sin\theta)} = e^{iR\cos\theta} e^{-R\sin\theta}$$

$$= [\cos(R\cos\theta) + i\sin(R\cos\theta)]e^{-R\sin\theta} .$$

When $R \to \infty$, the factor in the brackets is bounded and the real exponential behind it tends to zero. In addition, the integrand has another R, but it also has an R^2 in the denominator and therefore tends to zero. Then only the integral over the little circle is left, and we proceed as follows:

$$2H = \lim_{r\to 0} \int_{\pi/2}^{5\pi/2} \frac{e^{-a} e^{ir\cos\phi} e^{-r\sin\phi}}{a^2 - a^2 + 2iare^{i\phi} + r^2 e^{2i\phi}} rie^{i\phi} d\phi$$

$$= ie^{-a} \lim_{r\to 0} \int_{\pi/2}^{5\pi/2} \frac{e^{ir\cos\phi} e^{-r\sin\phi}}{2ia + re^{i\phi}} .$$

In the numerator each factor approaches in the limit $e^0 = 1$, and in the denominator the second term vanishes. The integrand is then a constant, and we arrive at the result

$$H = \frac{1}{2} \frac{e^{-a}}{2a} \cdot 2\pi = \frac{\pi}{2a} e^{-a} .$$

This we now apply to our original problem with $z = \omega t$, $a = \lambda t = q_0 t/q_1$ to obtain

$$J(t) = \frac{1}{q_0} - \frac{2t}{\pi q_1} \cdot \frac{\pi q_1}{2q_0 t} e^{-q_0 t/q_1} = \frac{1}{q_0}\left(1 - e^{-q_0 t/q_1}\right),$$

which is the correct result. It is suggested that the reader try to use (5.26b) in a similar way. This is more difficult, since an additional singularity at $z = 0$ turns up that needs special handling. The result confirms without further incident the one just obtained.

With this example we terminate our study of the oscillatory behavior of viscoelastic materials and now turn our attention to vibrations of mechanical systems endowed with mass and containing a viscoelastic spring.

5.5 The Simple Spring-Mass System

Figure 5.5a shows the prototype of all oscillators of one degree of freedom: a mass M connected by a spring to a fixpoint. However, our spring is not elastic, but is a viscoelastic bar of cross section A. The displacement u of the mass is measured from a position in which the system had been at rest before the vibration began.

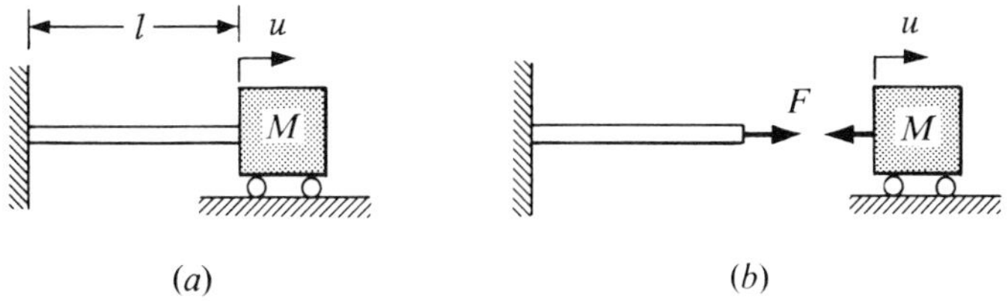

Figure 5.5. Simple oscillator.

To find the possible motions of the system, we have three equations, the dynamic equation

$$M\ddot{u} + F = 0\,, \tag{5.27a}$$

a kinematic relation

$$\epsilon = u/l \tag{5.27b}$$

and the constitutive equation of the spring material. Postulating an oscillatory motion

$$u = u_0 e^{i\omega t}\,, \tag{5.28}$$

we use the form (5.6).

From (5.27) we derive

$$\epsilon = \frac{u_0}{l} e^{i\omega t}, \quad A\sigma = F = -M\ddot{u} = Mu_0\omega^2 e^{i\omega t},$$

hence

$$\epsilon_0 = u_0/l, \quad \sigma_0 = Mu_0\omega^2/A .$$

When this is introduced into (5.6), the complex amplitude u_0 drops out and we have

$$\omega^2 G(\omega) = \frac{A}{Ml} . \tag{5.29}$$

This is the frequency equation of our oscillator. For all truly viscoelastic materials (excluding the limiting case of the elastic solid), $G(\omega)$ is complex valued for real ω, and, therefore, (5.29) cannot have real solutions. This was to be expected, since an oscillator containing a viscoelastic element cannot make undamped vibrations.

Let us consider a few examples. For a Maxwell material we have

$$G(\omega) = \frac{p_1}{q_1} - \frac{i}{q_1\omega}$$

and hence the frequency equation

$$\frac{1}{q_1}(p_1\omega^2 - i\omega) = \frac{A}{Ml} .$$

This is a quadratic equation for ω and it has the roots

$$\omega = \frac{i}{2p_1} \pm \sqrt{\frac{Aq_1}{Mlp_1} - \frac{1}{4p_1^2}} .$$

If the mass is small or the spring stiff (large $E_0 = q_1/p_1$), the root has a real value, let us say $= \nu$, and we have

$$i\omega = -\frac{1}{2p_1} \pm i\nu ,$$

hence

$$u = e^{-t/2p_1}(C_1 e^{i\nu t} + C_2 e^{-i\nu t}) = e^{-t/2p_1}(B_1 \cos \nu t + B_2 \sin \nu t) .$$

This is a damped vibration.

If the mass is large or the spring soft, the square root will be imaginary, let us say $= i\nu$, and we have

$$i\omega = -\frac{1}{2p_1} \pm \nu = -\omega_{1,2}, \quad \omega_{1,2} > 0 ,$$

and

$$u = C_1 e^{-\omega_1 t} + C_2 e^{-\omega_2 t} ,$$

that is, the case of aperiodic damping, as known from vibration theory. Our system, however, is not the one commonly used to study a damped oscillator (see Problem 5.1).

If the spring is made of a three-parameter solid, we arrive at an interesting paradox. From the last two columns of Table 1.2 we extract

$$G(\omega) = \frac{q_0 + p_1 q_1 \omega^2}{q_0^2 + q_1^2 \omega^2} - i \frac{(q_1 - q_0 p_1)\omega}{q_0^2 + q_1^2 \omega^2} ,$$

and when we introduce this into the frequency equation (5.29) and multiply by the common denominator, we obtain a fourth-degree equation for ω:

$$(q_0 + p_1 q_1 \omega^2)\omega^2 - i(q_1 - q_0 p_1)\omega^3 - \frac{A}{Ml}(q_0^2 + q_1^2 \omega^2) = 0 . \qquad (5.30a)$$

It has four roots, and this makes us expect that there are four different modes of vibration. However, if we use (5.7) to calculate $G(\omega)$, we find

$$G(\omega) = \frac{1 + p_1 i\omega}{q_0 + q_1 i\omega} ,$$

and when this is inserted into (5.29), the resulting equation is only of the third degree:

$$(1 + p_1 i\omega)\omega^2 - \frac{A}{Ml}(q_0 + q_1 i\omega) = 0 . \tag{5.30b}$$

We must conclude that either in (5.30b) we have missed something, or that (5.30a) contains an extraneous root. The latter is true. G_1 and G_2 are defined by the third member of (5.7). They were meant to be the real and imaginary parts of G, and this is the case as long as ω is real. The splitting of G into the two parts was achieved by multiplying the numerator and the denominator of the fraction in (5.7) by $\Sigma q_k(-i)^k \omega^k$. This increases the degree of the numerator (in this case by one), and the ω that makes this factor vanish is the root which (5.30a) has and (5.30b) does not have. It has nothing to do with the mechanical problem.

Instead of using the frequency equation (5.29) to find the possible motions of the oscillator, we might equally well formulate its differential equation and then solve it. To do this, we use again (5.27), but as the constitutive equation of the material we now use the differential equation (1.23c). On its right side we introduce ϵ from (5.27b) and on the left

$$\sigma = \frac{F}{A} = -\frac{M}{A}\ddot{u}$$

from (5.27a) to obtain the equation

$$-\frac{M}{A}\mathbf{P}(\ddot{u}) = \frac{1}{l}\mathbf{Q}(u) . \tag{5.31}$$

Since $\mathbf{P}$ is an operator of the mth order, and since the order of $\mathbf{Q}$ is $n < m + 2$, (5.31) is a differential equation of $(m + 2)$nd order. Upon inspecting the differential equations in Table 1.2, we see that for the viscous fluid and the Kelvin solid the problem is of the second order, exactly as for an elastic spring; that for the Maxwell fluid, both three-parameter materials, and the four-parameter solid it is of the third order; and for the four-parameter fluid, it is of the fourth order. A unique solution requires a corresponding number of initial conditions, and we ask where we may find them. As in every problem of dynamics, the initial values of u and $\dot{u}$ should certainly be known, but what else should be known, and why?

We find the key to an answer when we inspect the simplest case, the Maxwell spring. Fig. 5.6 shows the oscillator in three positions, the Maxwell bar being replaced by the proper model. In Fig. 5.6a the system is in the undisturbed position. The state of Fig. 5.6b can be obtained by pulling the mass very suddenly down. Then the dashpot has

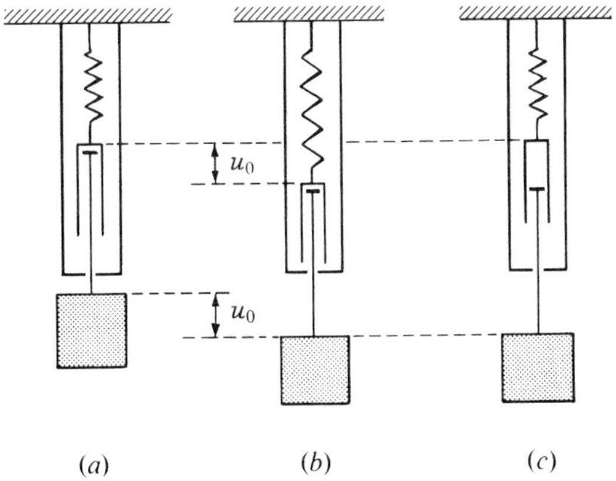

Figure 5.6. Simple oscillator with a Maxwell spring.

had no time to deform, and the spring is stretched. When the mass is held just long enough to make sure that $\dot{u} = 0$ and then released, a vibration will ensue which begins like an elastic vibration, the dashpot deforming as time permits and gradually draining energy from the system.

The system of Fig. 5.6a may be brought in the state of Fig. 5.6c by pulling the mass down very slowly. Then almost no force is needed and the entire deformation comes from the dashpot. When we again make sure that $\dot{u} = 0$ and then release the mass, nothing will happen. The oscillator is in a state of equilibrium, and it will remain there.

In both cases we have at $t = 0$ the initial conditions $u = u_0$ and $\dot{u} = 0$, and the difference lies in the position of the internal joint between the spring and the dashpot. If we know this, we know enough to choose the correct motion among the solutions of the differential equation. In an actual viscoelastic material, however, there is no spring and no dashpot, and a statement about the internal joint is not available. We must then formulate the difference between the two initial states in terms of the acceleration $\ddot{u}$. In the case of Fig. 5.6b, the sudden strain $\epsilon_0 = u_0/l$ leads to a stress $\sigma_0 = E_0\epsilon_0$ and hence to an accelaration $\ddot{u} = E_0 A\epsilon_0/M$. In Fig. 5.6c, there is no force at all and hence $\ddot{u} = 0$. Which of the two conditions applies depends on what has been done to the system before the vibration started, and there are, of course, infinitely many possibilities to produce different starting values of $\ddot{u}$.

On p. 114 the materials have been enumerated that lead to a third-order or a fourth-order equation, and if we now check in Table 1.2 the corresponding models, we see that for the third-order problems they have one internal joint and that the four-parameter fluid has two.

5.6 Forced Vibrations

As we have seen, the free vibrations of a viscoelastic oscillator are damped, that is, the solution ω of the frequency equation (5.29) is always complex with a positive imaginary part. We shall now apply to the same mass an external force

$$P = P_0 e^{i\omega_0 t}$$

with an arbitrary, real frequency ω_0 (Fig. 5.7). The amplitude P_0 of this "driving force" may be complex, that is, the real part of P may contain a sine as well as a cosine.

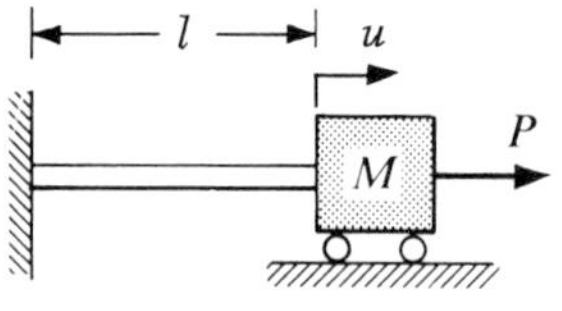

Figure 5.7. Forced vibration of a simple oscillator.

The presence of this force modifies the dynamic equation (5.27a), which now reads

$$M\ddot{u} + F = P_0 e^{i\omega_0 t} . \qquad (5.32)$$

When we combine this equation with (5.27b) and (1.23c), we arrive at a differential equation, which is the inhomogeneous counterpart to (5.31). The free vibrations studied before are its complementary solution, and besides this it has a particular solution of the form

$$u = u_0 e^{i\omega_0 t} .$$

It describes the steady state that develops after the free vibrations have died down. At present we are interested only in this solution. With this in mind, we may bypass the differential equation and combine (5.32) with (5.27b) and (5.6). After dropping a factor $e^{i\omega_0 t}$, (5.27b) and (5.32) yield

$$\epsilon_0 = u_0/l, \quad A\sigma_0 = Mu_0\omega_0^2 + P_0 ,$$

and upon introducing this into (5.6) we find

$$\frac{u_0}{l} = \frac{G(\omega_0)}{A}(Mu_0\omega_0^2 + P_0),$$

which may be solved for the displacement amplitude

$$u_0 = \frac{P_0 l G(\omega_0)}{A - Ml\omega_0^2 G(\omega_0)} .$$

Because of (5.29), this may be written in the form

$$u_0 = \frac{P_0}{M} \frac{G(\omega_0)}{\omega^2 G(\omega) - \omega_0^2 G(\omega_0)} . \tag{5.33a}$$

The velocity

$$\dot{u} = v = v_0 e^{i\omega_0 t}$$

has the amplitude

$$v_0 = \frac{iP_0}{M} \frac{\omega_0 G(\omega_0)}{\omega^2 G(\omega) - \omega_0^2 G(\omega_0)} . \tag{5.33b}$$

We describe the response of an oscillator to a periodic driving force by its **admittance**, which is the amplitude of the velocity per unit of driving force:

$$\mathfrak{A} = \mathfrak{A}_1 + i\mathfrak{A}_2 = \frac{v_0}{P_0} = \frac{1}{M}\,\frac{i\omega_0 G(\omega_0)}{\omega^2 G(\omega) - \omega_0^2 G(\omega_0)} . \tag{5.34}$$

The reciprocal of this quantity, the force needed per unit of velocity, is known as the **impedance** or **complex resistance** of the oscillator. When actually splitting a given $\mathfrak{A}$ into its real and imaginary parts, the reader should note that ω is complex, but that the expression $\omega^2 G(\omega)$ is real.

Problems

5.1. Assume that the spring in Fig. 5.5 obeys the Kelvin law. Formulate the frequency equation and discuss its solution.

5.2. A torsion bar (Fig. 5.8) consists of a viscoelastic core and an elastic outer shell. The stress laws are

for the core: $\tau + p_1\dot{\tau} = q_1\dot{\gamma}$,

for the shell: $\tau = G\gamma$.

An oscillating torque $M_t = M_0 e^{i\omega t}$ is applied. Calculate the complex compliance defined by the relation

$$\theta = M_0 G(\omega) e^{i\omega t},$$

where θ is the twist of the bar.

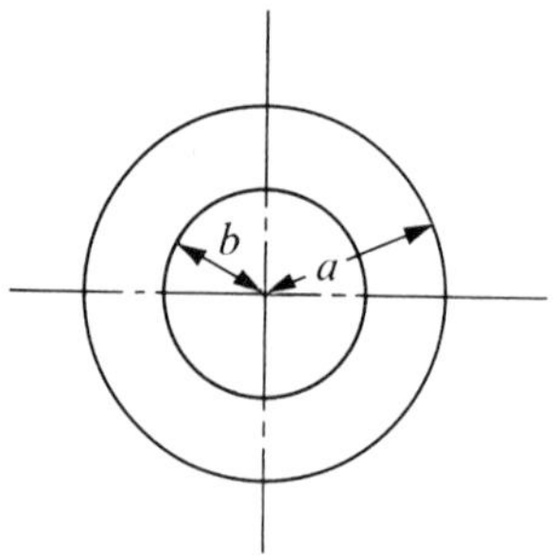

Figure 5.8.

5.3. A viscoelastic beam (Fig. 5.9) is simply supported at both ends and has at the midspan point a mass m attached to it. The mass of the beam is negligible. The beam material is characterized by its complex compliance $G(\omega)$. Find the natural frequency of the system. Calculate the forced vibrations caused by the load $P = P_0 e^{i\omega t}$. Calculate the impedance of the system and plot it as a function of the frequency ω of the driving force, using any one of the materials listed in Table 1.2.

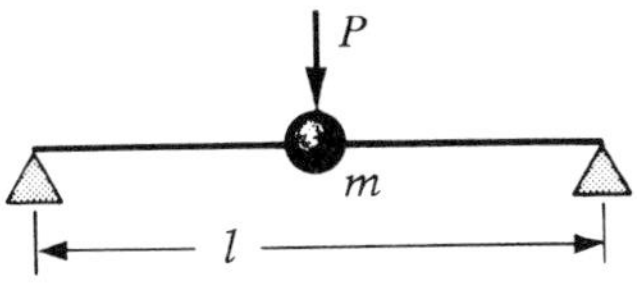

Figure 5.9.

5.4. The beam shown in Fig. 5.10 is made of a viscoelastic material and rests on two viscoelastic springs. The beam material is described by the relation $\mathbf{P}_a(\sigma) = \mathbf{Q}_a(\epsilon)$ and the springs by $\mathbf{P}_b(R) = \mathbf{Q}_b(\delta)$, where R is the reaction of the support and δ the deflection of the spring under this force.

At the midspan point a mass m is attached that is large enough to permit neglecting the mass of the beam. Find the frequency equation for lateral vibrations of the beam.

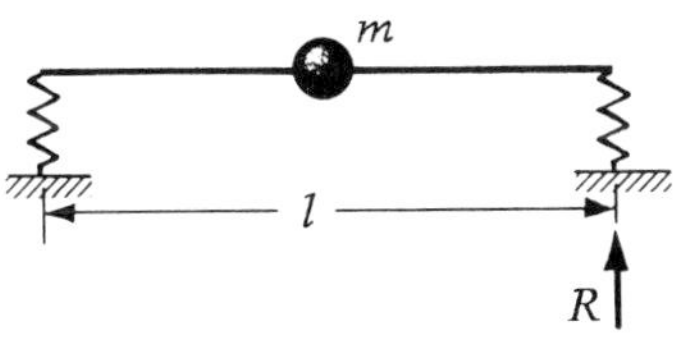

Figure 5.10.

For a numerical evaluation the following special case may be considered: beam: a three-parameter solid, constants

$$q_{0a} = q_0, \quad p_{1a} = p_1, \quad q_{1a} = 3q_0p_1 ;$$

springs: Kelvin law,

$$q_{0b} = 5lq_0, \quad q_{1b} = 5lq_0p_1 .$$

References

The complex compliance and its reciprocal, the complex modulus, may be found in many papers, e.g. [1], p. 463, and

26. E.H. Lee: Stress Analysis in Viscoelastic Materials. J. Appl. Phys., 27 (1956), 665-672.

The relations between the different compliances and the relaxation modulus are discussed in the following monograph:

27. B. Gross: Mathematical Structure of the Theories of Viscoelasticity (Paris, Hermann, 1953).

Equation (5.23) can easily be derived from the basic principles of the Fourier integral. It may be found at the following places:

28. G.A. Korn and T.M. Korn: Mathematical Handbook for Scientists and Engineers (New York, McGraw-Hill, 1961), p. 29.9-2, eq. (21.9-8). (Note a slight change in the integration domain.)

29. A. Papoulis: The Fourier Integral and its Applications (New York, McGraw-Hill, 1962), p. 39.

The definition of the sine integral may be found in reference [28], p. 21.3-1, eq. (21.3-1). For more detail consult

30. W. Flügge: Four-Place Tables of Transcendental Functions (London, Pergamon, 1954), pp. 115-116, 131, 133. (Contains the basic formulas needed for using the sine integral and a table of numerical values.)

The Cauchy theorem is one of the fundamental theorems of complex variable theory and may be found in all texts on the subject, for example:

31. R.V. Churchill: Complex Variables and Applications (2nd ed.) (New York, McGraw-Hill, 1960), pp. 106-111. (There this theorem is called the Cauchy-Goursat theorem.)

32. C.R. Wylie, ref. [9], p. 561.

Chapter 6

Wave Propagation

In this chapter we shall study a straight cylindrical bar which extends from x = 0 to infinity. At its end we wish either to apply a time-dependent tensile or compressive force or to enforce a time-dependent axial displacement. Changes in these quantities are to be so rapid that inertia of the material becomes an important element in the analysis.

For an elastic bar it is well known [33] that any such change in the prescribed force or displacement produces a stress wave which runs with a definite speed c along the bar. We shall study the corresponding phenomenon in a viscoelastic bar.

6.1 The Differential Equation

The bar is shown in Fig. 6.1a. Its cross section has the area A and may have any compact shape. Since there will be only axial forces, $\sigma_x = \sigma$ is the only nonvanishing stress component and the deformation is described by the displacement component u in axial direction. Because of the lateral contraction of the material, there are also displacements

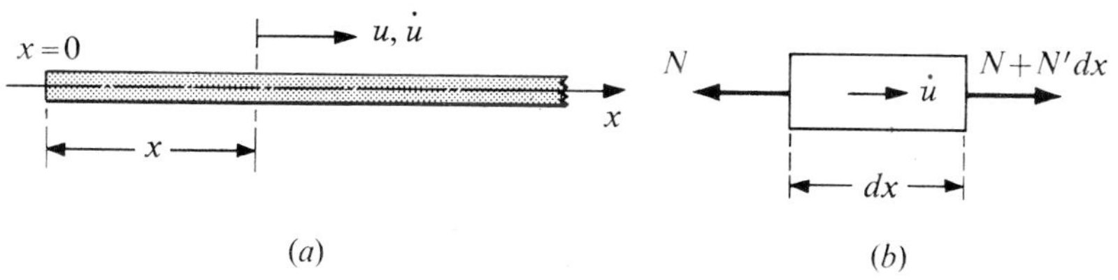

Figure 6.1. Semi-infinite viscoelastic bar - a: the bar; b: element.

v and w, but they are much smaller and will here be neglected. Their essential effect is to blur the sharpness of the discontinuity at wave fronts.

In Fig.6.1b a bar element is shown. At its left end the force $N = A\sigma$ is acting, which is a function of x and t. Let dots again indicate time derivatives and primes, derivatives with respect to x. Then the force at the right end of the element is $N + N'dx$, and the difference between these forces produces an acceleration $\ddot{u}$ of the element of mass $\rho A\,dx = \mu\,dx$, where ρ is the mass density of the material and μ is the mass per unit length of the bar. This yields the dynamic equation

$$\mu\ddot{u} = N'. \tag{6.1}$$

If at a certain time the displacement of the left end is u and that of the right end $u + u'dx$, then the strain, that is, the difference between the two divided by the length dx of the element, is

$$\epsilon = u'. \tag{6.2}$$

This is the kinematic relation. As the constitutive relation we use (1.23b), which we multiply at once by A to obtain

$$\sum_0^m p_k \frac{\partial^k N}{\partial t^k} = A \sum_0^n q_k \frac{\partial^k u'}{\partial t^k}. \tag{6.3}$$

In this equation we have already made use of (6.2). We differentiate it once more with respect to x and then use (6.1) to express N' by $\ddot{u}$:

$$\frac{\mu}{A} \sum_0^m p_k \frac{\partial^{k+2} u}{\partial t^{k+2}} - \sum_0^n q_k \frac{\partial^{k+2} u}{\partial x^2 \partial t^k} = 0. \tag{6.4}$$

This is the differential equation of our problem, a partial differential equation for the displacement u.

On the following pages, we shall find solutions of this equation for two cases, prescribing N(0,t) or u(0,t) either as a step function or as a harmonic oscillation. From what is known for an elastic bar, we might expect to find in the first case a wave front running from left to right along the bar, separating the part before it, which does not yet "know" that something has happened at $x = 0$, from the part behind it, which is under stress and in motion. We shall see in the next sections how this expectation must be modified when we are dealing with viscoelastic materials.

We have derived the differential equation (6.4) for a thin cylindrical bar, but it may also be applied to simple wave propagation problems in two and three dimensions, if we replace the viscoelastic coefficients by the proper quantities.

6.2 The Wave Front

For all the materials listed in Table 1.2, there is either $m = n$ or $m = n - 1$. In both cases (6.4) is of the order $(n + 2)$. If $m = n$, there are two terms of order $(n + 2)$. They are the second space and time derivatives of $\partial^n u/\partial t^n$, and since all coefficients p_k, $q_k > 0$, the minus sign in (6.4) indicates that our equation is of the hyperbolic type. Therefore, any discontinuity in the prescribed boundary values will manifest itself in the solution as a discontinuity along certain lines in the x, t plane, the characteristics of the differential equation [43-46]. In our case, such a discontinuity represents a shock wave running along the bar. As we have seen on p. 25, the materials for which $m = n$ are those which have an impact modulus $E_0 = q_n/p_n$.

If $m = n - 1$, there is only one term of order $(n+2)$, and (6.4) is of the parabolic type, like the heat conduction equation. In this case, there are no shock waves.

For the study of the propagation of shock waves, the impulse-momentum theorem is a very important tool. Although (6.6) can be derived from the differential equation and, therefore, does not represent new physical information, it is easier to derive it directly from basic mechanical principles, and this we shall now do.

When we speak of waves in this context, we do not mean anything oscillatory, but rather a sharp discontinuity in stress or velocity, or any other mechanical quantity, traveling along the bar at a finite speed c. We consider now an element dx of the bar which contains such a moving discontinuity or *wave front* (Fig.6.2). Before the wave front, the axial force and the velocity are N_1, $\dot{u}_1$; and behind it they are N_2, $\dot{u}_2$. The differences

$$\Delta N = N_2 - N_1, \qquad \Delta\dot{u} = \dot{u}_2 - \dot{u}_1 \tag{6.5}$$

are finite quantities describing the intensity of the wave front.

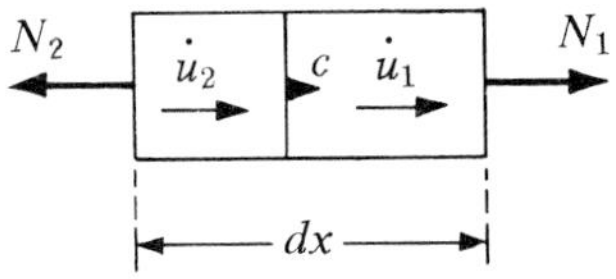

Figure 6.2. Bar element with wave front.

Before the wave front enters the element from the left, the velocity of all points is $\dot{u}_1$ and the forces at both ends differ at most by an infinitesimal amount. After the wave front has left, near-equilibrium has again been restored, but the velocity is now $\dot{u}_2$. During the time $dt = dx/c$, which the wave front needed to pass through the element, the forces were in unbalance and produced an impulse $(N_1 - N_2)dt = -\Delta N\,dt$, which is responsible for the increase in momentum $\mu\,dx \cdot \Delta\dot{u}$. The impulse-momentum theorem states that

$$\mu\,dx\,\Delta\dot{u} = -\Delta N\,dt\,,$$

whence

$$\Delta\dot{u} = -\frac{1}{\mu c}\,\Delta N\,. \tag{6.6}$$

The quantity μc is the force step needed to produce a unit step in velocity. It is called the *impedance* or *wave resistance* of the bar.

In an x,t plane, a wave front traveling with the constant speed c is represented by a straight line (Fig.6.3). This wave line separates a space-time region 1 from a region 2. For a fixed x, region 1 represents the time before the wave front passes; for a fixed time t, it contains that part of the bar where the wave front has not yet been. Certain quantities, like the jump ΔN of the axial force or $\Delta\dot{u}$ of the velocity, are defined only on the wave front, that is, on the boundary between the regions 1 and 2. Consequently, they have only a derivative along this line.

For any function f(x,t), we may write the difference df of its values for two adjacent points as

$$df = f'\,dx + \dot{f}\,dt\,.$$

In particular, if both points are on a wave line, we have $dt = dx/c$ and hence

$$df = \left(f' + \frac{1}{c}\dot{f}\right) dx\,.$$

Since the coordinates x and t do not have the same dimension, there is no such thing as a line element on the wave line. We therefore can-

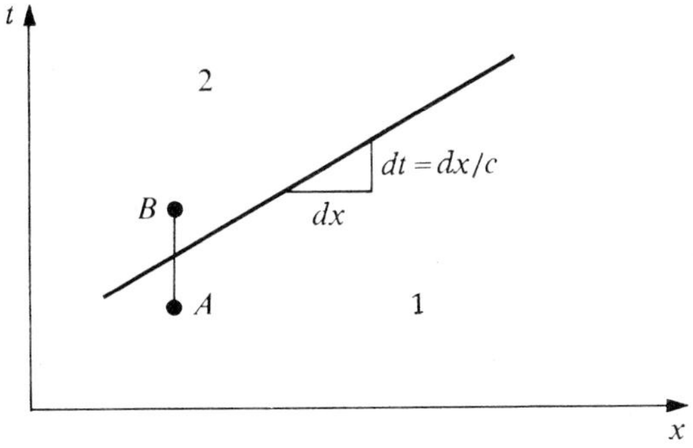

Figure 6.3. Wave propagation in the x,t-plane.

not form a differential quotient by dividing df by such a line element, but must resort to using either dx or dt to measure the distance of these points. We decide arbitrarily for x and write

$$\frac{df}{dx} \equiv \frac{Df}{Dx} = f' + \frac{1}{c}\dot{f}\,. \tag{6.7}$$

We shall use D to keep reminded that Dx is not the distance between the x,t points compared, but only a standardized measure for it.

Since the bar does not fall apart, the displacement u must be a continuous function of x and t, and even on the wave front there is

$$\Delta u = u_2 - u_1 \equiv 0\,.$$

Differentiating this identity along the wave line, we see that

$$\frac{D\Delta u}{Dx} = \Delta u' + \frac{1}{c}\,\Delta\dot{u} = 0\,,$$

whence

$$\Delta\dot{u} = -c\,\Delta u'. \tag{6.8}$$

We may combine this with the momentum equation (6.6) to find that

$$\Delta u' = \frac{1}{\mu c^2}\,\Delta N\,. \tag{6.9}$$

This may be interpretated as a relation between strain and stress, which does not depend on the constitutive law.

When this law, (6.3) is introduced, we arrive at a formula for the wave velocity c. The procedure is as follows: The differential equation (6.3) is integrated with respect to t, starting from a fixed point below the wave line and ending at a variable point below or above it. Any term of the sums in (6.3) is then a function of the upper integration limit and may again be integrated. This operation is repeated to a total of n integrations and the limits of the last integral are the points A and B in Fig.6.3. Most of the terms are then continuous functions of the t values at A and B. When we now let A and B approach the wave line, these integrals vanish.

There are two exceptions to this statement. The highest term on the right yields after n integrations

$$\lim_{A\to B}\int_A^B \frac{\partial u'}{\partial t}\,dt = \lim_{A\to B}\,(u'_B - u'_A) = \Delta u',$$

and if, but only if, $m = n$, also the highest term on the left makes a non-vanishing contribution:

$$\lim_{A\to B}\int_A^B \frac{\partial N}{\partial t}\,dt = \lim_{A\to B}\,(N_B - N_A) = \Delta N\,,$$

and there results the relation

$$p_n \Delta N = Aq_n \Delta u' . \tag{6.10}$$

If $m < n$, then $p_n = 0$, and the same relation holds true, but its left-hand side is zero.

When we now compare (6.9) and (6.10), we see that

$$c^2 = \frac{Aq_n}{\mu p_n} . \tag{6.11a}$$

With $\mu = A\rho$ and $q_n/p_n = E_0$ equal to the impact modulus, we may write our result also in the form

$$c^2 = E_0/\rho . \tag{6.11b}$$

Evidently, a finite wave velocity exists only in materials which have an impact modulus E_0. In other materials $p_n = 0$ leads to $c = \infty$.

In an infinite elastic bar, a wave once set in motion propagates without change in form or intensity. In a viscoelastic material we must expect that the wave front loses intensity as it travels. To find out what really happens, we go back to the impulse-momentum equation (6.6) and differentiate it along the wave line:

$$-\frac{D\Delta\dot{u}}{Dx} = \frac{1}{\mu c}\frac{D\Delta N}{Dx} = \frac{1}{\mu c}\Delta N' + \frac{1}{\mu c^2}\Delta\dot{N} .$$

When we still apply (6.1) to N', we may bring this into the following form:

$$\frac{D\Delta\dot{u}}{Dx} + \frac{1}{c}\Delta\ddot{u} + \frac{1}{\mu c^2}\Delta\dot{N} = 0 . \tag{6.12}$$

We shall later make out of this a differential equation for $\Delta\dot{u}$. To do so, we need the viscoelastic law of the material.

6.3 Maxwell Material

The Maxwell material is defined by the relation

$$p_1\dot{\sigma} + \sigma = q_1\dot{\varepsilon}. \tag{6.13}$$

Although its long-range behavior characterizes it as a fluid, it does have initial elasticity and therefore permits stress waves of finite velocity

$$c = \sqrt{q_1/\rho p_1}. \tag{6.14}$$

To find the law of decay of the step height of a wave, we must introduce information drawn from (6.13) into (6.12). To begin with, we write (6.13) for two adjacent points like A and B in Fig. 6.3 and form the difference (in other words, we apply the Δ operator to this equation). The result is

$$p_1\Delta\dot{\sigma} = -\Delta\sigma + q_1\Delta\dot{\varepsilon}\ .$$

Multiplying by A and using (6.6) and (6.2) on the right-hand side, we may write this as

$$p_1\Delta\dot{N} = \mu c\,\Delta\dot{u} + Aq_1\,\Delta\dot{u}'\ ,$$

and this may now be introduced in the last term of (6.12) to yield

$$\frac{D\Delta\dot{u}}{Dx} + \frac{1}{c}\Delta\ddot{u} + \frac{1}{p_1 c}\Delta\dot{u} + \frac{Aq_1}{p_1\mu c^2}\Delta\dot{u}' = 0\ .$$

Because of (6.11a), the coefficient of the last term equals unity, and the second and fourth terms can be combined into $D\Delta\dot{u}/Dx$, so that we arrive at a first-order differential equation for the velocity step:

$$2\frac{D\Delta\dot{u}}{Dx} + \frac{1}{p_1 c}\Delta\dot{u} = 0\ . \tag{6.15}$$

It has the solution

$$\Delta\dot{u} = Ce^{-x/2p_1c}. \tag{6.16a}$$

According to (6.6), this discontinuity in the velocity is accompanied by a step in the axial force

$$\Delta N = -C\mu c e^{-x/2p_1 c}. \qquad (6.16b)$$

Both decay as the wave moves on toward increasing x.

Of course, a wave front may also move from right to left. In this case the wave velocity is negative and all our formulas apply to such waves as well.

To obtain further information about stress and motion of the bar, we must solve (6.4). For the Maxwell material it reads

$$\rho(\ddot{u} + p_1\dddot{u}) - q_1\dot{u}'' = 0. \qquad (6.17)$$

We wish to solve it for the case that for $t < 0$ the bar is at rest and free of stress and that for all $t > 0$ either u or N is prescribed at the end $x = 0$.

When (6.17) is subjected to the Laplace transformation, all the terms in (1.18) which contain initial values do not appear, and we have simply

$$q_1 s\bar{u}'' - \rho(p_1 s^3 + s^2)\bar{u} = 0. \qquad (6.18)$$

Contrary to what is often said and written, this is a partial differential equation for a function $\bar{u}(x,s)$. However, it contains only a derivative with respect to x and therefore can be solved by familiar methods from the theory of ordinary differential equations. It is satisfied by

$$\bar{u} = B(s)e^{\lambda x} \qquad (6.19a)$$

with

$$\lambda = \pm\frac{1}{c}\sqrt{s(s + 1/p_1)}. \qquad (6.19b)$$

The positive value of λ, though acceptable for a solution of (6.18), must be rejected because every Laplace transform must, for $s \to \infty$, tend to zero. Mechanically speaking, this means that we are excluding waves running from right to left, since these would be incompatible with complete rest for $t < 0$. In fluid dynamics a similar exclusion is known as the "rule of forbidden signals" (no signals coming to us from $x = \infty$).

As might be expected of a solution of a partial differential equation, $\overline{u}(x,s)$ contains a free function $B(s)$, which we now shall determine from the initial condition. We choose the case that at $t = 0$ a constant tensile force is suddenly applied to the bar:

$$N(0,t) = P\,\Delta(t), \qquad \overline{N}(0,s) = Ps^{-1}. \tag{6.20}$$

Then the first element dx of the bar is exactly in the condition used for defining the creep compliance $J(t)$, and its strain is

$$\varepsilon(0,t) = u'(0,t) = \frac{P}{A}J(t), \qquad \overline{u}'(0,s) = \frac{P}{A}\overline{J}(s). \tag{6.21}$$

This is our initial condition. For a Maxwell material we have

$$J(t) = \frac{p_1 + t}{q_1}, \qquad \overline{J}(s) = \frac{1}{q_1}\left(\frac{p_1}{s} + \frac{1}{s^2}\right)$$

and, therefore,

$$\overline{u}'(0,s) = \lambda B(s) = \frac{P}{Aq_1}\left(\frac{p_1}{s} + \frac{1}{s^2}\right).$$

From this equation we find $B(s)$ and hence the final form of $\overline{u}$:

$$\overline{u}(x,s) = -\frac{P}{\mu c}\,\frac{\sqrt{s + 1/p_1}}{s^2\sqrt{s}}\exp\left(-\frac{x}{c}\sqrt{s(s + 1/p_1)}\right). \tag{6.22}$$

This must now be transformed back into the x,t plane.

We start from the transformation pair (7) in Table 1.1. As a first step, we let $a = i\alpha$ and introduce the modified Bessel function $I_0(x) = J_0(ix)$. This yields the pair

$$f(t) = I_0\left(\alpha\sqrt{t^2 - b^2}\right)\cdot\Delta(t-b),$$

$$\overline{f}(s) = \frac{1}{\sqrt{s^2 - \alpha^2}}\exp\left(-b\sqrt{s^2 - \alpha^2}\right).$$

Then we replace s by $(s + \alpha)$ in $\bar{f}$ and apply the shifting theorem [42], which says that the corresponding change of f is the appearance of a factor $e^{-\alpha t}$:

$$f(t) = I_0\left(\alpha\sqrt{t^2 - b^2}\right)e^{-\alpha t}\Delta(t - b),$$

$$\bar{f}(s) = \frac{1}{\sqrt{s(s + 2\alpha)}}\exp\left(-b\sqrt{s(s + 2\alpha)}\right).$$

When we now let $2\alpha = 1/p_1$ and $b = x/c$, we have a pair that can be used with (6.22):

$$f_1(t) = I_0(\zeta)e^{-t/2p_1}\Delta(t - x/c),$$

$$\bar{f}_1(s) = \frac{1}{\sqrt{s(s + 1/p_1)}}\exp\left(-\frac{x}{c}\sqrt{s(s + 1/p_1)}\right),$$

where the abbreviation

$$\zeta = \frac{1}{2p_1}\sqrt{t^2 - x^2/c^2}$$

has been used. Another necessary pair is found by differentiating f_1:

$$\dot{f}_1(t) = f_2(t) = \frac{1}{2p_1}\left[-I_0(\zeta) + \frac{t}{2p_1\zeta}I_1(\zeta)\right]e^{-t/2p_1}\Delta(t - x/c),$$

$$\bar{f}_2(s) = \frac{s}{\sqrt{s(s + 1/p_1)}}\exp\left(-\frac{x}{c}\sqrt{s(s + 1/p_1)}\right).$$

With the last two pairs, we can handle the transformation of $s^2\bar{u}(x,s)$, which yields $\ddot{u}(x,t)$:

$$\ddot{u}(x,t) = -\frac{P}{\mu c}\left[\frac{1}{p_1}f_1(t) + f_2(t)\right]$$

$$= -\frac{P}{\mu c}\cdot\frac{1}{2p_1}\left[I_0(\zeta) + \frac{t}{2p_1\zeta}I_1(\zeta)\right]e^{-t/2p_1}, \qquad (6.23)$$

valid for $t > x/c$.

From (6.1) we find immediately N', and now we may calculate N, $\dot{u}$, and u by numerical integration. For N we have to integrate N' in x direction, starting from the prescribed value N(0,t) = P, and for $\dot{u}$ and u we need two consecutive integrations in t direction starting at the wave front x = ct, where initial values are known. They are

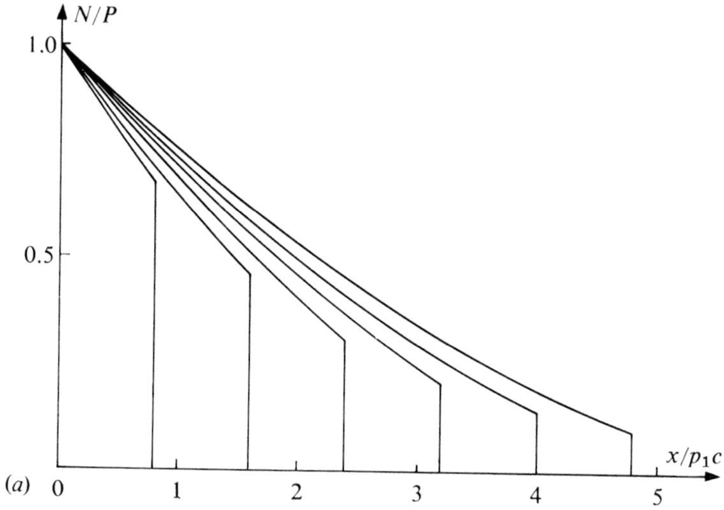

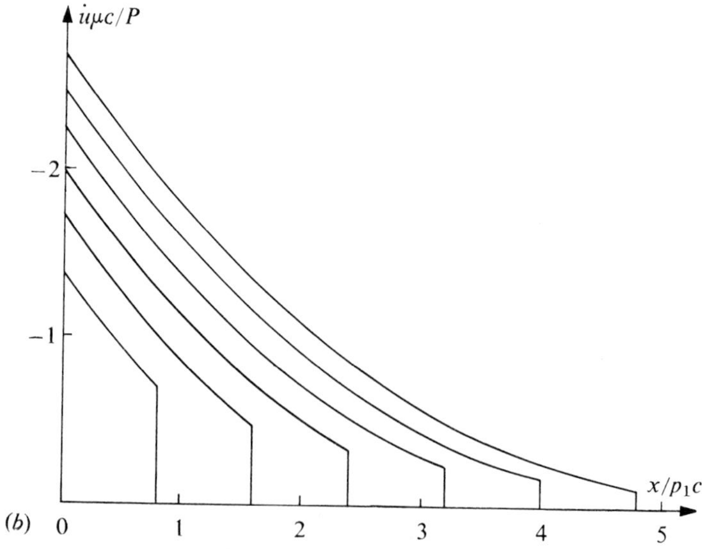

Figure 6.4. Wave propagation in a Maxwell bar - a: axial force; b: velocity.

$u(x,ct^+) = 0$ and $\dot{u}(x,ct^+) = \Delta\dot{u}$ from (6.16a). The constant C in this equation follows from the fact that for $x = 0, t = 0^+$ the velocity is

$$\dot{u} = -P/\mu c ,$$

as may be seen from (6.6).

Figure 6.4 shows the results of numerical work. The six curves in each diagram belong to values $t/p_1 = 0.8, 1.6, 2.4, 3.2, 4.0, 4.8$. Both diagrams show the presence of a wave front which runs at a constant velocity, and it may be seen how the step height decreases as the wave travels along the bar. In Fig. 6.4a, the value of N at the left end is, of course, constant, and at any other point N jumps to a finite value when the wave front arrives and then continues to grow slowly, never reaching P.

For a positive (tensile) force P, the velocity $\dot{u}$ is necessarily negative. We have already seen that at the end of the bar it jumps to $-P/\mu c$ when the load is applied. Figure 6.4b shows that it keeps growing, in contrast to what happens in an elastic bar.

At the end of the bar, (6.23) simplifies to read

$$\ddot{u}(0,t) = -\frac{P}{\mu c}\frac{1}{2p_1}[I_0(\zeta) + I_1(\zeta)]e^{-\zeta} .$$

For large arguments, I_0 and I_1 are approximately represented by the same expression

$$I_0(\zeta) \approx I_1(\zeta) \approx \frac{e^{\zeta}}{\sqrt{2\pi\zeta}}$$

and, therefore,

$$\lim_{t\to\infty} \ddot{u}(0,t) \approx -\frac{P}{\mu c}\sqrt{\frac{1}{\pi p_1 t}}$$

and its integral, the velocity $\dot{u}(0,t)$, increases like $t^{1/2}$. The result of a computation is shown in Fig. 6.5.

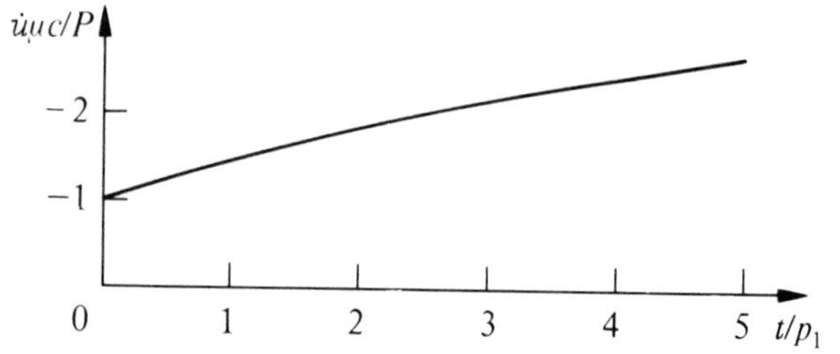

Figure 6.5. End velocity of a Maxwell bar, subjected to a constant tensile force applied at $t = 0$.

6.4 Viscous Material

In the limit $p_1 \to 0$ the Maxwell material degenerates into a viscous fluid. As may be seen from (6.14), the wave velocity c goes then to infinity. This means that there is no marked wave front and that every point of the bar "knows" at once when something is happening at the end. However, the product $c^2 p_1 = q_1/\rho$ remains finite, and this must be used when performing the limiting process.

This is most easily done on the Laplace transform $\bar{u}$, (6.22), writing

$$\bar{u}(x,s) = -\lim \frac{P}{A\rho c} \frac{\sqrt{p_1 s + 1}}{\sqrt{p_1}\, s^2 \sqrt{s}} \exp\left(-\frac{x}{c} \frac{\sqrt{s}\sqrt{p_1 s + 1}}{\sqrt{p_1}} \right)$$

$$= -\frac{P}{A\sqrt{\rho q_1}} \frac{1}{s^2\sqrt{s}} \exp\left(-x\sqrt{\frac{\rho}{q_1}}\sqrt{s} \right). \tag{6.24}$$

This expression looks quite different from (6.22) and needs another transform pair. It is listed as (8) in Table 1.1 and yields in this case the velocity

$$\dot{u}(s,t) = -\frac{P}{A\sqrt{\rho q_1}} \left\{ 2\sqrt{\frac{t}{\pi}} \exp\left(-\frac{x^2 \rho}{4 q_1 t} \right) - x\sqrt{\frac{\rho}{q_1}} \left[1 - \operatorname{erf}\left(\frac{x}{2}\sqrt{\frac{\rho}{q_1 t}} \right) \right] \right\}. \tag{6.25}$$

It is remarkable that in this case $\dot{u}/\sqrt{t}$ depends only on $x/\sqrt{t}$ and can be plotted over this variable as an abscissa. This has been done in Fig. 6.6, and in this diagram the results from Fig. 6.4b have been replotted. They yield, of course, different curves for different t, and it may be seen how these curves gradually approach the unique one for the viscous bar: The more time that has elapsed since the wave front has passed at a certain point, the closer the behavior of the Maxwell bar approaches that of viscous material.

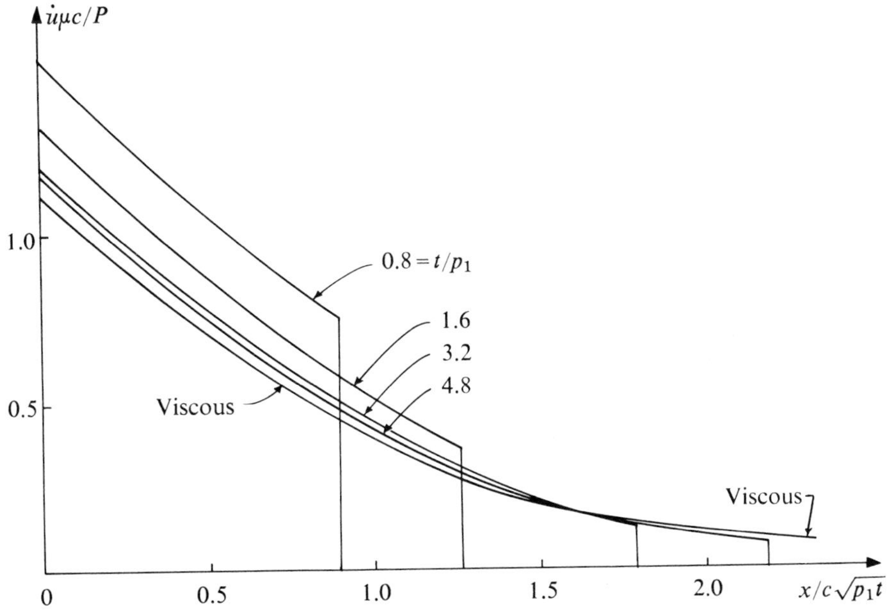

Figure 6.6. Wave propagation, comparison of Maxwell fluid and viscous fluid.

6.5 Oscillatory Load

We now turn to the second problem indicated in section 6.1. At the end $x = 0$ of a cylindrical bar either an oscillating axial displacement

$$u(0,t) = U \cos \omega t \tag{6.26a}$$

is enforced or an axial force

$$N(0,t) = P \cos \omega t \tag{6.26b}$$

is applied and it is assumed that either of these end conditions has been in force for a long time. Using the operators **P** and **Q** defined in (1.24) also here where partial time derivatives are needed, we rewrite the differential equation (6.4) in the form

$$\rho \mathbf{P}(\ddot{u}) - \mathbf{Q}(u'') = 0 \tag{6.27}$$

and restate for later use the constitutive equation (6.3) in the operator form

$$\mathbf{P}(N) = A\mathbf{Q}(u') . \tag{6.28}$$

In view of the end condition (6.26) we are interested in a solution of the form

$$u = C e^{i(\omega t - \lambda x)} . \tag{6.29}$$

We then have

$$\mathbf{Q}(u') = -i\lambda \mathfrak{Q}(i\omega) u$$

and

$$N = -i\lambda A \frac{\mathfrak{Q}(i\omega)}{\mathfrak{P}(i\omega)} u = -\frac{i\lambda A}{G(\omega)} u , \tag{6.30}$$

where the polynomials $\mathfrak{P}$ and $\mathfrak{Q}$ defined in (1.26) and the complex compliance $G(\omega)$ defined in (5.7) have been used. Introducing the solution (6.29) into (6.27), we see that C is a free constant, while ω and λ are related to each other by the equation

$$\lambda^2 = \rho \omega^2 G(\omega) . \tag{6.31}$$

It yields two values of λ of opposite sign. Reserving the notation λ for one among them, we may write the solution (6.29) as

$$u = e^{i\omega t}(C_1 e^{-i\lambda x} + C_2 e^{+i\lambda x}) \tag{6.32}$$

with

$$\lambda = \lambda_1 - i\lambda_2 = \omega \sqrt{\rho G(\omega)} = \omega \sqrt{\rho(G_1(\omega) + i G_2(\omega))} \tag{6.33}$$

where

$$\lambda_1 > \lambda_2 > 0 .$$

Separating real and imaginary parts, we may write (6.32) in the alternate form

$$u = C_1 e^{-\lambda_2 x} e^{i(\omega t - \lambda_1 x)} + C_2 e^{+\lambda_2 x} e^{i(\omega t + \lambda_1 x)} \tag{6.34}$$

This shows that there will be two sinusoidal waves running in opposite directions along the bar, and that each of them decreases exponentially in amplitude as it proceeds on its way. It may also be seen that there exists a solution of this kind for any of the materials listed in Table 1.2 and for any other material which can be described by a Kelvin chain. There is no essential difference between those materials which have an impact modulus E_0 and those which do not, and none between solids and fluids.

As an example let us consider a bar of finite length l. At $x = 0$, we impose an oscillatory displacement with an arbitrary frequency ω. The other end is fixed. Thus, we have the end conditions

$$x = 0 : u = U e^{i\omega t}, \qquad x = l : u = 0 . \tag{6.35a,b}$$

When we introduce here the solution (6.32), we obtain two linear equations for C_1 and C_2:

$$\begin{aligned} C_1 \qquad + C_2 \qquad &= U, \\ C_1 e^{-i\lambda l} + C_2 e^{+i\lambda l} &= 0 . \end{aligned} \tag{6.36}$$

Their solution is easily found to be

$$C_1 = \frac{1}{2} U(1 - i \cot \lambda l), \quad C_2 = \frac{1}{2} U(1 + i \cot \lambda l).$$

None of these constants ever vanishes and there are always two waves running along the bar and interfering with each other, one emanating from the disturbed end $x = 0$ and a reflected wave originating at the fixed end $x = l$.

When the expressions for C_1 and C_2 are introduced into (6.32), the solution assumes a very compact form, but the two running waves are no longer discernible:

$$u = Ue^{i\omega t}\frac{\sin\lambda(l-x)}{\sin\lambda l}. \tag{6.37}$$

The trigonometric functions have complex arguments. Separating their quotient into real and imaginary parts takes some trigonometric algebra. After this has been performed, we may drop the imaginary part and thus arrive at a solution to a problem in which the boundary condition (6.35a) has been replaced by (6.26a). It is

$$u = \frac{U}{\operatorname{Cosh} 2\lambda_2 l - \cos 2\lambda_1 l}\,[(\cos\lambda_1 x \operatorname{Cosh}\lambda_2(2l-x) +$$

$$+ \cos\lambda_1(2l-x)\operatorname{Cosh}\lambda_2 x)\cos\omega t +$$

$$+ (\sin\lambda_1 x \operatorname{Sinh}\lambda_2(2l-x) - \sin\lambda_1(2l-x)\operatorname{Sinh}\lambda_2 x)\sin\omega t]. \tag{6.38}$$

Thus far, it has been possible to develop the theory without making reference to any particular material. Now the time has come to make a choice and to work out some details. We choose a three-parameter solid. Taking G_1 and G_2 from Table 1.2, we find

$$\lambda_1 - i\lambda_2 = p_1\omega\sqrt{\frac{\rho}{p_1 q_1}}\sqrt{\frac{[q_0p_1/q_1 + (p_1\omega)^2] - i[1 - q_0p_1/q_1]p_1\omega}{(q_0p_1/q_1)^2 + (p_1\omega)^2}}.$$

Obviously, $p_1\omega$ is the dimensionless frequency; the first of the square roots serves to dedimensionalize λ; and in the second square root, q_0p_1/q_1 is the dimensionless parameter characterizing the material. As is seen from the inequality listed in Table 1.2, it must be less than unity. As it approaches this limit, the material approaches an elastic solid. We choose the material, the frequency, and the length of the bar such that

$$\frac{q_0p_1}{q_1} = 0.860, \qquad p_1\omega = 1.5, \qquad \lambda_1 l = 7\pi.$$

Numerical results obtained for these data are shown in Fig. 6.7a. The curves represent u/U for $\omega t = 0, \frac{1}{4}\pi, \frac{1}{2}\pi, \frac{3}{4}\pi, \pi$. In the left third of the bar a running wave is clearly visible, but in the right third we find a standing wave. The wave crests decrease from left to right, but not substantially. Most surprising is the fact that, upon entering the bar on the left, the wave, far from being damped, first increases in amplitude.

The diagram becomes understandable if one realizes that an elastic bar of the same length would be in resonance with the load at the end

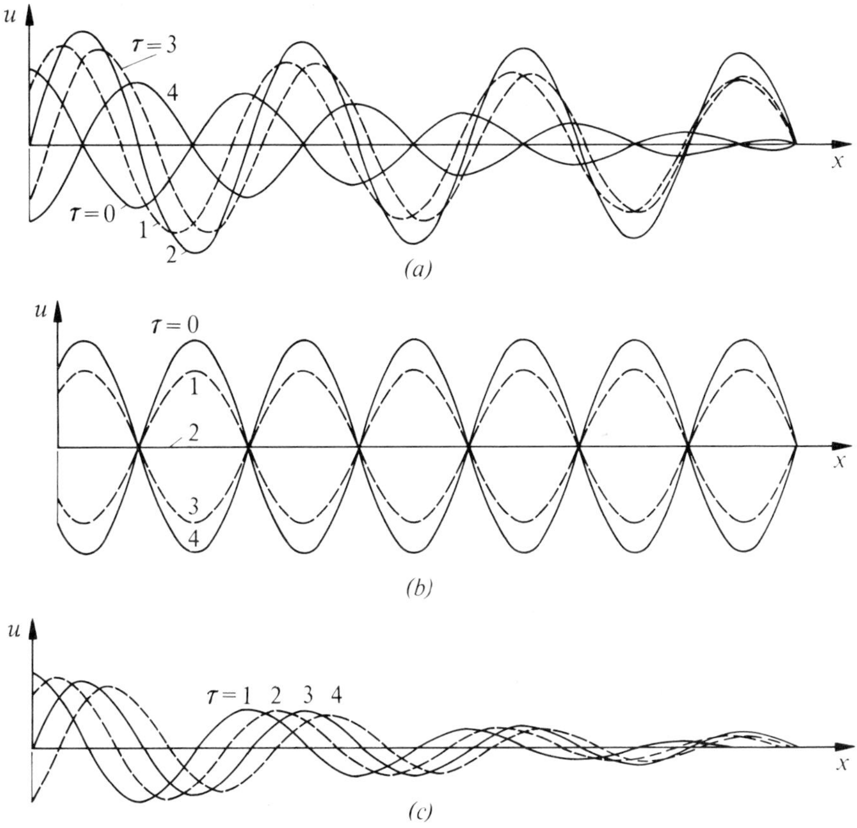

Figure 6.7. Running and standing waves in a bar of finite length - a and c: three-parameter solid; b: elastic material. $\tau = 4\omega t/\pi$.

and, therefore, would have standing waves of infinite amplitude. Figure 6.7b shows the solution for a slightly shorter elastic bar, which is not in resonance and vibrates with a finite amplitude.

Running waves become more pronounced when the damping of the material increases. For a comparison, we choose

$$\frac{q_0 p_1}{q_1} = 0.600, \qquad p_1 \omega = 1.5, \qquad \lambda_1 l = 7\pi .$$

The result is shown in Fig. 6.7c. One clearly recognizes a wave of decreasing amplitude running from the left to the right for almost the entire length of the bar. Only near the right end is the reflected wave strong enough to combine with the incoming wave to a standing wave, which obeys the condition $u \equiv 0$ at the end.

When we let $l \to \infty$, there is no longer a reflected wave. We see this most easily when we split the coefficients of C_1 and C_2 in (6.36) into their real and imaginary parts:

$$\lim_{l \to \infty} e^{-i\lambda l} = \lim e^{-i\lambda_1 l} e^{-\lambda_2 l} = 0 ,$$

$$\lim_{l \to \infty} e^{+i\lambda l} = \lim e^{i\lambda_2 l} e^{\lambda_2 l} = \infty .$$

Hence $C_2 = 0$ and $C_1 = U$ and only the first term in (6.34) survives.

6.6 Bar with Elastic Restraint

An interesting phenomenon appears when we consider a slightly more complicated case. In Fig. 6.8a we see again a cylindrical, viscoelastic bar extending along the x axis from zero to infinity. However, this time the bar is not free but surrounded by some elastic material, which is bonded to a rigid medium. If a bar element is displaced toward the right by the amount u, the elastic support exerts on it a restoring force

$$p\, dx = k\, u\, dx$$

in the direction of decreasing x, which enters the equation of motion of the element. To exclude the complicating phenomenon of waves propagating at a speed of their own in the elastic medium, we assume the support to consist of a kind of bristles similar to those of a pipe cleaner. We are then dealing with a model that has some similarity with the

Winkler medium explained on p. 000 and has similar drawbacks and advantages.

To establish the differential equation of the axial vibrations of the bar, we return to (6.1), the equation of motion of the bar element. Here $N'dx$ is the difference of the internal forces at the end of the

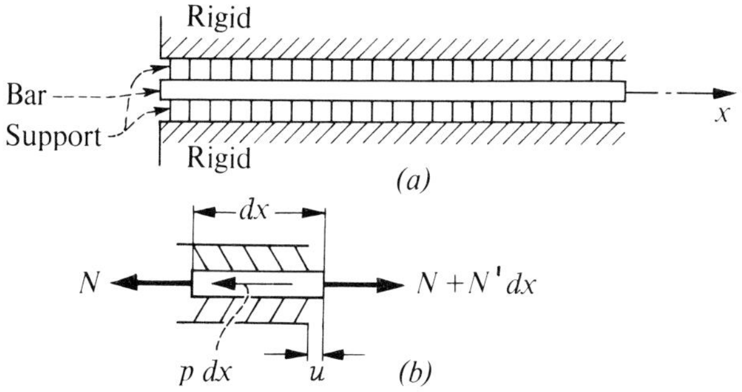

Figure 6.8. Viscoelastic bar with elastic restraint - a: the bar; b: element.

element, which produces the acceleration $\ddot{u}$. We must now add the restoring force $-ku\,dx$, and after dropping the factor dx we have

$$\mu\ddot{u} = N' - ku\,. \tag{6.39}$$

The kinematic relation (6.2) remains the same and so does the constitutive equation of the material. Proceeding as on p. 122, we find for u the differential equation

$$\rho\mathbf{P}(\ddot{u}) + \frac{k}{A}\mathbf{P}(u) - \mathbf{Q}(u'') = 0\,, \tag{6.40}$$

which takes the place of (6.27).

As in section 6.5, we want to prescribe an oscillatory displacement $u(0,t)$ or to apply an oscillating force $N(0,t)$ according to (6.26a,b) and, therefore, are interested in solutions of the type (6.29). Introduction of u from that equation into (6.40) leads to the relation

$$\left(\rho\,\omega^2 - \frac{k}{A}\right)\mathcal{P}(i\omega) = \lambda^2\mathcal{Q}(i\omega)$$

and, with (5.7) and the abbreviation

$$\omega_0^2 = k/\rho A = k/\mu$$

to

$$\lambda^2 = \rho(\omega^2 - \omega_0^2)G(\omega) . \tag{6.41}$$

Depending upon the frequency ω, the factor of $G(\omega)$ can be positive or negative. If $\omega = \omega_0$, λ vanishes and (6.29) simply reads

$$u = Ce^{i\omega t} .$$

In this case u does not depend on x and the bar makes a rigid-body vibration. With $u' \equiv 0$ we see from (6.3) that also $N \equiv 0$ and there cannot be a driving force at the end. We are dealing with the free vibration of a simple spring-mass system.

If $\omega \neq \omega_0$, we may again choose between the two problems described by (6.26a,b) and we consider, as before, the first one and write the end condition in the complex form (6.35a). If the bar extends to infinity, (6.35b) is to be replaced by the requirement than u tends to zero (or, at least, is bounded) for $x \to \infty$. Thus we have

$$x = 0 \quad : u = Ue^{i\omega t} ,$$
$$x \to \infty : u \to 0 . \tag{6.42a,b}$$

Condition (6.42b) requires that among the two values of λ which follow from (6.41), we must retain only the one with a negative imaginary part, and (6.42a) then leads to $C = U$.

It becomes now necessary to consider the two cases $\omega > \omega_0$ and $\omega < \omega_0$ separately. In the first one, the factor of $G(\omega)$ in (6.41) is positive. We write as before

$$\lambda = \lambda_1 - i\lambda_2 \quad \text{with} \quad \lambda_1 > \lambda_2 > 0$$

and retain in (6.32) only the C_1 term. The solution is then

$$u = Ue^{i\omega t}\, e^{-i\lambda x} = Ue^{i(\omega t - \lambda_1 x)}\, e^{-\lambda_2 x} . \tag{6.43a}$$

The corresponding axial force is found from (6.30) and (6.41):

$$N = -\frac{i\mu(\omega^2 - \omega_0^2)}{\lambda_1 - i\lambda_2} u . \qquad (6.43b)$$

This solution describes an outgoing wave, emanating from the end $x = 0$ of the bar and decreasing in amplitude as it proceeds. It is similar to the wave shown in Fig.6.7c.

A rather surprising result is found when $\omega < \omega_0$. In this case λ^2 lies in the second quadrant of the complex plane and it is useful to write

$$\lambda = \pm(\lambda_1 + i\lambda_2) \quad \text{with} \quad \lambda_2 > \lambda_1 > 0 . \qquad (6.44)$$

Since the end condition at infinity requires the imaginary part of λ to be negative, we must choose the minus sign in (6.44) and have

$$u = Ue^{i\omega t} e^{-i\lambda x} = Ue^{i(\omega t + \lambda_1 x)} e^{-\lambda_2 x} . \qquad (6.45a)$$

This is an incoming wave, running from right to left and increasing in amplitude like a surf wave. The axial force is

$$N = -\frac{i\mu(\omega_0^2 - \omega^2)}{\lambda_1 + i\lambda_2} u . \qquad (6.45b)$$

A surf wave is bringing energy from far away to the shore and its amplitude increases only when it runs into shallow water. In the case at hand such an energy transport is out of the question, but it seems astonishing that in the bar the energy should flow opposite to the wave.

To find out what is happening, we study the mechanism of the energy transport. In Fig.6.9 the bar has been cut at an arbitrary cross

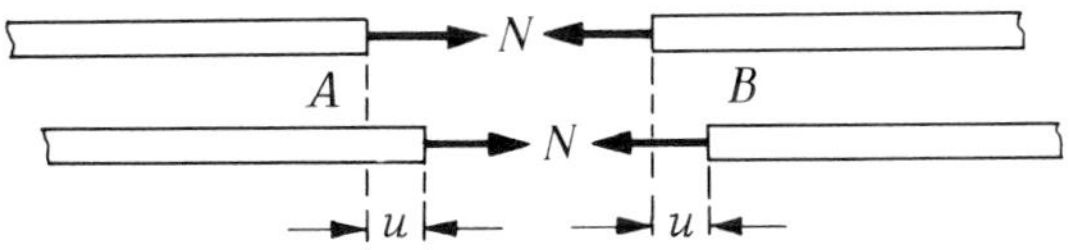

Figure 6.9. Bar cut at one cross section to demonstrate the energy flux.

section x. At both sides of the cut the internal forces N are acting, shown in their positive directions. If there is a positive displacement $du = \dot{u}\, dt$, the force at A does positive work $N\dot{u}\, dt$ on the left part of the bar, while the force at B takes an equal amount of energy out of the right part. We call the flow of energy per unit of time the energy flux Φ and count it positive in the direction of increasing x. We have then

$$\Phi = -N\dot{u} \; . \tag{6.46}$$

We shall now see that in our bar the energy flux is always positive, no matter in which direction the waves are running. As explained on p. 100, we have to give up the complex notation and must extraact the real parts of $\dot{u}$ and N before multiplying th e two quantities.

For $\omega > \omega_0$, we start from (6.43) and find

$$\dot{u} = U\omega \,\mathrm{Re}\left[i(\cos\omega t + i\sin\omega t)(\cos\lambda_1 x - i\sin\lambda_1 x)\, e^{-\lambda_2 x}\right.$$

$$= U\omega(\cos\omega t\,\sin\lambda_1 x - \sin\omega t\,\cos\lambda_1 x)\, e^{-\lambda_2 x}$$

and, after a few lines of calculation,

$$N = -\frac{U\mu(\omega^2-\omega_0^2)}{\lambda_1^2+\lambda_2^2}\left[\cos\omega t\,(\lambda_1\sin\lambda_1 x - \lambda_2\cos\lambda_1 x)\right.$$

$$\left. - \sin\omega t\,(\lambda_1\cos\lambda_1 x + \lambda_2\sin\lambda_1 x)\right] e^{-\lambda_2 x} \; .$$

We multiply these two expressions, consider any fixed value of x and integrate over one period $2\pi/\omega$:

$$\int_0^{2\pi/\omega} \Phi\, dt = -\int_0^{2\pi/\omega} N\dot{u}\, dt = \frac{U^2\mu(\omega^2-\omega_0^2)\pi}{\lambda_1^2+\lambda_2^2}\,\lambda_1\, e^{-2\lambda_2 x} \; .$$

This expression is obviously positive and the energy flows in the expected direction, from the end where it is pumped into the bar to infinity. However, the exponential factor shows that it gets quickly lost on its way through the viscoelastic damping of the bar material.

For $\omega < \omega_0$, we must use (6.45) and find that

$$\int_0^{2\pi/\omega} \Phi\,dt = \frac{U^2\mu(\omega_0^2 - \omega^2)\pi}{\lambda_1^2 + \lambda_2^2}\,\lambda_1\,e^{-2\lambda_2 x},$$

which, again, is positive indicating that, indeed, the energy is flowing toward the right, opposed to the incoming waves!

Problems

6.1. A tube of circular cross section is made of a viscoelastic material. It is filled with an incompressible, inviscid fluid of mass density ρ. In this fluid pressure waves can travel that are similar to the tension-compression waves in cylindrical rods. A theory of these waves can be formulated that parallels that of the rods. To obtain it, assume that the deformation of the tube in each cross section depends only on the local pressure p and not on the deformation of adjacent parts of the tube. Establish the differential equation, formulate the impulse-momentum equation, and find a formula for the wave velocity c.

6.2. The right end of a viscoelastic rod is connected to an elastic spring (spring stiffness k), which in turn is attached to a fixed abutment, Fig. 6.10. A stress wave arrives from the left and will be partially reflected when it reaches the end. Write the proper end condition in terms of the displacement u. Assume that the bar is made of a three-parameter solid.

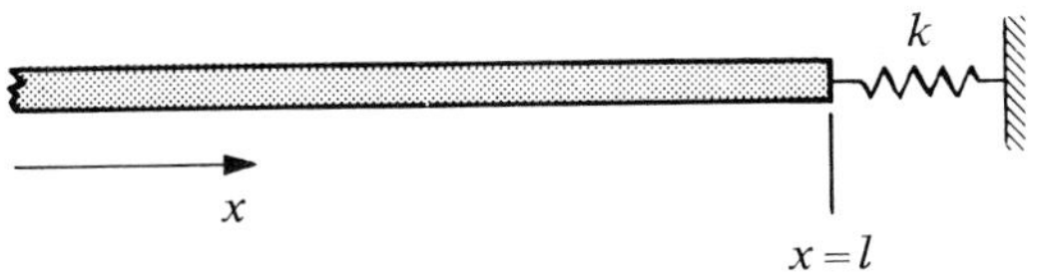

Figure 6.10.

References

A short outline of the theory of axial impact is found in

33. S. Timoshenko and J.N. Goodier: Theory of Elasticity (3rd ed.) (New York, McGraw-Hill, 1970), p. 492.

The presentation of the subject of viscoelastic impact in this book is based upon the author's work, done in 1944-1948 in Germany and France and, because of the world situation in those years, never published. The formalism used here has been developed in the following paper:

34. W. Flügge: Die Ausbreitung von Biegewellen in Stäben. Z. angew. Math. Mech., 22 (1942), 312-318.

The subject has found much attention in recent years. The following references [35] through [41] may be consulted for more detail:

35. E.H. Lee and I. Kanter: Wave Propagation in Finite Rods of Viscoelastic Material. J. Appl. Phys., 24 (1953), 1115-1122. (Maxwell solid, includes reflection of the wave at the far end of the bar.)

36. J.A. Morrison: Wave Propagation in Rods of Voigt Materials and Viscoelastic Materials with Three-Parameter Models. Qu. Appl. Math., 14 (1956), 153-169.

37. R.D. Glauz and E.H. Lee: Transient Wave Analysis in a Linear Time-dependent Material. J. Appl. Phys., 25 (1954), 947-953.

38. E.H. Lee and J.A. Morrison: A Comparison of Longitudinal Waves in Rods of Viscoelastic Materials. J. Polymer Sci., 19 (1956), 93-110. (Includes both three-parameter materials and the four-parameter fluid.)

39. D.S. Berry and S.C. Hunter: The Propagation of Dynamic Stresses in Viscoelastic Rods. J. Mech. Phys. Solids, 4 (1956), 72-95.

40. S.C. Hunter: Viscoelastic Waves, in I.N. Sneddon and R. Hill (eds.), Progress in Solid Mechanics, (New York, Interscience 1960), Vol. 1, pp. 1-57.

41. W. Flügge and J.R. Hutchinson: Axial Vibrations of a Semiinfinite Viscoelastic Rod with External Constraint. J. Acoust. Soc. Amer., 37, (1965), 14-18.

42. The shifting theorem is (under various names) found in the following books: [5], p. 15, [6], p. 4, [7], p. 6, [8], p. 74.

The classification of partial differential equations of the second order in elliptic, parabolic, and hyperbolic equations is explained in texts on partial differential equations, for example:

43. I.N. Sneddon: Elements of Partial Differential Equations, (New York, McGraw-Hill, 1957), pp. 108, 118.

44. F.B. Hildebrand: Advanced Calculus for Applications (Englewood Cliffs, N.J., Prentice-Hall, 1948), p. 409.

45. G. Hellwig: Partial Differential Equations (Waltham, Blaisdell, 1964) p. 60. (Translation from the German.)

46. P.W. Berg and J.L. McGregor: Elementary Partial Differential Equations (San Francisco, Holden-Day, 1964), p. 33.

Chapter 7

Buckling of Columns

Elastic Columns, plates, shells and some other structures can collapse at a modest stress level, due to an instability of the equilibrium. Viscoelastic structures display similar, but more complex phenomena, which we now shall study for the case of a simple column.

7.1 The Concept of Stability

Two definitions of stability are in common use:

First Definition – When a system in equilibrium is subjected to a small (infinitesimal) disturbance, it may happen that it returns to its original position when the disturbance is removed. In this case the system is in stable equilibrium.

If the system is endowed with mass and suddenly unloaded, it will not stop in the equilibrium position, but will vibrate about it. If there is no inertia, the return is immediate.

Second Definition – A system is in stable equilibrium if there does not exist any adjacent position for which its potential energy is smaller.

Both definitions are identical for conservative systems. For a nonconservative system, the second definition becomes meaningless, since a potential energy cannot be defined. But the first definition is also not of much use. A nonconservative system, when disturbed, may never return to its original position (for example, if dry friction or plastic deformation is involved), but if a small disturbance causes only a small displacement, it is for practical purposes as safe as a stable conservative system. Therefore the stability concept will be avoided altogether in the study of the behavior of viscoelastic columns.

7.2 Inverted Pendulum

Before approaching the column problem, let us have a look at a simpler problem of the same kind, the inverted pendulum shown in Fig.7.1. A rigid, massless, and weightless bar is supported by a frictionless hinge

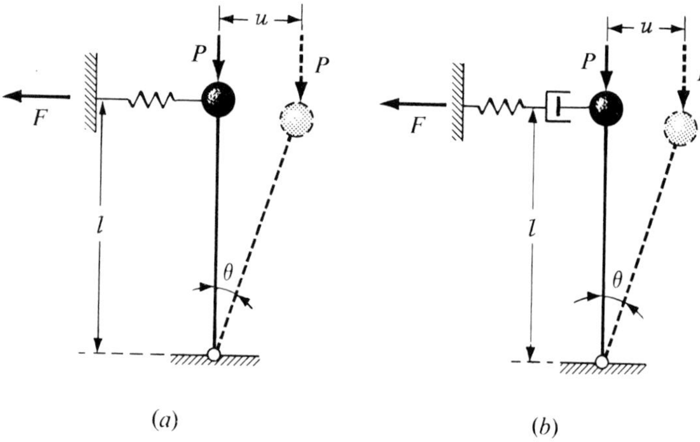

Figure 7.1. Inverted pendulum.

and carries at its upper end a rigid body of weight P. This body does, necessarily, have a mass P/g, but in true stability problems mass is irrelevant, and in the slow motion of viscoelastic creep its influence is negligibly small.

In Fig.7.1a the pendulum is braced laterally by a spring of stiffness k. In the undisturbed state the pendulum is vertical and the spring is undeformed. We disturb it by tilting it slightly as shown. This extends the spring by $u = \theta l$ and produces a spring force $F = ku$. The forces P and F have moments with respect to the hinge, and the resultant moment, positive when clockwise, is

$$M = Pl\theta - Fl = (P - kl)u . \qquad (7.1)$$

If $M < 0$, that is, counterclockwise, the pendulum will return to the upright position as soon as we release it: Its equilibrium is stable. If $M > 0$, that is, if $P > kl$, then P is stronger than F, and the pendulum will tip over as soon as we stop holding it in the deflected position. Its equilibrium is unstable. In the limiting case $P = kl$, the pendulum will remain indefinitely in the disturbed position. Its equilibrium is neutral or indifferent.

In Fig.7.1b the spring has been replaced by a viscoelastic element of the Maxwell type. The relation between the force and the displacement is now

$$F + p_1\dot{F} = q_1\dot{u} .$$

Since it contains time derivatives, it matters *how* we disturb the system.

In the undisturbed state the pendulum is again vertical and $F = 0$. We apply the same disturbance as before, and we apply it suddenly. Then the dashpot has no time to act, and $F = (q_1/p_1)u$. In the disturbed position there is a resultant moment

$$M = (P - q_1 l/p_1)u .$$

If $P < q_1 l/p_1$, the system will again return to the undisturbed position, and if $P > q_1 l/p_1$ it will collapse. The words "stable" and "unstable" seem meaningful. However, if $P < q_1 l/p_1$, a complete return is possible only if we release the pendulum at once. If we hold it in the deflected position for a finite time, the Maxwell element will begin to relax, and upon release the force F will be less than $q_1 u/p_1$. It may be that the system collapses immediately, and it may be that the force F is still strong enough to pull it toward the upright position, but no longer all the way. Moment equilibrium will be reached in a still slightly tilted position, in which F is still positive, and now creep will set in and the angle θ will slowly increase without bound. This indicates that the equilibrium of the pendulum is always precarious. If $P > q_1 l/p_1$, it collapses like an unstable elastic pendulum, and for smaller P the slightest disturbance will trigger a creeping collapse.

Now replace the Maxwell spring by a Kelvin spring, for which

$$F = q_0 u + q_1\dot{u} .$$

No matter how fast or slow we move the pendulum into the disturbed position, all that counts is the last time element Δt of this process. If we hold the pendulum for however short a time at θ, then $\dot{u} = 0$ and $F = q_0 u$. The stability decision is then the same as for an elastic spring, but even for a massless pendulum the return to $\theta = 0$ is not quick jerk, but a slow creep.

7.3 Elastic Column

Let us quickly review the buckling of an elastic column. We start from the beam-column problem, that is, we consider a column which carries in additio n to the axial load P a small lateral load p (Fig. 7.2). This

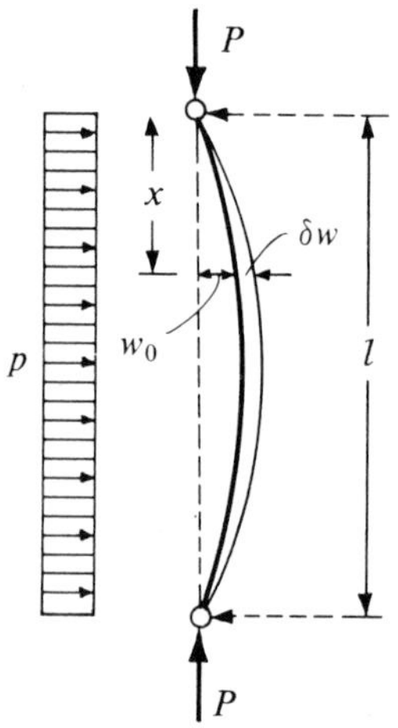

Figure 7.2. Beam-column.

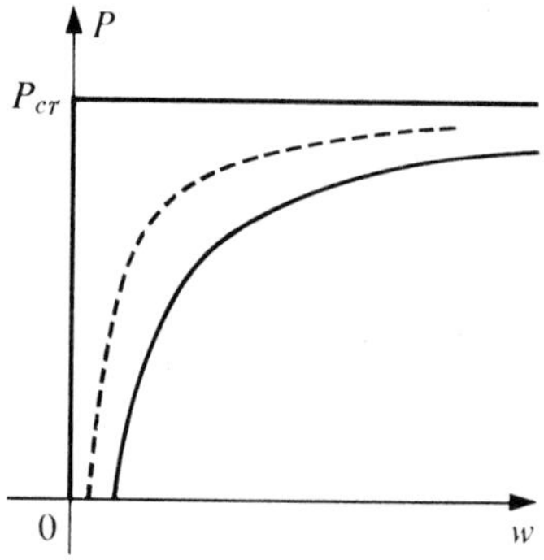

Figure 7.3. Deflection of an elastic beam-column.

lateral load and the reactions that go with it produce a certain bending moment M_0, the beam moment, and a deflection w_0, and there is an additional bending moment Pw_0 from the axial load acting on w_0 as its lever arm. This causes an additional deflection δw, which in turn increases the bending moment and hence the deflection, and so on *ad infinitum*. We ask whether this infinite process converges, that is, whether there exists a positive deflection w such that the moment $M_0 + Pw$ of the external forces is in equilibrium with the moment EIw'' of the stresses.

The answer is shown in Fig.7.3, which represents the relation between the load P and the deflection at $x = l/2$ for fixed p. Under increasing P the deflection increases slowly at first, and then faster, and tends to infinity as P approaches the critical load $P_{cr} = EI\pi^2/l^2$. If p is chosen smaller, the deflection follows the dotted line, and for $p = 0$ the curve degenerates into a vertical and a horizontal part, as indicated by heavy lines. They represent the ideal column, which carries only an axial load. It remains undeflected until $P = P_{cr}$, and then it is in neutral equilibrium. The critical load is usually calculated from this neutral equilibrium of the ideal column but it is used as a base of judgement for the safety of the actual column, which may have a small lateral load as shown, or may not be perfectly straight, or may be loaded with a slight eccentricity.

7.4 Viscoelastic Column

We consider again a straight column carrying an axial load P. Its deformation consists of an axial strain, which is unimportant for our problem and which will be disregarded. At $t = 0$ we apply in addition a lateral load, which we assume in the form

$$p(x,t) = q \sin \frac{\pi x}{l} \cdot \Delta(t) .$$

It produces the beam moment

$$M_0 = \frac{ql^2}{\pi^2} \sin \frac{\pi x}{l} \cdot \Delta(t) ,$$

and again there is an additional bending moment caused by the axial load. Let the total deflection be w; then the total bending moment is

$$M = \frac{ql^2}{\pi^2} \sin \frac{\pi x}{l} \cdot \Delta(t) + Pw , \tag{7.2}$$

and this must be introduced on the right-hand side of (3.11). This yields the differential equation of our problem:

$$I\mathbf{Q}(w'') + P\mathbf{P}(w) = -\frac{ql^2}{\pi^2} \sin \frac{\pi x}{l} \cdot \mathbf{P}\Delta(t) . \tag{7.3}$$

It is satisfied by the product solution

$$w(x,t) = W(t)\sin\frac{\pi x}{l}, \tag{7.4}$$

which reduces it to an ordinary differential equation for W:

$$\frac{I\pi^2}{l^2}\mathbf{Q}(W) - P\mathbf{P}(W) = \frac{ql^2}{\pi^2}\mathbf{P}\Delta(t), \tag{7.5}$$

or, in more detail,

$$\frac{I\pi^2}{l^2}\sum_0^n q_k \frac{d^kW}{dt^k} - P\sum_0^m p_k \frac{d^kW}{dt^k} = \frac{ql^2}{\pi^2}\sum_0^m p_k \frac{d^k\Delta(t)}{dt^k}. \tag{7.6}$$

The summation on the right-hand side contains the unit step function, the Dirac function, and its derivatives, that is, functions with singularities of increasing order at $t = 0$. For $t > 0$ all these functions except $\Delta(t)$ are zero, and the right-hand side is then a constant.

We have seen (p. 24) that viscoelastic materials may be classified as solids and fluids, and as those with and without an initial elastic response to the application of a load. For the solids $q_0 \neq 0$, for the fluids $q_0 = 0$. An initial elastic response occurs when $n = m$, and it is missing when $n = m + 1$. In (7.6), we may replace the summation limit m by n and still include all these cases if we reserve the right to let either $p_n = 0$ or $q_0 = 0$, or both.

When we integrate d^kW/dt^k from 0^- to some variable upper limit t, we obtain $d^{k-1}W/dt^{k-1}$ at t plus a constant of integration. When we integrate again and repeat the procedure to a total of k integrations, we obtain

$$W(t) + c_1t^{k-1} + c_2t^{k-2} + \dots + c_k.$$

Except for $W(t)$, which may have a step discontinuity at $t = 0$, this is a continuous function, and the next and any following integration will yield an entirely continuous function. Its value for $t = 0^-$ or 0^+ is the same, and when $t = 0^+$ is chosen as the upper integration limit, all these integrals equal zero. Therefore, when (7.6) is integrated n times, and, in the last integral, the upper limit made $t = 0^+$, in each of the sums only the term $k = n$ survives. Since $W(0^-) = 0$, this yields

$$\left(\frac{I\pi^2}{l^2} q_n - P p_n\right) W(0^+) = \frac{ql^2}{\pi^2} p_n \,, \tag{7.7}$$

and from this equation we find the initial value

$$W(0^+) = \frac{ql^2/\pi^2}{Iq_n\pi^2/p_n l^2 - P} \,. \tag{7.8}$$

Equation (7.8) is identical with that obtained for an elastic column with modulus $E_0 = q_n/p_n$, and the same conclusions can be drawn from it: If

$$P < P_i = \frac{E_0 I \pi^2}{l^2} \,, \tag{7.9}$$

then there is a finite positive deflection. If P comes very close to P_i, this deflection is rather large. If $P = P_i$, there exists no solution (within the limitations of the linearization underlying our equations), and the column will collapse immediately. We call this *instantaneous buckling*, and the critical load P_i is a kind of Euler load. For $P > P_i$ there exists a finite $W(0^+)$, but it is negative. It is of no practical interest, because (i) the load P will never get that high since the column will buckle before the load has reached the value P_i and because (ii) even if we could get the load high enough before applying the disturbing influence p, the column would never find this equilibrium but would bend in the positive direction, where there is no equilibrium possible.

To find out what happens if $P < P_i$, we might repeat the process which led us to (7.8), but integrate less than n times. This would yield starting values for the time derivatives of W and thus the initial conditions for a complete solution of the differential equation. In another context, this procedure has been demonstrated on pp. 26-27. We shall here avoid this tedious work and replace it by a second approach to the buckling problem, which will provide a deeper insight into what is happening to the column.

We subject (7.3) to the Laplace transformation and find a differential equation for $\overline{w}(s)$:

$$I\mathfrak{Q}(s)\,\overline{w}'' + P\,\mathfrak{P}(s)\,\overline{w} = -\frac{ql^2}{\pi^2 s}\,\mathfrak{P}(s)\sin\frac{\pi x}{l} .$$

Dividing by $\mathfrak{P}(s)$ and making use of the definition (1.32), we bring this into the form

$$I\mathcal{E}(s)\,\overline{w}'' + P\,\overline{w} = -\frac{1}{s}\,\frac{ql^2}{\pi^2}\sin\frac{\pi x}{l} . \tag{7.10}$$

This equation has a solution in the form

$$\overline{w} = \overline{W}(s)\sin\frac{\pi x}{l} ,$$

which satisfies the end conditions of simple support as shown in Fig. 7.2. When we introduce it into (7.10), we may solve for $\overline{W}(s)$:

$$\overline{W} = \frac{\dfrac{ql^2}{\pi^2}}{s\left(\dfrac{I\pi^2}{l^2}\,\mathcal{E}(s) - P\right)} . \tag{7.11}$$

From $\overline{W}(s)$ we may find $W(t)$ and hence

$$w(x,t) = W(t)\sin\frac{\pi x}{l}$$

by using the complex inversion theorem [5, 6, 7]. It states that

$$W(t) = \frac{1}{2\pi i}\int_{c-i}^{c+i}\overline{W}(s)\,e^{st}\,ds , \tag{7.12}$$

where c must be chosen such that all singularities of the integrand lie to the left of the integration path. In our case, there are two kinds of singularities. One stems from the factor s in the denominator of (7.11). It is a pole at $s=0$. The other singular points s_k $(k = 1, 2, \ldots m)$ are the roots of the equation

$$\mathcal{E}(s) = \frac{Pl^2}{I\pi^2} . \tag{7.13}$$

On p. 29 we have seen that all the roots of the similar equation $\mathscr{E}(s) = 0$ are real and nonpositive. We find an equal number (and hence all) of the solutions of (7.13) if we intersect any of the curves in Fig. 1.12 with a horizontal line. Also these roots are all real and at most one of them can be positive.

After these preliminaries we may proceed with the actual evaluation of the inversion integral. Fig. 7.4 shows the complex s plane and

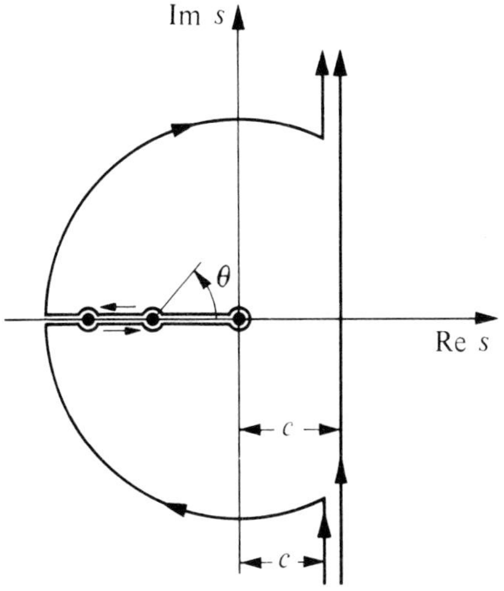

Figure 7.4. Integration path for the inversion integral.

the straight integration path suggested by (7.12). The shape of this path may be changed arbitrarily as long as it passes to the right of all the singular points of the integrand (Cauchy's integral theorem, see [31], [32]). We prefer to replace the straight path by a devious route, which swings far to the left until it reaches the real axis, then follows this axis toward the right making a small detour around every singular point of the integrand and, having surrounded the last one, returns in a similar fashion in the upper half-plane.

We leave it to the reader to verify that the contribution of the large circle to the integral vanishes if the radius is made larger and larger, and since the integrand is single-valued in the entire complex plane, the contributions of the real axis cancel each other. All that remains is a sum of counterclockwise integrals around the singularities:

$$W(t) = \frac{1}{2\pi i}\,\frac{ql^2}{\pi^2}\left[\frac{l^2}{I\pi^2\mathcal{E}(0) - Pl^2}\oint\frac{ds}{s}\right] + \sum_{k=1}^{m}\oint\frac{l^2 e^{st}\,ds}{s(I\pi^2\mathcal{E}(s) - Pl^2)} .$$

The first of the integrals is simply $2\pi i$. For each of the other ones we choose as integration path a circle of radius $r \to 0$ and may replace the denominator by

$$s_k I\pi^2\mathcal{E}'(s_k)\cdot(s - s_k) = s_k I\pi^2\mathcal{E}'(s_k) r e^{i\theta},$$

which leads us to

$$\oint\frac{l^2 e^{st}\,ds}{s(I\pi^2\mathcal{E}(s) - Pl^2)} = \int_{-\pi}^{+\pi}\frac{l^2 e^{s_k t}\, ri e^{i\theta}\,d\theta}{s_k I\pi^2\mathcal{E}'(s_k) r e^{i\theta}} = \frac{2\pi i l^2 e^{s_k t}}{s_k I\pi^2\mathcal{E}'(s_k)} .$$

Taking everything together, we obtain

$$W(t) = \frac{ql^4}{\pi^2}\left[\frac{i}{I\pi^2\mathcal{E}(0) - Pl^2} + \frac{1}{I\pi^2}\sum_{k=1}^{m}\frac{e^{s_k t}}{s_k\mathcal{E}'(s_k)}\right] . \qquad (7.14)$$

Now let us first consider the solid materials illustrated in Fig. 1.12a,c. If we choose P small enough, all the roots s_k of (7.13) are negative and, for $t \to \infty$, all the terms of the sum in (7.14) vanish. The deflection remains finite at all times and the column is safe in the same sense that an elastic column is safe if its axial load is below the Euler load. On the other hand, if P is larger than a critical value

$$P_c = \frac{I\pi^2}{l^2}\mathcal{E}(0) = \frac{E_\infty I\pi^2}{l^2}, \qquad (7.15)$$

then $s_1 > 0$ and one term in (7.14) contains an exponential function which grows beyond bounds as t increases. In this case the column will collapse. However, the collapse is not sudden like that of an elastic column or that of a viscoelastic column with the load P_i, but it is a creep process, which is called creep buckling. P_c is the critical load below which no creep buckling can take place.

When we now turn to fluid materials, we see from Fig. 1.12b, d that for any compressive load $P > 0$, no matter how small, $s_1 > 0$. Such columns will creep buckle under any load. This result is also contained in (7.15) since, for fluid materials, there is $E_\infty = 0$.

Since $E_0 > E_\infty$, the critical load for creep buckling is always lower than the one for instantaneous buckling. Never-the-less, the latter one is not without interest, because it signals a violent failure, while the creeping collapse may take a long time. It depends on the viscoelastic constants and on the kind and magnitude of the disturbance; and it may well be that a column, before it collapses, may fulfill a useful technical purpose.

Returning once more to the critical load for instantaneous buckling, we may now see that this can also be read from Fig. 1.12. It occurs only in materials which display instant elastic response with $E_0 \neq 0$, represented by Figs. 1.12a, b (one solid and one fluid). In these figures, the $\mathscr{E}$ curves have a horizontal asymptote at the level $\mathscr{E}(\infty) = E_0$. A horizontal line drawn at this level according to (7.13) corresponds to $P = P_i$ from (7.9) and leads to $s_1 \to \infty$. In this case the term $k = 1$ in (7.14) yields an infinite deflection as the limiting case of a very rapid, unbounded growth for a slightly smaller P. This, exactly, is the instantaneous collapse.

Problems

7.1. A rigid body of weight W (Fig. 7.5) rests on two viscoelastic supports, which are governed by a Maxwell law:

$$R + p_1\dot{R} = q_1\dot{u},$$

where R is the reaction exerted by the support and u the downward displacement of its upper end. Since the system has a vertical axis of symmetry, the rigid body will slowly sink. To find out whether this motion is sensitive to disturbances, add a small eccentric load W' and look for what happens. Are there any critical values of W or h?

7.2. Two straight bars AB and BC are connected and supported as shown in Fig. 7.6. At the point C a vertical load P is applied. Study the stability of the system for the following cases: (i) AB is viscoelastic, BC is rigid; (ii) AB is elastic, BC is viscoelastic; (iii) both bars are viscoelastic. Choose any of the standard laws for the viscoelastic parts.

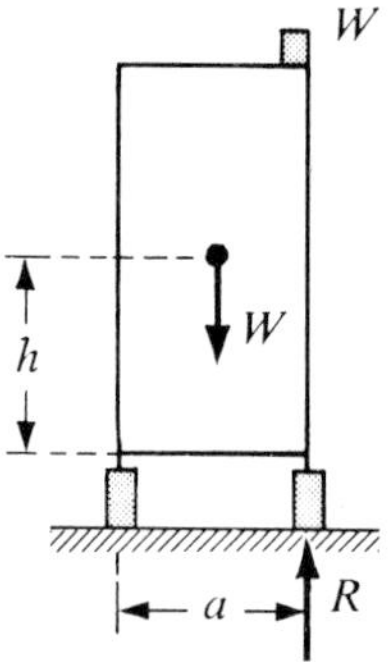

Figure 7.5.

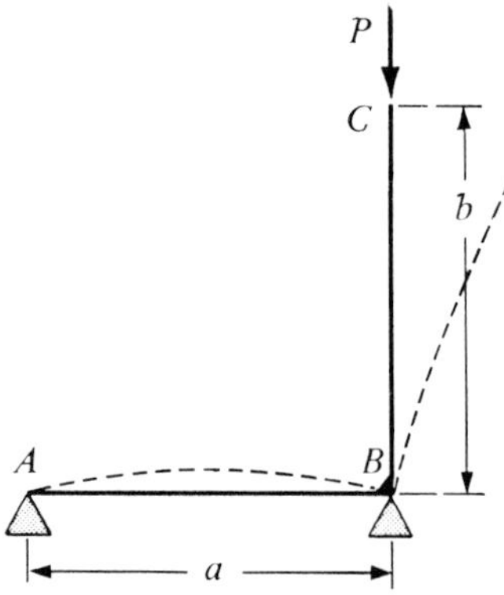

Figure 7.6.

References

A survey of the subject is found in the following handbook article:

47. J. Kempner: Viscoelastic Buckling, in W. Flügge (ed.), Handbook of Engineering Mechanics (New York: McGraw-Hill, 1962), Chap. 54.

The following paper deals with the main subject of the buckling of a straight column and the associated beam-column problem:

48. J. Kempner: Creep Bending and Buckling of Linearly Viscoelastic Columns. NACA, Techn. Note 3136 (1954). (Considers the four-parameter fluid and materials of lower order.)

The following paper gives an example of a buckling problem involving a linear viscoelastic material in a nonlinear kinematic setting:

49. J. Hult: Oil Canning Problems in Creep, in N.J. Hoff (ed.), Creep in Structures (Berlin: Springer-Verlag, 1962), pp. 161-173.

Chapter 8

Viscoelasticity in Three Dimensions

Thus far, we have restricted our attention to problems in which there was only one stress σ (or possibly τ) and one strain ϵ (or possibly γ), and the viscoelastic law (1.23) and its equivalents (2.6), (2.7), (5.6) were appropriate to describe the behavior of the material. When there is more than one stress component, we need a generalization of the viscoelastic law, which corresponds to the three-dimensional form of Hooke's law and contains it as a special case. We shall now find a logical approach to the general constitutive equations of viscoelastic materials and then apply them to a few typical cases.

8.1 Analysis of Stress and Strain

When a small rectangular block[1] is cut from a body, we can define on its sides six (or rather nine) stress components, which are shown in Fig. 8.1. It is well known that, for reasons of moment equilibrium, the shear stresses are equal in pairs, and we shall never have any reason to distinguish between τ_{xy} and τ_{yx}. The quantities σ_x, σ_y, ..., τ_{xz} are called *stress components*. Obviously, they are not the components of one vector, but of three vectors, and they form a physical entity, called the *stress tensor*. To display all the components of the stress tensor, we shall use matrix notation. However we shall not use in our formulas any matrix algebra beyond the addition of matri-

[1] Commomly called a parallelepipedon. It seems time that our language develop a word that is easier to pronounce and to spell than this monster.

ces and their multiplication by a numerical factor, and we shall not use any tensor calculus.

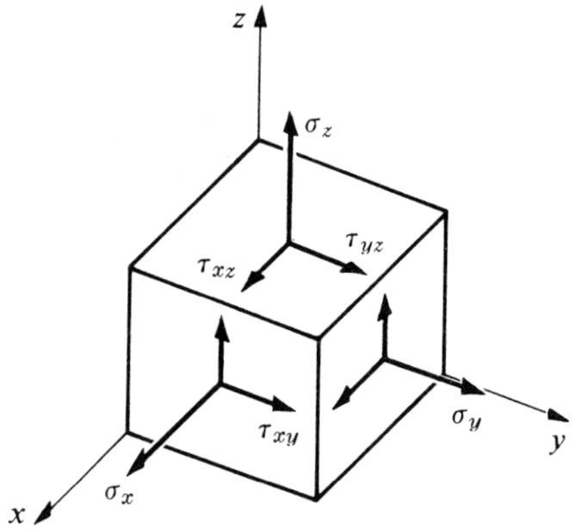

Figure 8.1. Infinitesimal element of a solid body.

As a first step in the analysis of the stress tensor, we split it into two parts:

$$\begin{bmatrix} \sigma_x & \tau_{xy} & \tau_{xz} \\ \tau_{xy} & \sigma_y & \tau_{yz} \\ \tau_{xz} & \tau_{yz} & \sigma_z \end{bmatrix} = \begin{bmatrix} s & 0 & 0 \\ 0 & s & 0 \\ 0 & 0 & s \end{bmatrix} + \begin{bmatrix} s_x & s_{xy} & s_{xz} \\ s_{xy} & s_y & s_{yz} \\ s_{xz} & s_{yz} & s_z \end{bmatrix}. \tag{8.1}$$

This matrix equation means that, for example,

$$\sigma_x = s + s_x, \qquad \tau_{xy} = 0 + s_{xy},$$

and so forth. The first stress system on the right-hand side consists of equal tensile (or compressive) stresses and no shear. The pressure inside an inviscid liquid or gas is of this kind, and therefore this stress system is called hydrostatic stress (also if s is a tension). The second term is, so far, simply what is left over after a hydrostatic stress has been subtracted from the given stress system. The question arises whether there is a special choice of s that would make the leftover meaningful.

We arrive at something useful when we choose

$$s = \frac{1}{3}(\sigma_x + \sigma_y + \sigma_z). \tag{8.2}$$

Then the sum of the three diagonal terms (the trace of the matrix) is the same for the first two matrices of (8.1) and, hence,

$$s_x + s_y + s_z = 0 . \tag{8.3}$$

A tensor of this peculiar kind is called a deviator. Its components are the stress deviations (that is, from the average normal

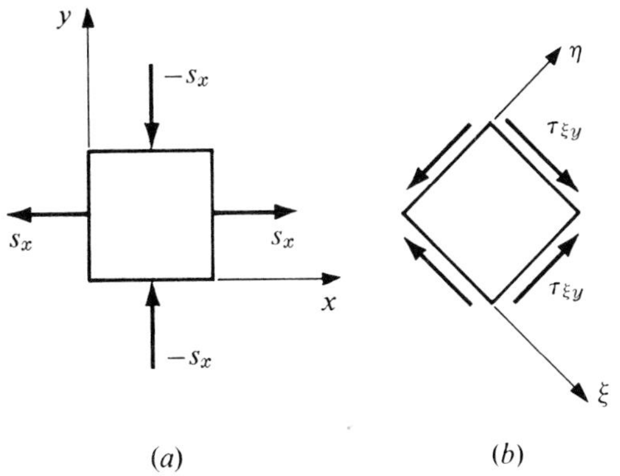

Figure 8.2. Pure shear stress in different reference frames.

stress). A stress deviator can be represented as a superposition of five simple shear-stress systems:

$$\begin{bmatrix} s_x & s_{xy} & s_{xz} \\ s_{xy} & s_y & s_{yz} \\ s_{xz} & s_{yz} & s_z \end{bmatrix} = \begin{bmatrix} 0 & s_{xy} & 0 \\ s_{xy} & 0 & 0 \\ 0 & 0 & 0 \end{bmatrix} + \begin{bmatrix} 0 & 0 & 0 \\ 0 & 0 & s_{yz} \\ 0 & s_{yz} & 0 \end{bmatrix} \tag{8.4}$$

$$+ \begin{bmatrix} 0 & 0 & s_{xz} \\ 0 & 0 & 0 \\ s_{xz} & 0 & 0 \end{bmatrix} + \begin{bmatrix} s_x & 0 & 0 \\ 0 & -s_x & 0 \\ 0 & 0 & 0 \end{bmatrix} + \begin{bmatrix} 0 & 0 & 0 \\ 0 & -s_z & 0 \\ 0 & 0 & s_z \end{bmatrix} .$$

The first three matrices on the right are obviously shear systems with $s_{xy} = \tau_{xy}$, and so forth. The fourth one is a plane stress system in the x,y plane, and it is well known that it is equivalent to shear stresses $\tau_{\xi\eta} = s_x$ in an element cut out as shown in Fig.8.2b. A similar interpretation is possible for the fifth term in (8.4).

We may now draw the following conclusions: The hydrostatic stress system has so high a degree of symmetry that the corresponding deformation can be only a change of size of the block shown in Fig. 8.1. If it was a cube it will remain a cube; and a sphere cut from the material will remain a sphere. On the other hand, each of the shear systems in (8.4) can produce only a shear deformation, be it the change of an angle between two faces of a block or between two of its diagonal planes; but none of these shear stress systems will change the volume. This is true whether the deformation is elastic or inelastic, as long as it is small enough to permit linear superposition, and as long as the material is isotropic, that is, as long as it does not have any preferential directions of deformation.

We now turn to a similar analysis of the strain. There are two kinds of strain, longitudinal strain and shear strain. The longitudinal strain describes the increase of length of a line element, like ϵ_x, ϵ_y, ϵ_z. The shear strain describes a change of an angle, for example, the small decrease of the right angle between line elements dx and dy, which is called the shear strain γ_{xy}. Our equations will turn out to be simpler when we use instead of γ_{xy} the quantity

$$\epsilon_{xy} = \frac{1}{2}\gamma_{xy} \tag{8.5}$$

to measure the shear deformation, and we shall use the word "shear" for it.

The quantities $\epsilon_x, \epsilon_y, \ldots, \epsilon_{xz}$ are the components of the *strain tensor*. We display them also as a matrix and split it just as we did for the stresses:

$$\begin{bmatrix} \epsilon_x & \epsilon_{xy} & \epsilon_{xz} \\ \epsilon_{xy} & \epsilon_y & \epsilon_{yz} \\ \epsilon_{xz} & \epsilon_{yz} & \epsilon_z \end{bmatrix} = \begin{bmatrix} e & 0 & 0 \\ 0 & e & 0 \\ 0 & 0 & e \end{bmatrix} + \begin{bmatrix} e_x & e_{xy} & e_{xz} \\ e_{xy} & e_y & e_{yz} \\ e_{xz} & e_{yz} & e_z \end{bmatrix} . \tag{8.6}$$

Again we choose

$$e = \frac{1}{3}(\epsilon_x + \epsilon_y + \epsilon_z), \tag{8.7}$$

that is, equal to one third of the volume strain (bulk strain). It follows that

$$e_x + e_y + e_z = 0\,, \tag{8.8}$$

which indicates that the second part of the strain system describes a change of shape without a change of volume. The meaning of (8.6) is, therefore, that we have split a general strain tensor into one part which represents a pure dilatation (without change of shape), and into another part which represents a distortion, that is, a change of shape at constant volume.

Just as we could resolve the stress deviator into a superposition of five simple shear stresses, we can resolve the strain deviator into five simple shear strains:

$$\begin{bmatrix} e_x & e_{xy} & e_{xz} \\ e_{xy} & e_y & e_{yz} \\ e_{xz} & e_{yz} & e_z \end{bmatrix} = \begin{bmatrix} 0 & e_{xy} & 0 \\ e_{xy} & 0 & 0 \\ 0 & 0 & 0 \end{bmatrix} + \begin{bmatrix} 0 & 0 & 0 \\ 0 & 0 & e_{yz} \\ 0 & e_{yz} & 0 \end{bmatrix}$$
$$+ \begin{bmatrix} 0 & 0 & e_{xz} \\ 0 & 0 & 0 \\ e_{xz} & 0 & 0 \end{bmatrix} + \begin{bmatrix} e_x & 0 & 0 \\ 0 & -e_x & 0 \\ 0 & 0 & 0 \end{bmatrix} + \begin{bmatrix} 0 & 0 & 0 \\ 0 & -e_z & 0 \\ 0 & 0 & e_z \end{bmatrix}. \tag{8.9}$$

The first three matrices on the right-hand side obviously represent simple shears. The fourth one is a deformation in the x,y plane, which

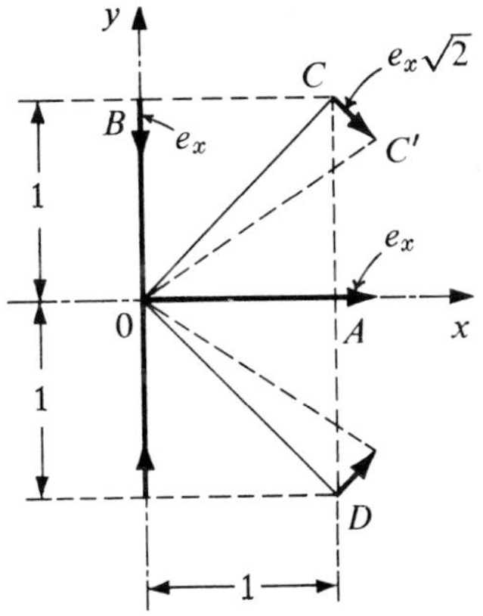

Figure 8.3. Pure shear strain in different reference frames.

is illustrated in Fig.8.3. To produce the deformation, we keep O at rest and let A move to the right by a distance e_x, while B moves as much downward. The point C has the vector sum of both these displacements and hence moves by a distance $CC' = e_x\sqrt{2}$ as shown. The diagonal OC rotates through the angle $e_x\sqrt{2}/\sqrt{2} = e_x$, and the right angle COD decreases by $2e_x$. In a coordinate system ξ, η (Fig.8.2) this is a simple shear with

$$\epsilon_{\xi\eta} = \frac{1}{2}\gamma_{\xi\eta} = e_x .$$

8.2 The Viscoelastic Law

If a viscoelastic material is isotropic, a hydrostatic stress must produce a dilatation and no distortion. The quantities s and e may be connected by a relation like (1.23) or any of its equivalents. We write

$$\sum_0^{m''} p_k'' \frac{d^k s}{dt^k} = \sum_0^{n''} q_k'' \frac{d^k e}{dt^k} \tag{8.10a}$$

or, shorter,

$$\mathbf{P}'' s = \mathbf{Q}'' e . \tag{8.10b}$$

On the other hand, each of the five shear stress systems in (8.4) must produce the shear strain represented by the corresponding matrix in (8.9), and isotropy of the material requires that the relation be the same for all these pairs. We write it in the form

$$\sum_0^{m'} p_k' \frac{d^k S}{dt^k} = \sum_0^{n'} q_k' \frac{d^k E}{dt^k} \tag{8.11a}$$

or

$$\mathbf{P}' S = \mathbf{Q}' E , \tag{8.11b}$$

where S and E stand for corresponding components of stress and strain deviators or, if we wish, for the entire matrices on the left-hand side of (8.4) and (8.9).

The operator pairs **P**'', **Q**'' and **P**', **Q**', which describe the viscoelastic material, are entirely independent of each other. To each pair Table 1.2 is applicable. We shall standardize them so that $p_0'' = p_0' = 1$.

The elastic solid is a limiting case of the viscoelastic materials. We may write the linear elastic law (that is, Hooke's law) in the form (8.10a), (8.11a). The cubic dilatation 3e is proportional to the hydrostatic part of the stress, and each shear component to the corresponding shear stress:

$$s = K \cdot 3e , \qquad \tau_{xy} = G \cdot 2\epsilon_{xy} . \tag{8.12}$$

Here K is the bulk modulus and G the shear modulus. We see that for the elastic solid the four operators are simple multiplicative constants:

$$\mathbf{P}'' = 1, \quad \mathbf{Q}'' = 3K, \quad \mathbf{P}' = 1, \quad \mathbf{Q}' = 2G .$$

Since all components of the stress deviator are subject to the same law, we have now

$$\begin{aligned}\sigma_x = s + s_x &= 3Ke + 2Ge_x \\ &= 3K \cdot \frac{1}{3}(\epsilon_x + \epsilon_y + \epsilon_z) + 2G\left[\epsilon_x - \frac{1}{3}(\epsilon_x + \epsilon_y + \epsilon_z)\right] \\ &= (K + \frac{4}{3}G)\epsilon_x + (K - \frac{2}{3}G)(\epsilon_y + \epsilon_z) .\end{aligned}$$

The usual formulation of this law reads

$$\sigma_x = \frac{E}{(1+\nu)(1-2\nu)} [(1-\nu)\epsilon_x + \nu(\epsilon_y + \epsilon_z)].$$

A comparison of the coefficients of both formulas leads to relations between the elastic modulus E and Poisson's ratio ν on the one side and K and G on the other:

$$E = \frac{9KG}{3K+G} , \qquad \nu = \frac{1}{2}\,\frac{3K-2G}{3K+G} . \tag{8.13}$$

8.3 Uni-axial Stress

The viscoelastic law (8.10), (8.11) is a new and more general formulation of the constitutive equations of materials. When applied to the special case of simple tension, it must lead back to (1.23) and to a relation between its operators **P**, **Q** and the four new ones.

In uni-axial tension we have only one stress, σ_x. From (8.2) we find $s = \frac{1}{3}\sigma_x$, and then the stress deviations

$$s_x = \frac{2}{3}\sigma_x, \qquad s_y = s_z = -\frac{1}{3}\sigma_x .$$

The strain has three components: the axial strain ϵ_x and the lateral contractions $\epsilon_y = \epsilon_z$. From (8.7) we have then

$$e = \frac{1}{3}(\epsilon_x + 2\epsilon_y)$$

and, hence,

$$e_x = \frac{2}{3}(\epsilon_x - \epsilon_y), \quad e_y = e_z = -\frac{1}{3}(\epsilon_x - \epsilon_y) .$$

To these quantities we apply (8.10b) and (8.11b):

$$\mathbf{P}''\left(\frac{1}{3}\sigma_x\right) = \mathbf{Q}''\left(\frac{1}{3}(\epsilon_x + 2\epsilon_y)\right),$$
$$\mathbf{P}'\left(\frac{2}{3}\sigma_x\right) = \mathbf{Q}'\left(\frac{2}{3}(\epsilon_x - \epsilon_y)\right) .$$

Since the operators are linear, we may pull the constant factors out and then cancel them, and we may also split the right-hand sides into sums:

$$\mathbf{P}''\sigma_x = \mathbf{Q}''\epsilon_x + 2\mathbf{Q}''\epsilon_y ,$$
$$\mathbf{P}'\sigma_x = \mathbf{Q}'\epsilon_x - \mathbf{Q}'\epsilon_y . \qquad (8.14a,b)$$

We now apply the operator $\mathbf{Q}'$ to the first equation and $2\mathbf{Q}''$ to the second and add:

$$(\mathbf{Q}'\mathbf{P}'' + 2\mathbf{Q}''\mathbf{P}')\sigma_x = (\mathbf{Q}'\mathbf{Q}'' + 2\mathbf{Q}''\mathbf{Q}')\epsilon_x + 2(\mathbf{Q}'\mathbf{Q}'' - \mathbf{Q}''\mathbf{Q}')\epsilon_y .$$

It is now important to know that the operators are not only linear, but that their coefficients p_k'', q_k'', p_k', q_k' are independent of time. Then

$$\mathbf{Q}''\mathbf{Q}'\epsilon_y = \mathbf{Q}'\mathbf{Q}''\epsilon_y ,$$

that is, the operators are commutative, and the ϵ_y term in our last equation vanishes. Thus we have

$$(\mathbf{P}''\mathbf{Q}' + 2\mathbf{Q}''\mathbf{P}')\sigma_x = 3\mathbf{Q}''\mathbf{Q}'\epsilon_x . \tag{8.15a}$$

This is identical with (1.23) if we set

$$\mathbf{P} = \mathbf{P}''\mathbf{Q}' + 2\mathbf{Q}''\mathbf{P}' , \qquad \mathbf{Q} = 3\mathbf{Q}''\mathbf{Q}' . \tag{8.16}$$

By a quite similar operation we may eliminate ϵ_x between (8.14) to obtain a relation governing the lateral contraction ϵ_y:

$$(\mathbf{P}''\mathbf{Q}' - \mathbf{Q}''\mathbf{P}')\sigma_x = 3\mathbf{Q}''\mathbf{Q}'\epsilon_y . \tag{8.15b}$$

Equations (8.15) are the viscoelastic equivalent of a complete statement of Hooke's law for uni-axial tension. To interpret them, we shall now inspect a number of special choices for the operators.

While the shear deformation may be rather large, the change of volume measured by e is always very limited. It seems, therefore, reasonable to neglect the latter completeley and to assume $e = 0$. This corresponds to $\mathbf{P}'' = 0$, $\mathbf{Q}'' = 1$. The constitutive equations for uni-axial stress are then

$$2\mathbf{P}'\sigma_x = 3\mathbf{Q}'\epsilon_x , \qquad -\mathbf{P}'\sigma_x = 3\mathbf{Q}'\epsilon_y .$$

They show that at all times $\epsilon_y = -\frac{1}{2}\epsilon_x$.

The next best approximation to a real material would be to assume that the dilatation is elastic:

$$s = 3Ke .$$

This corresponds to $\mathbf{P}'' = 1$, $\mathbf{Q}'' = 3K$, and (8.15) are now

$$(\mathbf{Q}' + 6K\mathbf{P}')\sigma_x = 9K\mathbf{Q}'\epsilon_x ,$$
$$(\mathbf{Q}' - 3K\mathbf{P}')\sigma_x = 9K\mathbf{Q}'\epsilon_y . \tag{8.17a,b}$$

The choice of the distortion operators $\mathbf{P}'$, $\mathbf{Q}'$ is still free, and we shall inspect two possibilities.

First, we assume a Maxwell law for the distortion, letting

$$\mathbf{P}' = 1 + p_1' \frac{d}{dt}, \qquad \mathbf{Q}' = q_1' \frac{d}{dt} . \tag{8.18}$$

When we introduce this in (8.17) and collect terms, we find the following pair of equations:

$$\begin{aligned} 6K\sigma_x + (q_1' + 6Kp_1')\dot{\sigma}_x &= 9Kq_1'\dot{\epsilon}_x , \\ -3K\sigma_x + (q_1' - 3Kp_1')\dot{\sigma}_x &= 9Kq_1'\dot{\epsilon}_y . \end{aligned} \tag{8.19a,b}$$

Both have the form of the Maxwell equation. In (8.19a) we divide by 6K and extract the coefficients

$$p_1 = p_1' + q_1'/6K , \qquad q_1 = \frac{3}{2} q_1' ,$$

and similarly from (8.19b)

$$p_1^* = p_1' - q_1'/3K , \qquad q_1^* = -3q_1' .$$

We may use these coefficients in all formulas which Table 1.2 gives for the Maxwell material. In particular for unit step loading $\sigma_x = \Delta(t)$, we can describe the strains by two creep compliances

$$\epsilon_x = J_x(t) , \qquad \epsilon_y = J_y(t) ,$$

formed from the coefficients according to the formula for $J(t)$ in Table 1.2. We find

$$\begin{aligned} J_x(t) &= \frac{p_1 + t}{q_1} = \frac{2p_1'}{3q_1'} + \frac{1}{9K} + \frac{2t}{3q_1'} , \\ J_y(t) &= \frac{p_1^* + t}{q_1^*} = -\frac{p_1'}{3q_1'} + \frac{1}{9K} - \frac{t}{3q_1'} . \end{aligned} \tag{8.20a,b}$$

These compliance have been plotted in Fig.8.4. The plot shows that the ratio $\epsilon_x/(-\epsilon_y)$ varies with time, which indicates that the concept of a Poisson ratio is not very meaningful for a viscoelastic material.

Now let us compare these results with those for another viscoelastic material. We again assume that it is elastic in dilatation, but postulate

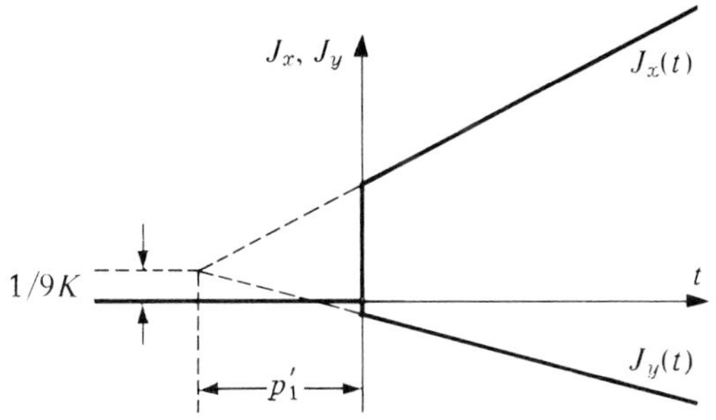

Figure 8.4. Creep compliances for a material with elastic dilatation and Maxwell distortion.

the Kelvin law for distortion. We have then to introduce in (8.17) the operators

$$\mathbf{P}' = 1\,, \qquad \mathbf{Q}' = q_0' + q_1' \frac{d}{dt}$$

and this leads to the following constitutive equations:

$$(q_0' + 6K)\sigma_x + q_1'\dot{\sigma}_x = 9K(q_0'\epsilon_x + q_1'\dot{\epsilon}_x)\,,$$

$$(q_0' - 3K)\sigma_x + q_1'\dot{\sigma}_x = 9K(q_0'\epsilon_y + q_1'\dot{\epsilon}_y)\,. \qquad (8.21a,b)$$

These equations are not of the Kelvin type; they have the same form as (1.19), which describes the three-parameter solid. This is understandable, since a material which has elastic dilatation must have an impact response, which the Kelvin solid is lacking.

After dividing each equation by the coefficient of σ_x and then comparing it with (1.19), we may read from it a set of coefficients. For (8.21a) they are

$$p_1 = \frac{q_1'}{q_0' + 6K}\,, \qquad q_0 = \frac{9Kq_0'}{q_0' + 6K}\,, \qquad q_1 = \frac{9Kq_1'}{q_0' + 6K}$$

and for (8.21b), which controls the transverse strain,

$$p_1^* = \frac{q_1'}{q_0' - 3K}\,, \qquad q_0^* = \frac{9Kq_0'}{q_0' - 3K}\,, \qquad q_1^* = \frac{9Kq_1'}{q_0' - 3K}\,.$$

With these we enter the formula for the creep compliance $J(t)$ of the three-parameter solid in Table 1.2 and find with $q_0/q_1 = q_0^*/q^*_1 = q_0'/q_1' = \lambda$ for the axial strain

$$J_x(t) = \frac{1}{9K} e^{-\lambda t} + \left(\frac{1}{9K} + \frac{2}{3q_0'}\right)(1 - e^{-\lambda t}) \tag{8.22a}$$

and for the transverse strain

$$J_y(t) = \frac{1}{9K} e^{-\lambda t} + \left(\frac{1}{9K} - \frac{1}{3q_0'}\right)(1 - e^{-\lambda t}) . \tag{8.22b}$$

These creep compliances are plotted in Fig. 8.5. The curves show that the material is solid; both strains tend asymptotically toward finite limits. In addtion, the curves show a rather surprising feature: For

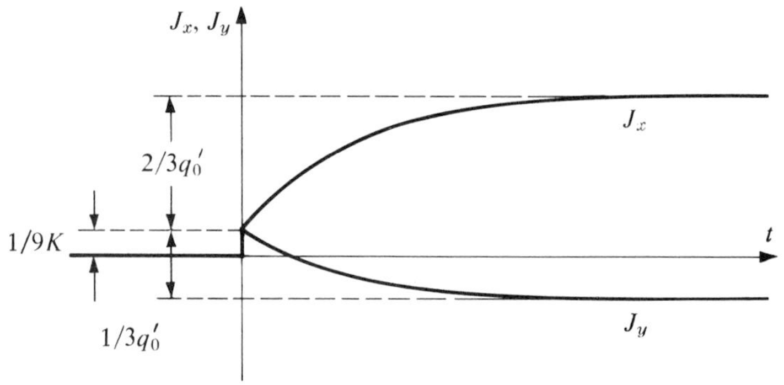

Figure 8.5. Creep compliances for a material with elastic dilatation and Kelvin distortion.

$t = 0^+$, both compliances are positive. This means that upon a sudden application of load to a tension bar, its first response is that it gets not only longer, but also thicker! This is a necessary consequence of the combination of elastic dilatation (with impact response) and Kelvin distortion (without it). The first thing the bar does is to increase its volume - equally in all directions - and then distortional creep sets in, which makes the bar longer and thinner without further change of its volume. Although the "negative lateral contraction", if we may call it so, looks improbable, there seems to be no physical law standing against it.

8.4 Viscoelastic Cylinder in a Rigid Die

We are now prepared to solve a simple problem. A cylindrical sample of an arbitrary viscoelastic material is inserted in a die and loaded by a pressure p as shown in Fig. 8.6. The axis of the cylinder is the x axis, and there are y and z axes in some horizontal plane. If we assume that there is no friction between the cylinder and the die, the

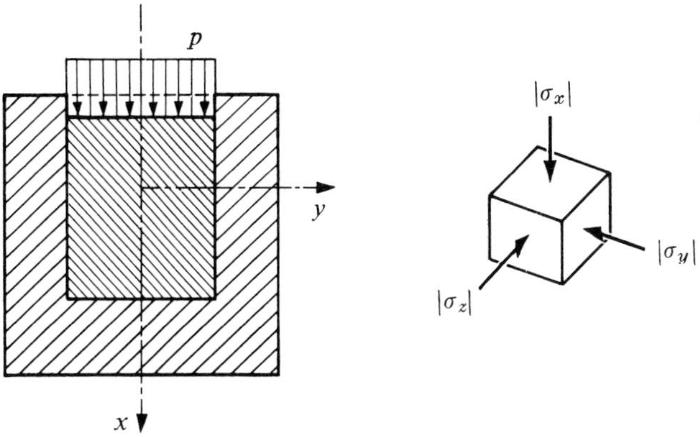

Figure 8.6. Viscoelastic cylinder in a rigid die.

stresses are the same at all points. They consist of a compression $\sigma_x = -p$ and of equal, but still unknown, stresses $\sigma_y = \sigma_z$. The die confines the sample horizontally so that $\epsilon_y = \epsilon_z = 0$, but there is, of course, a strain ϵ_x, which we expect to be negative. The unknowns of our problem are σ_y and ϵ_x.

We formulate differential equations by expressing each of the strains as the superposition of contributions caused by σ_x, σ_y, and σ_z, that is by applying repeatedly (8.15).

If there were only the stress σ_x, then ϵ_x would be related to it by (8.15a). For a stress σ_y, acting alone, ϵ_x is a transverse strain and the relation between the two is (8.15b), modified by interchanging the subscripts x and y. The stress σ_z makes another contribution of the same magnitude. Adding the three contributions to $3\mathbf{Q}''\mathbf{Q}'\epsilon_x$ obtained in this way, we have

$$(\mathbf{P}''\mathbf{Q}' + 2\mathbf{Q}''\mathbf{P}')\sigma_x + 2(\mathbf{P}''\mathbf{Q}' - \mathbf{Q}''\mathbf{P}')\sigma_y = 3\mathbf{Q}''\mathbf{Q}'\epsilon_x \,. \quad (8.23a)$$

In the same way we obtain an equation for ϵ_y, noting that now σ_y is the stress that acts in the same direction, while for σ_x and σ_z, ϵ_y is a transverse strain. We find

$$(\mathbf{P}''\mathbf{Q}' + 2\mathbf{Q}''\mathbf{P}')\sigma_y + (\mathbf{P}''\mathbf{Q}' - \mathbf{Q}''\mathbf{P}')(\sigma_x + \sigma_z) = 3\mathbf{Q}''\mathbf{Q}'\epsilon_y ,$$

which, with $\sigma_z = \sigma_y$, may be simplified to read

$$(2\mathbf{P}''\mathbf{Q}' + \mathbf{Q}''\mathbf{P}')\sigma_y + (\mathbf{P}''\mathbf{Q}' - \mathbf{Q}''\mathbf{P}')\sigma_x = 3\mathbf{Q}''\mathbf{Q}'\epsilon_y .$$

Since we know that $\epsilon_y = 0$, this is a differential equation for our first unknown, σ_y:

$$(2\mathbf{P}''\mathbf{Q}' + \mathbf{Q}''\mathbf{P}')\sigma_y = (\mathbf{Q}''\mathbf{P}' - \mathbf{P}''\mathbf{Q}')\sigma_x . \qquad (8.23b)$$

After it has been solved, (8.23a) may be used to find ϵ_x.

To actually solve these equations, we subject them to the Laplace transformation. If we assume that all the initial values appearing in (1.18) are zero, this amounts to replacing the time-dependent stresses and strains by their Laplace transforms $\bar{\sigma}$ and $\bar{\epsilon}$ and the differential operators $\mathbf{P}'$, $\mathbf{Q}'$, $\mathbf{P}''$, $\mathbf{Q}''$ by polynomials in the Laplace variable $\mathscr{s}$ defined as indicated in (1.26)[2]:

$$3\mathcal{Q}''\mathcal{Q}'\bar{\epsilon}_x = (\mathcal{P}''\mathcal{Q}' + 2\mathcal{Q}''\mathcal{P}')\bar{\sigma}_x + 2(\mathcal{P}''\mathcal{Q}' - \mathcal{Q}''\mathcal{P}')\bar{\sigma}_y ,$$
$$(2\mathcal{P}''\mathcal{Q}' + \mathcal{Q}''\mathcal{P}')\bar{\sigma}_y = (\mathcal{Q}''\mathcal{P}' - \mathcal{P}''\mathcal{Q}')\bar{\sigma}_x . \qquad (8.24a,b)$$

Since in these equations everything is simple algebra, we may divide each one by the coefficient on its left-hand side [we could not have divided (8.23) by operators!] and find, after some algebra,

$$\bar{\sigma}_y = \frac{\mathcal{Q}''\mathcal{P}' - \mathcal{P}''\mathcal{Q}'}{2\mathcal{P}''\mathcal{Q}' + \mathcal{Q}''\mathcal{P}'}\bar{\sigma}_x , \qquad \bar{\epsilon}_x = \frac{3\mathcal{P}''\mathcal{P}'}{2\mathcal{P}''\mathcal{Q}' + \mathcal{Q}''\mathcal{P}'}\bar{\sigma}_x . \qquad (8.25a,b)$$

---

[2] The reader will notice that here the symbol for the Laplace variable has been changed from s to $\mathscr{s}$. This has been necessary, because we shall soon (p. 177) find in the same equation the Laplace variable $\mathscr{s}$ and the hydrostatic stress s and it does not seem wise to depart in the choice of symbols for either one very far from generally accepted usage.

Before we can complete the solution, we have to specify how σ_x is to depend on time, and we have to choose a viscoelastic material. We apply σ_x as a step load

$$\sigma_x = -p\,\Delta(t)\,,$$

which has the transform

$$\bar{\sigma}_x = -p/s\,, \tag{8.26}$$

and we consider now two typical materials.

Since, in this case, no deformation is possible without a change of volume, it would make no sense to consider an incompressible material. We begin, therefore, with assuming elastic behavior in dilatation and the Maxwell law for distortion, that is, $\mathbf{P}'' = 1$, $\mathbf{Q}'' = 3K$, and (8.18). The corresponding polynomials are

$$\mathcal{P}'' = 1, \quad \mathcal{Q}'' = 3K, \quad \mathcal{P}' = 1 + p_1' s, \quad \mathcal{Q}' = q_1' s\,,$$

and when we insert these in (8.25), we find

$$\bar{\sigma}_y = -\frac{p}{s}\,\frac{3K(1 + p_1' s) - q_1' s}{3K(1 + p_1' s) + 2q_1' s}\,,$$

$$\bar{\epsilon}_x = -\frac{p}{s}\,\frac{3(1 + p_1' s)}{3K(1 + p_1' s) + 2q_1' s}\,.$$

With the abbreviations

$$1/\alpha = 3K\,, \qquad 1/\lambda = p_1' + 2\alpha q_1'$$

these expressions may be rewritten in the following form:

$$\bar{\sigma}_y = -\lambda p\left[\frac{1}{s(s+\lambda)} + \frac{p_1' - \alpha q_1'}{s+\lambda}\right],$$

$$\bar{\epsilon}_x = -\frac{\lambda p}{K}\left[\frac{1}{s(s+\lambda)} + \frac{p_1'}{s+\lambda}\right],$$

and now we may use the transform pairs (3) and (4) of Table 1.1 to find the physical quantities σ_y and ϵ_x. They are, for $t > 0$,

$$\sigma_y = -p\left[1 - \frac{3q_1'}{3Kp_1' + 2q_1'} e^{-\lambda t}\right],$$

$$\epsilon_x = -\frac{p}{K}\left[1 - \frac{2q_1'}{3Kp_1' + 2q_1'} e^{-\lambda t}\right]. \qquad (8.27a,b)$$

The stress $-\sigma_y$ is the pressure which the sample exerts on the cylindrical surface of the die. It is shown in Fig. 8.7 as a function of time.

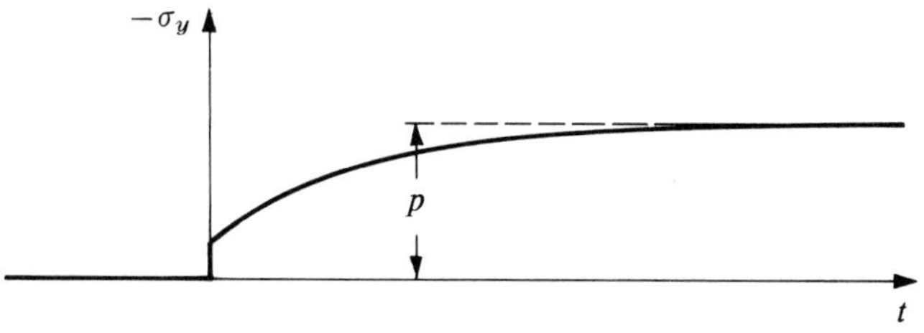

Figure 8.7. Lateral pressure in a die, elastic dilatation, Maxwell distortion.

At $t = 0^+$ it begins with the value

$$-\sigma_y(0^+) = p\,\frac{3Kp_1' - q_1'}{3Kp_1' + 2q_1'},$$

which is less than p, and it increases asymptotically to p. The strain ϵ_x behaves similarly. Although the material is a fluid (see Fig. 8.4), the strain ϵ_x is bounded, quite naturally so since even water would not show much deformation under the present circumstances. At the outset the interplay of the elastic responses in dilatation and distortion makes the material behave similar to an elastic solid, developing a lateral pressure less then p, but in the course of time the stresses approach those in an inviscid fluid with $\sigma_x = \sigma_y = \sigma_z = -p$.

As another choice, we consider now a material which combines Kelvin dilatation with Maxwell distortion:

$$\mathcal{P}'' = 1, \qquad \mathcal{Q}'' = q_0'' + q_1''\mathcal{s}, \qquad \mathcal{P}' = 1 + p_1'\mathcal{s}, \qquad \mathcal{Q}' = q_1'\mathcal{s}.$$

When this and $\bar{\sigma}_x$ from (8.26) are introduced in (8.25a), there comes

$$\bar{\sigma}_y = -p\left[\frac{1}{s} - \frac{3q_1'}{p_1'q_1''s^2 + (p_1'q_0'' + q_1'' + 2q_1')s + q_0''}\right].$$

Now, let $s = -\lambda_1$ and $s = -\lambda_2$ be the roots of the denominator. Then it may easily be seen that λ_1 and λ_2 are always positive, and after resolution into partial fractions, transform pairs (1) and (3) of Table 1.1 may be applied to yield for $t > 0$ the stress

$$\sigma_y = -p\left[1 - \frac{3q_1'}{p_1'q_1''}\cdot\frac{1}{\lambda_1 - \lambda_2}\left(e^{-\lambda_2 t} - e^{-\lambda_1 t}\right)\right].$$

This has been plotted in Fig.8.8. At $t = 0$ the lateral pressure jumps at once to p, but then it decreases and recovers ultimately again to the

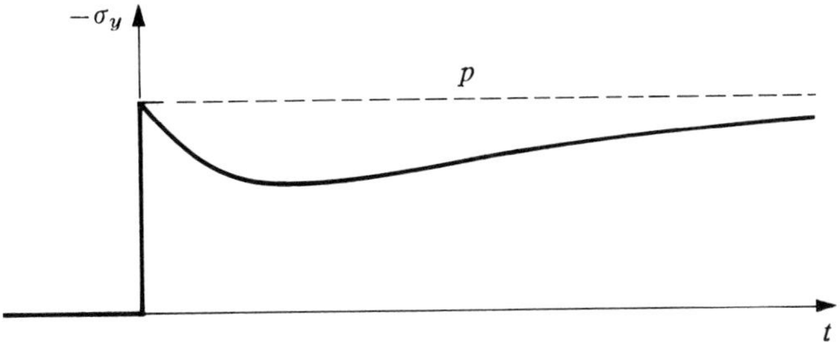

Figure 8.8. Lateral pressure in a die, Kelvin dilatation, Maxwell distortion.

full hydrostatic value. This may be understood by reasoning along the following lines: Since in this system any deformation must include a change of volume, and since the Kelvin law assumed for the dilatation does not permit an immediate response, $\epsilon_x(0^+) = 0$. Now, the Maxwell law assumed for the distortion would require an immediate response, which can be avoided only if the stress deviator vanishes at $t = 0^+$, that is, when $\sigma_y = \sigma_x$. Then, as the deformation begins, it cannot be a change of volume alone and therefore stress deviations are now needed, whence $\sigma_y \neq \sigma_x$. Ultimately the presence of a Maxwell part in the deformation law requires fluid behavior, that is, $\sigma_y \to \sigma_x$.

It is left to the reader to work out the formula for $\epsilon_x(t)$. The transform pairs (3) and (4) of Table 1.1 will be needed, and the result will confirm the statements just made.

8.5 Correspondence Principle

To formulate an arbitrary stress problem, three kinds of equations are needed: the equilibrium conditions, the kinematic relations, and the constitutive law of the material. The first two of these are common to elastic and viscoelastic materials and may be found in any book on the theory of elasticity [21, 57, 58]. The equilibrium conditions describe the force equilibrium for an element dx dy dz cut from the material:

$$\frac{\partial\sigma_x}{\partial x} + \frac{\partial\tau_{xy}}{\partial y} + \frac{\partial\tau_{xz}}{\partial z} + X = 0, \qquad \frac{\partial\tau_{xy}}{\partial x} + \frac{\partial\sigma_y}{\partial y} + \frac{\partial\tau_{yz}}{\partial z} + Y = 0,$$

$$\frac{\partial\tau_{xz}}{\partial x} + \frac{\partial\tau_{yz}}{\partial y} + \frac{\partial\sigma_z}{\partial z} + Z = 0, \tag{8.28}$$

where X, Y, and Z are the components of the external force per unit of volume. The kinematic relations express the strains in terms of the components u, v, and w of the displacement vector:

$$\epsilon_x = \frac{\partial u}{\partial x}, \qquad \epsilon_y = \frac{\partial v}{\partial y}, \qquad \epsilon_z = \frac{\partial w}{\partial z},$$

$$\epsilon_{xy} = \frac{1}{2}\left(\frac{\partial u}{\partial y} + \frac{\partial v}{\partial x}\right), \qquad \epsilon_{yz} = \frac{1}{2}\left(\frac{\partial v}{\partial z} + \frac{\partial w}{\partial y}\right), \qquad \epsilon_{xz} = \frac{1}{2}\left(\frac{\partial w}{\partial x} + \frac{\partial u}{\partial z}\right). \tag{8.29}$$

The constitutive equations do, of course, depend on the material. For an elastic body we have stated them in (8.12) and restate them here in the notation used in (8.11b):

$$s = 3Ke, \qquad S = 2GE. \tag{8.30a,b}$$

For viscoelastic materials, we use instead (8.10b) and (8.11b).

In an elastic body under constant load, nothing depends on time. In a viscoelastic body all the stresses, strains, and displacements occurring in (8.28), (8.29), (8.10b), and (8.11b) are time dependent, and we may subject these equations to the Laplace transformation. In (8.28) and (8.29) this amounts to replacing $\sigma_x, \ldots \epsilon_x, \ldots u, \ldots$ by $\bar{\sigma}_x, \ldots \bar{\epsilon}_x, \ldots \bar{u}, \ldots$, but in (8.10b) and (8.11b) we must also replace the differential operators **P**, **Q** by the polynomials $\mathcal{P}(s)$, $\mathcal{Q}(s)$ and, hence, have the following equations

$$\mathcal{P}''(s) \cdot \bar{s} = \mathcal{Q}''(s) \cdot \bar{e}, \qquad \mathcal{P}'(s) \cdot \bar{S} = \mathcal{Q}'(s) \cdot \bar{E}. \tag{8.31a,b}$$

These are algebraic relations, and they become identical with their elastic counterparts (8.30) if we make the following substitutions:

$$3K \to \frac{\mathcal{Q}''(s)}{\mathcal{P}''(s)}, \qquad 2G \to \frac{\mathcal{Q}'(s)}{\mathcal{P}'(s)}. \tag{8.32a,b}$$

This leads us to the following, most general, form of the correspondence principle: If the solution of an elastic problem is known, the Laplace transform of the solution to the corresponding viscoelastic problem may be found by replacing the elastic constants K and G according to (8.32) by quotients of operator polynomials, and the actual loads by their Laplace transforms.

Since in most cases the solutions of elastic problems are not written in terms of the bulk modulus K and the shear modulus G, but rather in terms of Young's modulus E and Poisson's ratio ν, we introduce the right-hand sides of (8.32a,b) into the right-hand sides of (8.13) to find the substitutions

$$E \to \frac{3\mathcal{Q}'\mathcal{Q}''}{2\mathcal{P}'\mathcal{Q}'' + \mathcal{Q}'\mathcal{P}''}, \qquad \nu \to \frac{\mathcal{P}'\mathcal{Q}'' - \mathcal{Q}'\mathcal{P}''}{2\mathcal{P}'\mathcal{Q}'' + \mathcal{Q}'\mathcal{P}''}. \tag{8.32c,d}$$

If several viscoelastic materials are involved, the corresponding elastic problem has several elastic materials with different elastic constants.

This form of the correspondence principle is of a sweeping generality, but it does have its limitations. There are cases in which a Laplace transformation is not possible, in particular the following two:

(i) It may be that a point on the boundary of a viscoelastic body is first kept free of stress, while loads are being applied elsewhere, and that after some time a device is applied which makes this point undergo a prescribed displacement. Then neither the surface traction nor the displacement is known at all times $t > 0$, and neither of these functions can be subjected to the Laplace transformation.

(ii) The boundaries of a viscoelastic body may be changing in the course of time. Examples are a burning mass of rocket fuel, a melting body, or one solidifying from a melt. A body extruded from an orifice (see Problem 4.8) also belongs in this class.

The fact that in most cases a correspondence to an elastic problem exists, does not mean, of course, that one has to use the correspondence principle when dealing with a stress problem in viscoelasticity. If the elastic solution is not readily available, a direct approach may be preferable.

8.6 Two-Dimensional Problems

As an example for the application of the correspondence principle, we shall now derive the constitutive equations for two-dimensional stress problems. There are two such problems, commonly known as plane stress and plane strain.

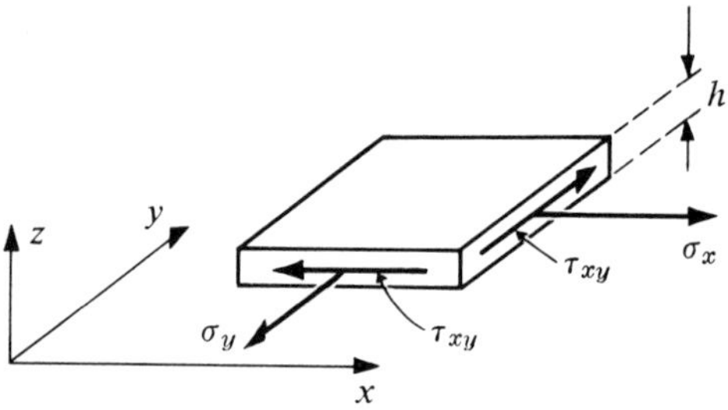

Figure 8.9. Slab element, plane stress.

In plane stress we are dealing with a thin slab (thickness h), which is exposed to forces lying in its middle plane. Let this be the x,y plane, then the stresses σ_z and τ_{xz}, τ_{yz} are all zero, and we have only the stresses shown in Fig. 8.9. Hooke's law reads then as follows:

$$E\epsilon_x = \sigma_x - \nu\sigma_y, \quad E\epsilon_y = \sigma_y - \nu\sigma_x, \quad G\gamma_{xy} = 2G\epsilon_{xy} = \tau_{xy} \, . \qquad (8.33a\text{-}c)$$

When we solve (8.33a,b) for the stresses, we have

$$\sigma_x = \frac{E}{1-\nu^2}(\epsilon_x + \nu\epsilon_y), \qquad \sigma_y = \frac{E}{1-\nu^2}(\epsilon_y + \nu\epsilon_x). \tag{8.34}$$

We use the correspondences (8.32b-d) to translate these equations into relations between the Laplace transforms of the stresses and strains:

$$3\mathcal{Q}'\mathcal{Q}''\bar{\epsilon}_x = (2\mathcal{P}'\mathcal{Q}'' + \mathcal{Q}'\mathcal{P}'')\bar{\sigma}_x - (\mathcal{P}'\mathcal{Q}'' - \mathcal{Q}'\mathcal{P}'')\bar{\sigma}_y ,$$

$$\mathcal{P}'(\mathcal{P}'\mathcal{Q}'' + 2\mathcal{Q}'\mathcal{P}'')\bar{\sigma}_x = \mathcal{Q}'[(2\mathcal{P}'\mathcal{Q}'' + \mathcal{Q}'\mathcal{P}'')\bar{\epsilon}_x + (\mathcal{P}'\mathcal{Q}'' - \mathcal{Q}'\mathcal{P}'')\bar{\epsilon}_y],$$

$$\mathcal{Q}'\bar{\epsilon}_{xy} = \mathcal{P}'\bar{\tau}_{xy}. \tag{8.35}$$

When in these equations the polynomials $\mathcal{Q}(s), \ldots,$ are replaced by the differential operators $\mathbf{Q}, \ldots,$ and $\bar{\epsilon}$, $\bar{\sigma}$ by the time-dependent physical quantities ϵ, σ, one has differential equations of the same type as (1.23c), and these are the constitutive relations of plane stress.

In plane strain we start from a very long cylinder or prism extending in z direction (Fig.8.10), and we postulate that all external forces are uniformly distributed in that direction. This applies not only to the

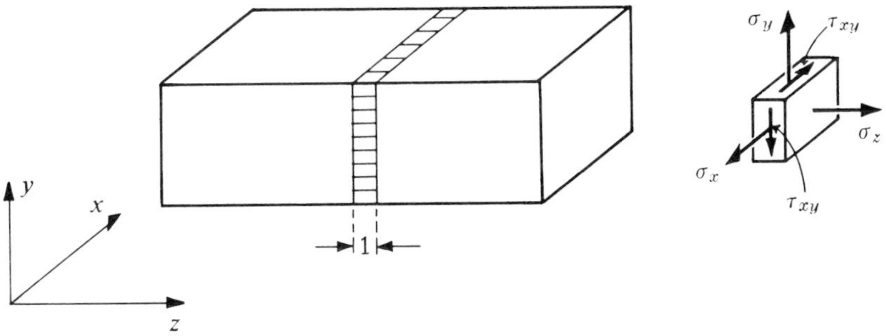

Figure 8.10. Element in plane strain.

loads, but also to reactions at supports. Then all stresses, strains, and displacements must be independent of z, and there is, in particular, no strain ϵ_z. When we cut a slice from the cylinder, we find in it the same stresses σ_x, σ_y, τ_{xy} in Fig.8.9, but also a stress σ_z

needed to keep

$$\epsilon_z = \frac{1}{E}(\sigma_z - \nu\sigma_x - \nu\sigma_y) = 0 .$$

When one solves this equation for σ_z and introduces the result into its companion equations for ϵ_x and ϵ_y, he finds

$$E\epsilon_x = (1 - \nu^2)\sigma_x - \nu(1 + \nu)\sigma_y ,$$
$$E\epsilon_y = (1 - \nu^2)\sigma_y - \nu(1 + \nu)\sigma_x \tag{8.36a,b}$$

and, solving for the stresses:

$$\sigma_x = \frac{E}{(1 + \nu)(1 - 2\nu)}[(1 - \nu)\epsilon_x + \nu\epsilon_y] . \tag{8.37}$$

The correspondence principle may again be used to find the corresponding relations for viscoelastic materials. For the physical quantities they are

$$(2\mathbf{P}'\mathbf{Q}'' + \mathbf{Q}'\mathbf{P}'')\mathbf{Q}'\epsilon_x = (\mathbf{P}'\mathbf{Q}'' + 2\mathbf{Q}'\mathbf{P}'')\mathbf{P}'\sigma_x - (\mathbf{P}'\mathbf{Q}'' - \mathbf{Q}'\mathbf{P}'')\mathbf{P}'\sigma_y , \tag{8.38}$$

and

$$3\mathbf{P}'\mathbf{P}''\sigma_x = (\mathbf{P}'\mathbf{Q}'' + 2\mathbf{Q}'\mathbf{P}'')\epsilon_x + (\mathbf{P}'\mathbf{Q}'' - \mathbf{Q}'\mathbf{P}'')\epsilon_y \tag{8.39}$$

and similar equations for ϵ_y and σ_y. The relation between τ_{xy} and ϵ_{xy} is the same as in plane stress.

8.7 Thick-walled Tube

As an example for plane strain, we choose the thick-walled tube (Fig. 8.11). In the plane of the cross section we use a polar coordinate system r, θ and normal to it we have a z axis. Continuity of the deformation demands that $\epsilon_z = 0$. The theory of elasticity yields the following formulas for the stresses defined in Fig. 8.11 and for the radial displacement u:

$$\sigma_r = A - Br^{-2}, \qquad \sigma_\theta = A + Br^{-2} ,$$
$$u = \frac{1 + \nu}{E}[A(1 - 2\nu)r + Br^{-1}] . \tag{8.40a-c}$$

We use these formulas to solve two problems.

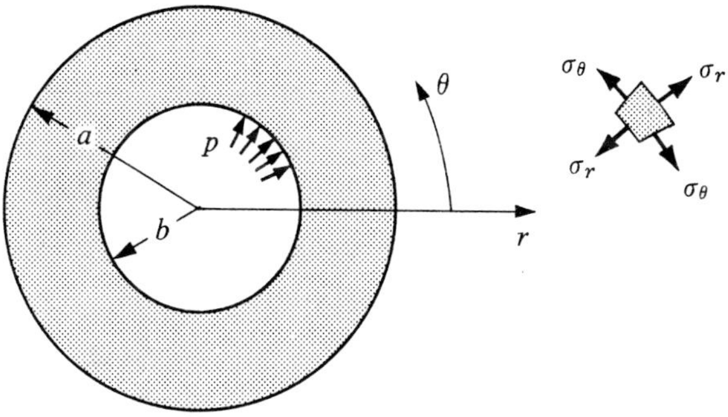

Figure 8.11. Thick-walled tube.

First, we apply an internal pressure p while keeping the outside of the tube free from stress. We have then the boundary conditions

$$r = b: \quad \sigma_r = -p ,$$

$$r = a: \quad \sigma_r = 0 .$$

Upon inserting σ_r from (8.40a) into them, we find

$$A = \frac{pb^2}{a^2 - b^2}, \qquad B = \frac{pa^2b^2}{a^2 - b^2},$$

and hence

$$\sigma_r = \frac{pb^2}{a^2 - b^2}\left(1 - \frac{a^2}{r^2}\right), \qquad \sigma_\theta = \frac{pb^2}{a^2 - b^2}\left(1 + \frac{a^2}{r^2}\right),$$

$$u = \frac{(1+\nu)pb^2}{E(a^2 - b^2)}\left[(1 - 2\nu)r + \frac{a^2}{r}\right]. \tag{8.41a-c}$$

The stresses do not depend on the elastic constants and therefore are the same when the tube is made of a viscoelastic material. To find the displacement u of a viscoelastic tube, we apply the general correspondence principle. The substitutions (8.32c,d) lead to

$$\bar{u} = \frac{\bar{p}b^2}{a^2 - b^2}\,\frac{\mathcal{P}'}{\mathcal{Q}'}\left[\frac{3\mathcal{Q}'\mathcal{P}''}{2\mathcal{P}'\mathcal{Q}'' + \mathcal{Q}'\mathcal{P}''}\,r + \frac{a^2}{r}\right]. \tag{8.42}$$

We now apply this relation to specific materials and begin with one that is elastic in dilatation and shows Kelvin behavior in distortion:

$$\mathcal{P}'' = 1, \quad \mathcal{Q}'' = 3K, \quad \mathcal{P}' = 1, \quad \mathcal{Q}' = q_0 + q_1 s \, . \tag{8.43}$$

Assuming step function loading, $p(t) = p\Delta(t)$, $\bar{p} = p/s$, we have then

$$\bar{u}(x,s) = \frac{pb^2}{a^2 - b^2}\,\frac{1}{s}\left[\frac{3}{6K + q_0 + q_1 s}\,r + \frac{a^2}{q_0 + q_1 s}\,\frac{1}{r}\right],$$

and with the help of Table 1.1 we find easily the actual radial displacement

$$u(r,t) = \frac{pb^2}{a^2 - b^2}\left\{\frac{3r}{6K + q_0}\left[1 - \exp\left(-\frac{(6K + q_0)t}{q_1}\right)\right]\right.$$

$$\left. + \frac{a^2}{q_0 r}\left[1 - \exp\left(-\frac{q_0 t}{q_1}\right)\right]\right\} . \tag{8.44}$$

For $t = 0$ there is no deformation at all, since, with $\epsilon_z = 0$, there can be no deformation without distortion and the Kelvin law does not admit an immediate elastic response. For $t \to \infty$, there is a finite deformation, described by the displacement

$$u(r,\infty) = \frac{pb^2}{a^2 - b^2}\left[\frac{3r}{6K + q_0} + \frac{a^2}{q_0 r}\right],$$

corresponding to that of an elastic material with bulk modulus K and shear modulus $G_\infty = \frac{1}{2} q_0$.

We consider a second material, which is again elastic in dilatation, but which follows the Maxwell law in distortion:

$$\mathcal{P}'' = 1, \quad \mathcal{Q}'' = 3K, \quad \mathcal{P}' = 1 + p_1 s, \quad \mathcal{Q}' = q_1 s \, . \tag{8.45}$$

Assuming step loading as before, we have now

$$\bar{u}(r,s) = \frac{pb^2}{a^2 - b^2}\,\frac{1 + p_1 s}{s}\left[\frac{3r}{9K + (9Kp_1 + q_1)s} + \frac{a^2}{q_1 s}\,\frac{1}{r}\right].$$

Transformation into the r,t plane can be done with the pairs (3), (4), and (6) of Table 1.1, yielding the following result:

$$u(r,t) = \frac{pb^2}{a^2 - b^2}\left\{\frac{r}{3K}\left[1 - \frac{q_1}{9Kp_1 + q_1}\exp\left(-\frac{9Kt}{9Kp_1 + q_1}\right)\right] + \frac{a^2(p_1 + t)}{q_1 r}\right\}. \tag{8.46}$$

In this case, there is a finite initial response $u(r,0^+)$, depending on the moduli K and $G_0 = q_1/2p_1$, and for increasing time the deformation is unbounded, since with respect to distortion the material behaves like a fluid. There is, of course, a limit to the applicability of our results, since the deformation will ultimately get so large that our linear, small-displacement theory is no longer correct.

We turn now to a second problem, assuming that the tube is again subjected to an internal pressure p, but that its outer surface is in contact with a surrounding medium so rigid that its deformation may be neglected. We have then the following boundary conditions:

$$r = b: \quad \sigma_r = -p,$$

$$r = a: \quad u = 0.$$

When we introduce the general solution (8.40) here and solve for the constants, we find

$$A = -\frac{pb^2}{(1 - 2\nu)a^2 + b^2}, \qquad B = -(1 - 2\nu)Aa^2,$$

and when we introduce this into (8.40), we have the solution of the elastic problem (where the upper sign is for σ_r and the lower for σ_θ):

$$\sigma_{r,\theta} = -\frac{pb^2}{(1 - 2\nu)a^2 + b^2}\left[1 \pm (1 - 2\nu)\frac{a^2}{r^2}\right],$$

$$u = \frac{pab^2(1 + \nu)(1 - 2\nu)}{E[(1 - 2\nu)a^2 + b^2]}\left(\frac{a}{r} - \frac{r}{a}\right). \tag{8.47}$$

In this case the elastic constants appear not only in u, but also in the stresses. Therefore, when we apply the general correspondence principle, we shall find that the stresses in a viscoelastic tube are time dependent. Indeed, the substitutions (8.32) yield:

$$\bar{\sigma}_{r,\theta} = -\frac{\bar{p}b^2}{r^2}\,\frac{(2\mathcal{P}'\mathcal{Q}'' + \mathcal{Q}'\mathcal{P}'')r^2 \pm 3\mathcal{Q}'\mathcal{P}''a^2}{(2\mathcal{P}'\mathcal{Q}'' + \mathcal{Q}'\mathcal{P}'')b^2 + 3\mathcal{Q}'\mathcal{P}''a^2},$$

$$\bar{u} = \bar{p}ab^2\,\frac{\mathcal{P}'\mathcal{P}''}{(2\mathcal{P}'\mathcal{Q}'' + \mathcal{Q}'\mathcal{P}'')b^2 + 3\mathcal{Q}'\mathcal{P}''a^2}\left(\frac{a}{r} - \frac{r}{a}\right). \qquad (8.48)$$

It will suffice to evaluate these formulas for only one specific material, the one described by (8.45). For step loading we find:

$$\bar{\sigma}_{r,\theta} = -\frac{pb^2}{r^2}\,\frac{1}{s}\,\frac{6Kr^2 + [(6Kp_1 + q_1)r^2 \pm 3q_1a^2]s}{6Kb^2 + [(6Kp_1 + q_1)b^2 + 3q_1a^2]s},$$

$$\bar{u} = pab^2\,\frac{1}{s}\,\frac{1 + p_1 s}{6Kb^2 + [(6Kp_1 + q_1)b^2 + 3q_1a^2]s}\left(\frac{1}{r} - \frac{r}{a}\right).$$

Again the transformation to the x,t plane can be achieved with the help of the pairs (3) and (4) of Table 1.1. After some lengthy arithmetic the following expressions may be found:

$$\sigma_{r,\theta} = -p\left[1 - \frac{\lambda q_1 a^2(a^2 \pm b^2)}{2Kb^2r^2}\,e^{-\lambda t}\right],$$

$$u = \frac{pa}{6K}\left(\frac{a}{r} - \frac{r}{a}\right)\left[1 + \frac{\lambda q_1(3a^2 - b^2)}{6Kb^2}\,e^{-\lambda t}\right]$$

with

$$\lambda = \frac{6Kb^2}{6Kp_1b^2 + q_1(3a^2 + b^2)}.$$

The radial displacement appears in the form $f(r) \cdot g(t)$, that is, its radial distribution is always the same while its magnitude inreases with time. However, the deformation is bounded, although in the preceding example the material displayed fluid behavior. This difference is caused by the external constraint, which here is exerted by the surrounding rigid medium.

The fluid character of the material manifests itself in the stresses. For $t = 0^+$, the stress distribution is similar to that in an elastic tube, while for $t \to \infty$ it tends to a simple hydrostatic stress system $\sigma_r = \sigma_\theta = -p$. Exactly as in the structure of Figs. 4.8 and 4.12, this tube behaves like a system made of two materials, but here the "two materials" are the two aspects of the deformation of the only material present: its dilatation and its distortion.

Problems

8.1. Consider a long, thin-walled cylinder that is closed at its ends by two bulkheads. Restrict your attention to that part of the cylinder which is not affected by the local stress disturbances caused by the bulkheads. (i). Analyze stress and strain in the cylinder wall in terms of an average and a deviator. (ii). Writing operator equations for these parts, derive from them a similar equation connecting an internal pressure p and the radial displacement w.

8.2. The elastic law (8.33), (8.34) for plane stress may be used in polar coordinates by simply replacing the subscripts x, y by r, θ. This may be used for solving the following problem: An infinite plane sheet is subjected to a uni-axial stress system $\sigma_x = \text{const}$, $\sigma_y = \tau_{xy} = 0$. This stress system is disturbed by (i) a small circular hole or (ii) a small rigid inclusion of radius a. Find stresses and displacements using polar coordinates and, possibly, the solution of the corresponding elastic problem. Suggested material: elastic in dilatation, Maxwell law for distortion.

8.3. A thin spherical shell of radius a_0 and thickness h is subjected to a pressure $p = p_0 \Delta(t)$. The dilatation of the material is elastic and its distortion follows the Kelvin law. How does the radius a increase with time?

8.4. Use (8.38) and the kinematic relation $\epsilon_\theta = u/r$ to derive (8.42) from equations (8.41a,b).

8.5. In plane strain there is a stress σ_z which helps making $\epsilon_z \equiv 0$. When one calculates σ_z connected with (8.41), one finds that it is independent of r. Therefore, even a very long tube, if not constrained at its ends, will actually develop a plane s t r e s s system with $\sigma_z \equiv 0$

and ϵ_z = const. The stresses σ_r, σ_θ are the same as in plane strain, but the displacement u is different. Calculate it and specialize the result for the material described by (8.43).

8.6. A thick-walled viscoelastic tube (the core) is enclosed in a thin elastic shell (the mantle), see Fig.8.12. For the core material assume elastic dilatation (bulk modulus K) and Maxwell distortion (p_1, q_1). For the mantle, use E and ν as its elastic constants. An internal pressure $p(t) = p\Delta(t)$ is applied at r = b. Find σ_r, σ_θ, and u in the core and the hoop stress σ_θ in the mantle. Assume plane strain.

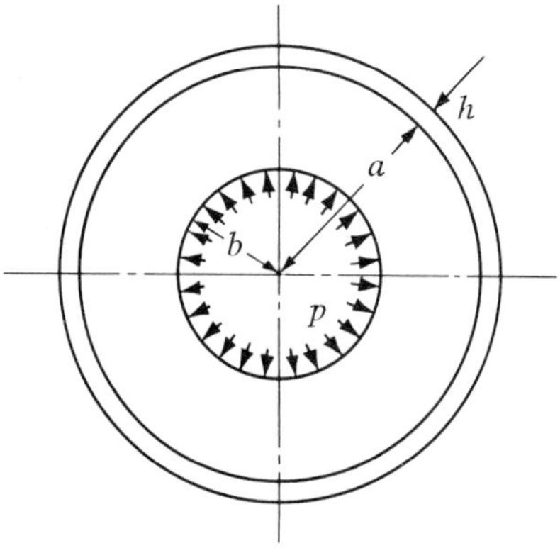

Figure 8.12.

References

Papers on stress analysis in three dimensions have been numerous in recent years. The following are recommended for collateral reading:

50. E.H. Lee: Viscoelasticity in W. Flügge (ed.), Handbook of Engineering Mechanics, (New York: McGraw-Hill, 1962), Chap. 53. (General survey.)

51. E.H. Lee, J.R.M. Radok, and W.B. Woodward: Stress Analysis for Linear Viscoelastic Materials. Trans. Soc. Rheology, 3 (1959), 41-59. (Contains several cases of thickwalled cylinders.)

52. J.R.M. Radok: Viscoelastic Stress Analysis. Qu. Appl. Math., 15 (1957), 198-202.

The correspondence principle seems to have emerged gradually, being formulated by several authors with different, unessential limitations to its generality:

53. T. Alfrey: Nonhomogeneous Stress in Viscoelasticity. Qu. Appl. Math., 2 (1944), 113-119. (Contains the principle for tri-axial stress and strain, but limited to an incompressible material.)

54. W.T. Read: Stress Analysis for Compressible Viscoelastic Materials. J. Appl. Phys., 21 (1950), 671-674. (Contains the principle for compressible materials, but with reference to the Fourier transform.)

55. M.A. Biot: Theory of Stress-Strain Relations in Anisotropic Viscoelasticity and Relaxation Phenomena. J. Appl. Phys., 25 (1954), 1385-1391. (A very general operator formulation.)

56. E.H. Lee: Stress Analysis in Viscoelastic Bodies. Qu. Appl. Math., 13 (1955), 183-190. (General formulation using the Laplace transformation.)

The equilibrium conditions and the kinematic relations in three-dimensional elasticity are found in Reference [21], pp. 235 and 7, respectively, and in the following books:

57. A.E.H. Love: A Treatise on the Mathematical Theory of Elasticity (4th ed.), (Cambridge, Cambridge University Press, 1927 and New York, Dover Publications, 1944), pp. 85 and 38.

58. I.S. Sokolnikoff: Mathematical Theory of Elasticity (2nd ed.), (New York, McGraw-Hill, 1956), pp. 41 and 22.

Index